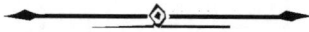

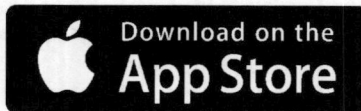

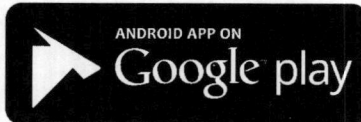

ISBN 978-1-330-98230-3
PIBN 10129573

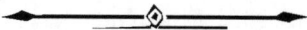

English
Français
Deutsche
Italiano
Español
Português

www.forgottenbooks.com

Mythology Photography **Fiction**
Fishing Christianity **Art** Cooking
Essays Buddhism Freemasonry
Medicine **Biology** Music **Ancient**
Egypt Evolution Carpentry Physics
Dance Geology **Mathematics** Fitness
Shakespeare **Folklore** Yoga Marketing
Confidence Immortality Biographies
Poetry **Psychology** Witchcraft
Electronics Chemistry History **Law**
Accounting **Philosophy** Anthropology
Alchemy Drama Quantum Mechanics
Atheism Sexual Health **Ancient History**
Entrepreneurship Languages Sport
Paleontology Needlework Islam
Metaphysics Investment Archaeology
Parenting Statistics Criminology
Motivational

HORSE-SHOES

AND

HORSE-SHOEING

THEIR ORIGIN,
HISTORY, USES, AND ABUSES.

BY

GEORGE FLEMING, F.R.G.S., F.A.S.L.

MEMBER OF COUNCIL OF THE ROYAL COLLEGE OF VETERINARY SURGEONS; VETERINARY
SURGEON, ROYAL ENGINEERS;
AUTHOR OF 'TRAVELS ON HORSEBACK IN MANTCHU TARTARY,' ETC.

WITH 210 ILLUSTRATIONS.

LONDON ·
CHAPMAN AND HALL,
193, PICCADILLY.
1869.

Por un clavo se pierde una herradura, por una herradura un Cavallo, por un Cavallo un Cavallero —*Old Spanish Proverb.*

A little neglect may breed great mischief. For want of a nail the shoe was lost ; for want of a shoe the horse was lost ; and for want of a horse the rider was lost, being overtaken and slain by the enemy ; all for want of a little care about a horse-shoe nail.—*Benjamin Franklin.*

A proper mode of shoeing is certainly of more importance than the treatment of any disease, or perhaps of all the diseases incident to horses. The foot is a part that we are particularly required to preserve in health ; and if this art be judiciously employed, the foot will not be more liable to disease than any other organ.—*Professor E. Coleman.*

JOHN CHILDS AND SON, PRINTERS

PREFACE

To all who possess an interest in or a love for the horse, but little apology will be required in offering for their acceptance a work like the present. The result of much labour and research, it is an attempt to trace, for the first time in England, the origin and history of the art of shoeing horses. Since the publication, in 1831, of Bracy Clark's essay 'On the Knowledge of the Ancients respecting the Art of Shoeing the Horse,' the science of ethnological archæology has made wonderful progress in throwing light upon much that was obscure, or altogether lost, in the darkness of pre-historic, and even historic times, and the manners and customs of ancient peoples have been largely elucidated by it. Some of its rays have been incidentally shed upon the early condition of this apparently humble handicraft, tending considerably to modify, or altogether disprove, the opinions held by various authorities as to the antiquity of horse-shoeing.

Though but of minor importance in archæology, yet the discussion of this subject has attracted much notice at times, and engaged a large share of attention on the part of men much celebrated as antiquarians and scholars. And the origin of the art, though of comparatively little moment in an utilitarian point of view, is nevertheless one of those interesting subjects which will always prove interesting to the anthropologist and archæologist.

To make this portion of the work complete, every discovery of relics connected with the subject has been inquired into, when possible, and no pains have been spared in the investigation of its unwritten story.

With regard to the Middle Ages, much original research has, I trust, satisfactorily brought the history forward to a period when authentic records become abundant, and these have been made sufficiently available for the purpose; while, for the succeeding centuries, and up to our own time, the principal kinds of shoeing introduced, and their various defects, have been noticed in detail.

The importance of the farrier's art to civilization, and to the welfare of the horse, with its evils and how to remedy them, have been considered in separate chapters. It is, perhaps, scarcely necessary to assert, that if the progress of this craft, as it has been practised in Europe, had been carefully studied, and the teachings of its most notable exponents kept in view, the modern patent offices would have been much less patronized, the equine species would have been benefited to an extent which those who abhor cruelty to animals little dream of, and a large aving in horse-power and horse-life would have been the result. It is to be hoped that the investigations now published may prove useful in this respect, and that the latter portions of the work may attract attention to the great injury done to the horse by the barbarous treatment its feet are generally subjected to, so that the lessons afforded by history may not be without advantage to the noble animal and his master.

For many years the anatomy, functions, and management of the horse's limbs and feet have been made the object of careful observation. The present treatise contains a portion of the results arrived at ; the remainder will appear, I trust, at no distant day.

The assignment of the diversely-shaped antique shoes to certain ages—a matter of much difficulty—resulted from the examination and comparison of specimens found in various parts of Great Britain and the Continent of Europe, and the remains discovered with them.

Nothing has been omitted, so far as I am aware, that might prove useful or interesting in this inquiry into the origin, progress, traditions, and utility of an art to which our Western civilization owes so much. The drawings have been most carefully prepared to illustrate its various phases, and, whenever possible, photography has been resorted to for greater correctness.

For obliging assistance in my labours, I gratefully beg to acknowledge the kind services of Messrs Mayer, F.S.A., Morgan, Moor, and Picton, of Liverpool, in furnishing me with information relative to specimens in the free Museum of that city ; Mr C. Roach Smith, F.S.A., Strood, for much assistance in obtaining specimens, and in aiding me in every possible way ; Mr Murray, British Museum ; and M. Megnin, veterinary surgeon to the Horse Artillery of the Imperial Guard, at Versailles, for a copy of his excellent treatise on French farriery. .

Brompton Barracks,
Chatham, June 1, 1869.

CONTENTS.

Saxons. Domes-day Book. Monkish Smith. St Dunstan and the Evil One. St Eloy and Highworth Church. Zurich. Abyssinia. Arabia. Persia. Java. Acadie. Mysteries of Samothrace and Druidism. First of November. Reasons for Roman Ignorance of Shoeing. The Caledonian Wall. 'Horse-shoe' Medal. Change in Designation of the Farrier. Early Marechals and their Rank. Age of Chivalry. Apprenticeship of a Chevalier. Archbishop Hughes of Besançon. Rights of the Marechal. Normans in France. Origin of Marshall and Farrier. Fleta. The London Marescallis. Seal of Ralph. The Marshall Ferrer. Superstitions concerning Horse-shoes in various Countries. German Legends. Moonwort.

ERRATA.

Page 334, line 19, *for* brass' *read* ' bronze
,, 454, line 5. *for* ' 1763 *read* ' 1673 '

HORSE-SHOES

AND HORSE-SHOEING.

CHAPTER I.

THE VALUE OF THE HORSE AS A LIVING MACHINE DEPENDS TO A GREAT EXTENT UPON HIS FEET. THE CARE OF THEM BY ANCIENT PEOPLE. XENOPHON AND HIS ADVICE. THE NECESSITY FOR SOUND FEET. HISTORY OF THE ART OF SHOEING. THE HOOF IN A NATURAL STATE. EFFECTS OF DOMESTICATION AND CLIMATE. THE PERSIANS, ETHIOPIANS, ABYSSINIANS, TARTARS, MONGOLS, AND OTHER NATIONS. THE GREEKS. DIFFICULTY IN TRACING THE ORIGIN OF SHOEING. SCRIPTURAL TIMES. HOMER, AND 'BRAZEN-FOOTED. TRYPHIODORUS. BRONZE SHOES, AND SHOELESS HOOFS. XENOPHON ON THE MANAGEMENT OF HORSES' FEET. ARISTOTLE. POLYDORE VERGIL. THE GREEK MARBLES. CLIMATE OF GREECE. EFFECTS OF MARCHING. TRANSLATORS' AND COMMENTATORS' MISTAKES. ARRIAN AND ARTEMIDORUS. THE COIN OF TARENTUM.

THE horse is justly considered, even in these days, when the application of steam power has to a certain extent limited some of his more important functions, one of the most tractable and serviceable living machines, viewing him as a motor, ever pressed into slavery by man, and consequently ranks high above all those creatures which have submitted themselves to domestication and toil for the benefit of the human species.

The varied uses to which he has been subjected, since taken from a wild state, and the willing and cheerful manner with which he has undergone fatigue, and performed duties which are, one would think, quite foreign to his nature, have all been owing to his combined and unequalled qualities of strength, courage, speed, fidelity, and obedience, as well as docility; and though his great value depends essentially upon a just disposition of these, yet more especially is it as a living machine, capable of moving or producing motion, and communicating it to inert masses at all times and in nearly all situations, that he is to be prized.

Where, and at what period of the world's history, he was first brought into a state of servitude; whether at one or more points of the earth's surface man commenced to utilize his noble attributes, we know not. Certain it is, however, that some of the pre-historic races of the human family sought his aid; and the ancient Aryans, more than three thousand years ago, as we learn from the Riga-Veda, in their home towards the upper valley of the Indus, loved and bred the horse, harnessed him to their chariots with spoked-wheels, and made him assume the principal part in their greatest religious sacrifices.

The history of mankind abundantly testifies, that every possible use and application of this animal, whether in war, commerce, or pleasure, seems to have been anticipated by the most ancient peoples; proving the earliest sense and conviction of his immense importance to man. Those old-world nations which, long ages ago, most largely employed the horse, were the great centres of antique civilization; and it may safely be asserted, that, without him, the human race could not have reached its present state of refinement, or have been able to contend against the numerous obstacles to comfort and happiness which have surrounded it; indeed, it has been said, that next to the want of iron, the want of horses would have been, perhaps, one of the greatest physical barriers to the advancement of the arts of civilized life.

Doubtless, what might be termed the moral qualities of the horse, had largely conduced to make him so serviceable in all ages, but by far the largest share must be attributed to those of a physical kind. Strength, speed, endurance, and astonishing alacrity have endowed him with his most useful characteristics, and given him the pre-eminence over all other domesticated animals; and these qualities again depend upon a marvellous adaptation of the organs and textures of which he is composed to the most varied requirements.

Cuvier has somewhere said of the horse, that but for the space of bare gum between the incisor and molar teeth which affords space for the insertion and action of the bit, it would never have been subjected to the power of man. Far rather with truth may it be said, that but for the horse being endowed with a hoof which covers and protects the most beautiful and delicate of structures, and which being solid and a slow conductor of heat and cold, fits it for travelling in snow and ice during the winter of northern regions, and in the burning sands of tropical climates, he would scarcely have proved himself worth the trouble of domesticating. Means could have been employed to ride and drive him without a bit in his mouth, but no invention or device of man could have compensated for the absence of his solid, hoof-cased foot. From the earliest ages, the attention of horsemen and horse-loving nations has been directed to the conservation or perfectioning of those attributes which make this ever-willing slave so worthy of our admiration and gratitude; and those horses which had the best conformation, and proved themselves fleetest and hardiest, were ever selected as models for breeding and purchasing. And curiously enough, though it was not to be wondered at, nearly every one of the ancient writers, when speaking of the horse, centre their attention on his feet; no matter how beautifully formed the other *points* of his conformation may have been, if his feet were defective, all was bad. The excellent horseman and gallant soldier, Xenophon, to whose extant treatises on the horse we are indebted for so much of what we know of equestrian matters in the ancient world, tersely specifies how essential even in his day, when the uses of this animal were more limited, it was that he have good feet, or there was no profit in him. He says: ' In respect to the horse's body, then, we assert that we must first examine the feet; for as there would be no use in a house, though the upper parts were extremely beautiful, if the foundations were not laid as they ought to be, so there would be no profit in a war-horse, even if he had all his other parts excellent but was unsound in his feet; for then he would be unable to render any of his other good qualities effective.' [1]

And from the days of Xenophon to the present, when

[1] De Re Equestri.

the uses of the horse have been so multiplied and so much more necessary for our business or pleasure, the truth of this advice has been daily receiving confirmation, until the aphorism ' No foot, no horse,' has become a painful reality in modern days, though it is but a re-echo of what was enunciated centuries beyond two thousand years ago.

For the manifestation of his strength and the due performance of his useful qualities, the horse must, therefore, rely upon the soundness of his feet, as in them are concentrated the efforts created elsewhere; and on them depend not only the sum total of these propulsive powers being properly expended, but also the solidity and just equilibrium of the whole animal fabric. So that it is wisely considered that the foot of the horse is one of the most, if not *the* most, important part of all the locomotory apparatus; and that all the splendid qualities possessed by the noble creature may be diminished in value or hopelessly lost, if through disease or accident, natural or acquired defects, or other causes, this organ fails to perform its allotted task.

Seeing, then, the great interest which attaches to this animal, in its being of all creatures most concerned with man in promoting a progressive and long-continued civilization, and to the means and appliances which the lord of the creation has from time to time brought to bear in increasing the utility (would I could say comfort and happiness!) of this devoted servant, I have entered on the present inquiry into the origin and early history of what is generally looked upon as a humble art; for the simple reason that it affords us a glimpse, or rather a faint idea, of an obscure occupation, a modest handicraft, in-

creasing a hundred-fold the value of the horse, and testifies to what an apparently insignificant operation very
much of our immense progress in civilization has depended. I refer to the art of shoeing, by which, in arming that portion of the horse's hoof coming in contact
with the ground, and sustaining the whole weight, while
it receives the full force of the propelling power, would
(in our northern climate, at least) under the strain of load-
bearing or draught, soon be destroyed, and the animal
rendered useless, injury is not only averted, but the utility
and power of the horse are largely increased.

An art which has exerted some influence on the des-
tinies of man, and lent its aid to the restless wave of
human action, deserves some notice from those who care
to note the sources and influences on which improvement
and increased communication have relied; and if this be a
modest one, it is at least endowed with all the more interest in consequence of its being so closely related to the
conservation of the best qualities of the noblest quadruped
on earth.

In a state of nature the hoof requires no protection.
The solidity and toughness of its inferior border; the absence of artificial roads; nothing but the weight of the
body to be supported; and the matter of which the
horny case is composed never being subjected to any
other influences than those which it is naturally adapted
to resist, all tend to obviate any injurious amount of attrition in the roaming-at-will life of the feral horse. But in
connection with climate, domestication alters, more or
less, the conditions on which the horn depends for its integrity as an efficient protection to the highly sensitive

and vascular textures it encloses. In eastern countries, where the climate is dry and the earth elastic and soft, and where the equine species is usually wiry and firm in its organization, with dense inflexible hoofs, an armature of any kind is seldom, if ever, required. Not unfrequently, however, we learn that the care and attention of the people who so employ horses is bestowed on the quality and resistance of the hoof; and as this has an important bearing on our inquiry, we will notice a few of the authorities who mention the fact. Thevenot informs us that the Persians cared little for shoes for their horses;[1] the Ethiopians, in the time of Ludolphus, although they seldom rode, did not employ any defence for the hoofs, and when they had to travel over rough and stony ground, they dismounted and sat on the backs of mules, leading their horses in hand, so that these might tread lighter, and do their hoofs less damage. 'They do not defend their horses' hoofs with iron shoes; if they travel over rough and uneven ground, they lead them, and ride mules.'[2] The same authority asserts that the Tartars, who ride so much, never shod their steeds. 'In the winter time, when, on account of the frost, roads are rough and hard, they cover their horses' feet with the recently flayed hide of cattle, if nothing else is at hand.'[3]

A recent traveller in Abyssinia states that the horses

---

[1] Voyages, vol. ii. p. 113. Paris, 1684.

[2] *Joh. Ludolphus.* Hist. Æthiopic., vol. i. cap. 10. 'Ideo nec ungulas eorum soleis ferreis muniunt : si per aspera et salebrosa loca eundum fit, eos ducunt, ipsi mulis insidentes.'

[3] Ibid. in Commentario, p. 149. 'Tempore vero hyemis, viis ob gelu asperis et duris, *corio boum, etiam recenti,* si-aliud non suppetat, pedes equorum suorum involvunt.

and mules of that country are not shod.[1]   The wandering
Mongols who roam between the Great Wall of China,
the desert of Gobi, and the Russian frontier, with their
flocks of sheep and droves of horses and cattle, do not
employ shoes for their hardy but uncouth solipedes, according to the account of my friend and fellow-traveller,
Mr Michie.   Whenever a pony selected from a drove has
become footsore from being ridden too long a time, the
rider dismounts, a fresh steed is caught from the crowd,
and the hoof-worn one is set at large again, to recover as
it best may the loss it has sustained.   So that a traveller
often requires to change his invaluable steed when crossing
these inhospitable wilds.   But in this there does not appear
to be any difficulty, as an exchange can be readily effected
by paying a slight difference to the nomadic owner of a
drove, who knows that by allowing the lame creatures to
pasture quietly for a few weeks, they will soon have replaced the lost horn, and be as serviceable as ever.

It would appear, however, that horses are sometimes
shod here, but they may only be Russian ones.   Tim
kowski in travelling through this country, and when at a
halting-place, writes: 'While the smith was *shoeing* our
horses, a lama, who kept walking about, and seemed very
attentive to what he was doing, suddenly mounted his
horse and galloped away.   It was afterwards discovered
that this priest had stolen one of the smith's tools.'[2]

Marco Polo, in the 13th century, travelling in Badak
shan, says: 'The country is extremely cold, but it breeds

---

[1] *Mansfield Parkyns.*   Life in Abyssinia, vol. ii.   See also *Baker,*
Nile Tributaries in *A*byssinia.   Proc. Roy. Geo. Soc., 1866.

[2] Travels through Mongolia to China, vol. i. p. 188.

very good horses, which run with great speed over these wild tracts without being shod with iron.' [1]

The *Tanghans*, or Tibetan ponies Hooker saw in the Himalayas, are described as wonderfully strong and endur- ing. ' *They are never shod,* and the hoof often cracks and they become pigeon-toed.' [2]

Horses are never shod in the Moluccas, or the Straits of Malacca. With regard to Java, Sir Stamford Raffles says : ' Horses are never shod in Java, nor are they secured in the stable as is usual in Europe and Western India. A separate enclosure is appropriated for each horse, within which the animal is allowed to move and turn at pleasure, being otherwise unconfined. These enclosures are erected at a short distance from each other, and with separate roofs. They are generally raised above the ground, and have a boarded floor.' [3] The same kind of floor is in use at Manilla.

Lichtenstein remarks of the Cape of Good Hope horses, that, owing to their being accustomed from their youth to seek their nourishment upon dry mountains, they are easily satisfied, and ' *grow so hard in the hoofs* that there is no occasion to shoe them.' [4]

Anderssen, describing some of his journeys in South Africa, says : ' On an after-occasion, I remember to have performed upwards of ninety miles at a very great pace, only once or twice removing the saddle for a few minutes. And be it borne in mind that the animals were young, in-

---

[1] Narrative of the Travels of Marco Polo. London, 1849. p. 234.
[2] Himalayan Journals, vol. ii. p. 131.
[3] History of Java, vol. ii. p. 319.
[4] Travels in Southern Africa, vol. ii. p. 27. London, 1812.

differently broken in, *unshod,* and had never been stall-fed.' [1]

Dr Browne reports of the horses in Jamaica: 'They are generally small, but very sure-footed and hardy, which renders them extremely fit for those mountainous lands; and their hoofs are so hard that they seldom require shoes; but this is the effect of the heat of the country and dryness of the land.' [2]

Iron shoes are not used for horses in Japan, and Head, in his ride across the Pampas of South America, tells us that shoes are utterly unknown to all the South American country horses. 'But even when unshod, the wear of their boundless plains, on which scarcely a stone is seen, is so insignificant, that to keep the hoofs of a proper length, they have even to be shortened by the hammer and chisel.' [3] Another traveller in that region asserts that the mule of the Peruvian Sierras, with its massy and well-rounded hoof, needs no shoes on hard or soft ground, in summer or in winter.

Clark says of the north of Sweden: 'Neither the men nor their horses are shod, but go bare-footed. In some parts of Sweden, as at Naples, the hinder feet only of the horses are left unshodden; but here horses of a beautiful breed were put to our waggon, without a shoe to any of their feet, as wild and fleet as Barbs;' and again, when entering Finland from Sweden, he writes: 'The horses are, as usual, small, but beautifully formed, and very fleet. The peasants take them from the forests when they are

[1] Lake Ngami, p. 339.
[2] The Civil and Natural History of Jamaica, p. 487. London, 1756.
[3] A Ride *A*cross the Pampas, p. 387.

wanted for travellers, and, with very little harness, fasten them to the carriage. In this state, *they are without shoes,* and seem perfectly wild; but it is surprising to observe how regularly and well they trot.'[1]   Brooke, however, remarks, that ' so dangerous are the wolves in some parts of Sweden that the peasants, on turning their horses out, generally tip their feet with iron, by which means of defence they are frequently enabled to beat off their ferocious assailants.'[2]

It is well known that in many southern regions there is but little need for any attempt at shoeing. The littoral of Libya, and some parts of Arabia and Persia, furnish examples. In Tartary, whole tribes ride horses without shoes of iron, and in Senegal the French squadron of Spahis have no farriers, for the simple reason that they have no shod horses.[3]   In the East Indies, among some races shoeing is far from general.

So we can easily understand, that in certain parts of the world, horses have been and can be made serviceable to a certain extent without employing an iron defence. If one may judge from the paintings of Ancient Egypt and the sculptures of Assyria, where we see the horse portrayed with great skill, and with that minute perception of his external form which seems to us even now very remarkable, no protection for the hoof was ever had recourse to, and no remains of anything bearing a resemblance to such an appliance have been found. And though these countries were acquainted with many arts,

[1] Travels in various countries of Scandinavia. London, 1838.
[2] Travels in Sweden, p. 19.
[3] *Megnin.* Ferrure du Cheval, p. 8.

and had attained a comparatively advanced state of civilization, in which the horse played no insignificant part, yet in the absence of this craft, even with their favourable climate and soil, the use of this animal must have been but limited, compared to what it is in our own days. It is only when we reach the period in which the ancient Greeks begin to figure in history, that doubts and inquiries arise among modern investigators with regard to a real iron or other metal shoe being employed ; and for nearly two hundred years, various writers have spared neither time nor patience in attempting to arrive at some definite conclusion as to whether or not the Greeks and Romans were cognisant of this art, or at what period it first became known.

With the spread of civilization, the demands upon the services of the horse became, doubtless, very much extended ; and the diversity of climate, as well as of races, would lead one to suppose that greater wear and modifications, more or less wrought in the nature and consistency of the hoof, must at an early period have rendered some kind of defence absolutely necessary ; and that this again would be mentioned in the writings of men who largely devoted their attention to the welfare of this animal. Nevertheless, the antiquity of shoeing, notwithstanding the well-directed labours of many learned men, is yet a subject admitting of considerable diversity of opinion, simply because of the absence of written documents, or records of a positive character, by which this art could be traced to its origin in any particular part of the world.[1]   True, there

[1] *A*mong the principal writers who have occupied themselves in this investigation may be mentioned the following :—

would not probably be much gain in finally deciding as to which race of the human family, or to what age, the successful utilization of the horse by arming its hoofs with a hard rim of metal is due; and it would, perhaps, be more satisfactory and instructive to trace briefly the progress of the art from its earliest known introduction into the social economy of civilized nations, up to the present time, than attempt to seek its inventors in the perplexing obscurity surrounding this subject. But, as before noticed, the interest which attaches to all that pertains to the horse, and particularly to the management of its feet, by those people who were among the first to discover the beauties and merits of that noble animal, and to press its strength, fleetness, courage, and endurance

Raphael Fabretti. Syntagma de Columna Trajani.

A. Winckelmann. Description des Pierres Antiques Gravées, p. 169. Florence, 1760.

I. Pegge. Archæologia, 1776.

Beckman. History of Discoveries and Inventions, vol. ii. London, 1797.

Bourgelat. Essai Théorique et Pratique sur la Ferrure.

Huzard. Théâtre d'Agriculture, vol. i. p. 630. Paris, 1804.

Bracy Clark. An Essay on the Knowledge of the Ancients respecting the Art of Shoeing the Horse. London, 1831.

T. D. Fosbrooke. Encyclopædia of Antiquities. London, 1840.

An anonymous writer in United Service Magazine, 1849.

C. H. Smith. The Naturalist's Library, vol. xii. p. 128.

H. Bouley. Dictionnaire Vétérinaire, vol. vi. *Art.* Ferrure.

H. S. Cuming. Journal Archæological Association, vol. vi. xiv.

F. Defays. Annales de Méd. Vétérinaire, p. 256. Brussels, 1867.

J. P. Megnin. De l'Origine de la Ferrure du Cheval. Paris, 1865.

La Maréchalerie Française. Paris, 1867.

Nickard. Mémoires de la Soc. Nationale des Antiquaires de France, 1866.

into their service, is a great inducement to review, in as graphic a manner as possible, all that has been said in relation to the existence, non-existence, or *status* of this art among them.   And in this inquiry the poet, painter, and sculptor have some interest, inasmuch as the correctness or incorrectness of their delineations, when this apparently trifling detail comes to be treated, will depend.   This will be exemplified hereafter.

It is a remarkable circumstance that, considering the mighty influence the horse has been called on to exercise on the destiny of nations and the progress of civilization from the earliest times,—at one period an important adjunct to luxury, as well as a mainspring of utility; at another, an essential element in the arts of peace, and a still more potent one in that of war,—the first written indication of horse-shoeing (as we now understand the term) is only found in the annals of a comparatively recent period.   The knowledge of being able to defend from undue wear and injury such an important organ as the horse's foot, and by such an efficacious, yet simple means, one would think indispensable to those who, in primitive times, so largely employed horses, and sought from them such important services.   Such is not the case, however, if an entire omission of the fact in their writings or on their monuments be received as proof; and though several authors of some weight have in recent years asserted that the ancients were acquainted with this art, and have adduced evidence which appears to substantiate their opinion, yet a careful examination of the times and the meaning of the texts has, in nearly every case, tended to lead others to the opposite conclusion.

That shoeing was not known to Old Testament people, no one has yet, so far as I am aware, offered a doubt. Deborah [1] (B.C. 1296) sings, ' Then were the *horse-hoofs broken* by the means of their prancings, the prancings of their mighty ones ; ' or, as it might perhaps more correctly be rendered, ' Then did the *horses' hoofs* smite the ground, and were broken from the haste of their riders.' Isaiah [2] (B.C. 760), in the grandly prophetic language in which he foreshadows the downfall of Jerusalem by the armies of Rome, mentions the hoofs of their horses and what was esteemed their best quality. He says, ' Whose arrows are sharp, and all their bows bent, *their horses' hoofs shall be counted like flint,* and their wheels like a whirlwind.' And Jeremiah [3] (B.C. 607), when foretelling the punishment of the Philistines, says : ' At the noise of the *stamping of the hoofs of his strong horses,* at the rushing of his chariots.'

It is in Homer (B.C. 1000) that we find some investigators contending for the first notice of a metallic foot defence. Among these appear Fabretti, Bourgelat, Montfauçon, Cuming, and a few others. In reality, however, it was Eustathius, who lived in the 12th century, who, in his Commentaries on Homer, first speaks of that poet mentioning horses as shod. In the ' Iliad ' (Book xi., lines 150-2) occurs the passage noted by Eustathius ·

πεζοὶ μὲν πεζοὺς ὄλεκον φεύγοντας ἀνάγκῃ
ἱππεῖς δ' ἱππῆας—ὑπὸ δέ σφισιν ὦρτο κονίη
ἐκ πεδίου, τὴν ὦρσαν ἐρίγδουποι πόδες ἵππων.

---

[1] Judges v. 22.   [2] Isaiah v 28.
[3] Jeremiah xlvii.

And this striking picture has been thus translated by a recent and celebrated scholar :

> ' Foot on foot, and horse on horse :
> While from the plain thick clouds of dust arose
> Beneath the *armèd* hoofs of clatt'ring steeds.

This it will be readily perceived is an error. The passage, literally rendered, ought to read something like the following : ' Foot on foot and horse on horse, they perished forcibly while flying ; and under them the dust arose from the plain, and the loud-sounding (crushing or thundering) feet of the horses raised it.'

The word is ἐρίγδουποι. Another translator of the Iliad renders this passage :

> ' Horse trod by horse lay foaming on the plain,
> From the dry fields thick clouds of dust arise,
> Shade the black host, and intercept the skies ;
> The *brass-hoof'd* steeds tumultuous plunge and bound,
> And the thick thunder beats the labouring ground.'

In another place (Book viii., lines 44-5) Bourgelat, Cuming, and others, found their opinion in favour of the Greeks having shod their horses at this early period, on the fact that Homer speaks of Jove's horses as

> ' The *brazen-footed* steeds
> Of swiftest flight, with manes of flowing gold.'

The translation of χαλχόποδ' ἵππω is correct, and is rendered so by Chapman, an old versifier :

> ' This said, his brasse-hou'd (brass-hoof'd) winged horse
> He did to chariot binde.'

The ' brass-hoof ' was undoubtedly used by Homer in a metaphorical sense to denote firmness and solidity, not a hoof shod with brass ; it was meant to convey an idea of the really good qualities of the horn in those days, and which, not being garnished with a defence of brass or bronze, was ever in danger of being destroyed when of a weak nature. Besides, brazen-footed and solid or strong-footed ($\chi\rho\alpha\tau\epsilon\rho\omega\nu\upsilon\xi$) appear to be synonymous terms ; thus (in Book xxii., lines 192-3) he sings of the time

> ‘ When the *solid-footed* horses fly
> Around the course, contending for the prize.’

And again (Book xxiv., line 331), strong-hoofed mules are mentioned. The terms were used for many purposes, but never as an indication of shod hoofs. Homer made Achilles and Stentor brazen-voiced.[1] Bulls, fabular stags, and horses, had solid or metallic feet. Thus Pindar[2] (B.C. 520) tells us that Bellerophon was enjoined to sacrifice a *strong-footed* bull to the mighty encircler of the earth before subduing the winged horse Pegasus; and we find that the Grecian heroes who went in search of the golden fleece would all have been destroyed by the *brazen-footed* bulls, from whose nostrils flames issued, had not Medæa interposed and driven away these taurine monsters belonging to King Ætes.[3] Virgil[4] frequently mentions animals of various kinds with metal feet, and Ovid[5] also alludes to them oftener than once. And an older authority than

---

[1] Iliad, book v. 785.   [2] Olymp. xiii.
[3] Ibid. Olymp. iv. :

> ‘ His furious bulls, whose nostrils bright
> Flames of consuming fire diffused,
> Battering the ground with. *brazen tread*.’

[4] Æneid, book vi. 803.
[5] Heroid. ep. xii. 93 : Metamorphosis vii. 105 : Apollonius, iii. 228.

either of these, and next to Homer himself, the prophet Micah (B. C. 710), exclaims · ' Arise and thresh, O daughter of Zion : for I will make thine horn iron, *and I will make thy hoofs brass:* and thou shalt beat in pieces many people.' [1]

So that really there is no foundation for supposing that the words quoted bear any reference whatever to shoeing. Homer is very minute in some of his descriptions of horses, chariots, armour, and equipment, but there is nothing particular in his poem to lead any one to suspect that the steeds of his warriors were shod. Had they been so, or had he been aware of the art, we can scarcely doubt but he would have introduced some notice of it ; entering as he does into so many particulars about horses, which were, next to man, the chief figures in his word-pictures. For instance, he speaks of the method of securing horses ; Neptune's team was stabled in a cave

' 'Twixt Tenedos and Imbro's rocky isle.'

After driving the brazen-footed steeds through the sea, skimming the waves of blue, Neptune takes them to his retreat, then

' Loosed from the chariot, and before them placed
*A*mbrosial provender ; *and round their feet
Shackles of gold,* which none might break nor loose,
That there they might await their lord's return.' [2]

As Homer's famous epic describes the misfortunes and the siege of Troy, occurring about twelve hundred years before our era, it is important that the words supposed to denote shoeing be properly understood.

[1] Chap. IV. 13.   [2] Iliad, xiii. 41-5.

A passage from the Greek poet Tryphiodorus has often been quoted to support the argument in favour of Homer's brazen-footed horses being provided with shoes; and it has been asserted from this passage that shoes of a description similar to those now in use were known at the siege of Troy, because this poet, when speaking of the fabrication of the Trojan horse, mentions that the artist did not forget to put the metal or iron on the hoofs of that wooden machine, in order to make the resemblance more complete. It must be remembered, however, that Tryphiodorus flourished at some period between the third and sixth centuries of our era, when, as will be shown hereafter, this art was not unknown; and as the poem is of comparatively modern date, he may have introduced imaginary shoes to make his picture more complete, just as some of the modern translators of the *Iliad* have done, but without the slightest authority, to prove that these were in use at the time of the war between the Greeks and Trojans.

In his verses, however, I can find no proof of any such intention, nor any mention of an iron rim for the wooden horse's hoofs.

A literal translation of the original Greek is as follows: 'Then at length he finished the work, the hoofs *appearing* not without brass, and shone forth, being covered with tortoise-shell.' Dr Merrick,[1] who furnishes a Latin and English version, renders the passage thus:

'To deck each hoof and grace the artist's skill,
The clouded tortoise yields her polished shell.'

There has been nothing more advanced, so far as I

[1] Tryphiodorus, by Merrick. Oxford, 1742.

am aware, to prove that the ancient Greeks were cognizant of hoof defences, as we now employ them, except the
finding of a horse's hoof (of stone?) in the ruins of the
Parthenon.   In alluding to this, Mr Syer Cuming, who
appears to have taken some interest in the subject, asks,
' Does not Homer allude to shoes when he speaks of
" brazen-footed horses?" (χαλκοποδες ιπποι). Mr Cureton
informs me that he has seen horse-shoes of bronze.' [1]

And at a later period he writes, ' Since the publication
of my paper a few facts have come to light, which tend
to prove in an eminent degree the assertion therein advanced, namely, that the horses of the classic ages were
shod in a similar way to those of our own day.   At the
time the paper was produced, we had little to countenance
the idea that the early Greeks protected the feet of their
steeds with metallic shoes, beyond the bare fact that some
ancient horse-shoes of bronze were known to be in existence, and the poetical mention of " brazen-footed horses"
in the Iliad (viii. 41, xiii. 23).   Within these few years,
however, Mr Charles Newton, while Vice-consul at My-
tilene, found among the fragments of the Parthenon, a
horse's hoof with holes all around the inside, clearly indicating where a metallic shoe had been fastened, and it is
quite unlikely that any such defence should appear upon
a statue if a similar article had not been in actual use at
the time.' [2]

It must be confessed that the discovery of a horse's
foot among the world-renowned ruins of the Parthenon,
with what appeared to be holes *all round the inside* only,

[1] Journal of the *Archæological Association*, vol. vi.
[2] Ibid. vol. xvi.

is no indication whatever that a metallic shoe had ever been fastened to it. Had such an article been used, the ancient Greeks would have left us more indisputable proof than a few holes *only round the inside* of the hoof of one of their statues. The holes were doubtless made for some other purpose, and it is to be regretted that no description beyond this is to be found. This, however, will be referred to hereafter.

An allusion to hoofs of horses is frequently discovered in the Greek poets and writers of a later date than the days of Homer, but all negative the idea that they had any brass, bronze, or iron protection. Aristophanes (B.C. 427), for example, in his Comedy of the ' Knights,' makes the chorus address Neptune as the god 'who loves the *noise of the hoofs of horses* and their neighing.' Further reference to the noise made by the hoofs of horses will be furnished when we speak of the Romans.

The strongest evidence that shoeing was not practised among the Greeks of this period, is to be found in the great attention paid to the nature and durability of the hoofs by horsemen and others, and this testimony one would think perfectly convincing. Of these we may select Xenophon, the celebrated Athenian General, in whose eloquent writings enough will be found to satisfy the most incredulous in this respect. This celebrated cavalry officer appears to have carefully studied that animal's character and habits, and all the precepts he gives in his treatise on horsemanship are dictated with an amount of wisdom and humanity which has not, perhaps, been excelled since his day. The safety and comfort of that animal and his rider were ever before him, and his teaching was principally directed to make the horse particularly adapted for war, as the importance of cavalry was beginning to be perceived by the Greeks in their contests with that nation of horsemen, the Persians. He displays great judgment when specifying the proper form and disposition of parts which collectively make up the nearest approach to a perfect horse, and markedly shows to what a high degree in that distant age this kind of knowledge was cultivated; indeed, from his writing, we are led to infer, that in his time, and perhaps for long before, there were accomplished horse-breakers and public riding masters, as well as men who were excellent judges of horses' qualities.

Xenophon's instructions are well worthy of a place in every treatise on horses and horsemanship, and as his chief experience was no doubt derived while following the profession of arms, and during his command of the cavalry in conducting and covering the glorious retreat of the Ten Thousand Greeks from the interior of Persia, abundant opportunities must have presented themselves to justify him in afterwards urging on the attention of those who had the care of horses, the most scrupulous circumspection in the preservation of their hoofs; thus strongly indicating that shoes were not in use.

In advising as to the good 'points' to be sought for in a horse, he employs the clearest terms to express his meaning. 'A person,' he says, 'may form his opinion of the feet by first examining the hoofs; for *thick* (or strong) hoofs are much more conducive to firmness than *thin* ones; and it must not also escape his notice whether the hoofs are high or low, as well before as behind; for high hoofs (that is, concave or hollow-soled hoofs) raise what is called the frog (χελιδούα) far above the ground; and low ones tread equally on the strongest and weakest parts of the foot, like in-kneed men, or like cripples among men, who limp on parts which were never intended by nature to support them.[1] Simo[2] says that horses which have good feet may be known by the *sound;* and he says this with great justice, for a *hollow hoof* rings against the ground like a cymbal.' It is somewhat strange to find Markham, in the 17th century, laying stress on this sounding property of a good hoof: 'If a horse's hoofs be rugged, and as it were seamed one seam over another, and many seams; if they be dry, full and crusty, or crumbling, it is a sign of very old age: and on the contrary part, a smooth, moist, *hollow, and well-sounding hoof* is a sign of young years.'[3]

Xenophon continues: 'As attention must be paid to the horse's food and exercise, that his body may be vigorous, so must care be likewise taken of his feet. Damp and smooth stable-floors injure even naturally good hoofs; and to prevent them from being damp, they ought to be sloping; to prevent them from being smooth, they should

---

[1] Οἱ γὰρ παχεῖς πολὺ τῶν λεπτῶν διαφέρουσιν εἰς εὐποδίαν. ἔπειτα οὐδὲ τοῦτο δεῖ λανθάνειν, πότερον αἱ ὁπλαί εἰσιν ὑψηλαὶ ἢ ταπειναὶ, καὶ ἔμπροσθεν, καὶ ὄπισθεν, ἢ χαμηλαί. αἱ μὲν γὰρ ὑψηλαὶ πόρρω ἀπὸ τοῦ δαπέδου ἔχουσι τὸν χελίδονα καλουμένην, αἱ δὲ ταπειναὶ ὁμοίως βαίνουσι τῷ τε ἰσχυροτάτῳ, καὶ τῷ μαλακωτάτῳ τοῦ ποδός, ὥσπερ οἱ βλαισοὶ τῶν ἀνθρώπων.—ΠΕΡΙ ἹΠΠΙΚΗΣ, Ed. Lennc. p. 932.

[2] Simo, an *A*thenian, mentioned by Suidas and cited by Pollux, was, according to Pliny, the first who wrote on horsemanship. Some reference to him is made in a fragment of Hierocles, which is inserted in the *De Re Veterinariâ* of Simon Grynæus. Basil, 1537.

[3] The Perfect Horseman, p. 129. London, 1655.

have irregularly-shaped stones inserted in the ground (or be paved), and close to one another, similar to a horse's hoofs in size; for such stable floors give firmness to the feet of horses that stand on them.'   In alluding to grooming a horse out of doors, he continues: 'The ground outside the stable may be put into excellent condition, and serve to strengthen the horse's feet, if a person throws down in it, here and there, four or five measures full of round stones, large enough to fill the two hands, and each about a pound (?) in weight; surrounding them with an iron rim, so that these may not be scattered; for as the horse stands on these, he will be in much the same condition as if he were to travel part of every day on a stony road.

Isaac Vossius observes on this passage, that Xenophon speaks of iron shoes περὶ ἱππιχῆς, where he directs the hoofs of horses to be protected with iron περιχηδῶσαι σίδηρου. This is the iron hoop to bind the stones. He also says that in an old manuscript of the Greek Hip piatrics in his possession, which was illustrated with paint ings, the *marks* and *traces* of the nails that pierced their hoofs were plainly seen. No reliance can be placed on this author's statements, unfortunately, for marks on a hoof in an old drawing are no great proofs of shoeing; and besides, the strange construction he puts on Xenophon's words, furnishes another instance of how little he could be received as an authority on such a subject. He was remarkable for believing the strangest inconsistencies, and almost anything but the truth; which caused Charles II. to say of him, 'This learned divine is a strange man; he believes everything but the Bible.'

The Greek warrior adds: 'A horse must also move his hoofs when he is rubbed down, or when he is annoyed with flies, as much as when he is walking; and the stones which are thus spread about strengthen the FROGS of the feet.' In another book he[1] repeats the suggestion as to the improvement of the feet by this kind of pavement, and adds, 'He that makes trial of this suggestion will give credit to others which I shall offer, and will see the feet of his horse become firm.' The word Στρογγύλους, here employed to denote firmness, has evidently the same signification as the Latin word *teres:* that is, something smooth, round, and of a proper shape, indicative of strength, soundness, and durability.

It is curious to note a similar expression in use at the present day among the Arabs of the Sahara. 'The hoof round and hard. The hoof should resemble the cup of a slave. They walk on hoofs hard as the moss-covered stones of a stagnant pool. The frogs hard and dry. The frogs concealed beneath the hoofs are seen when he lifts his feet, and resemble date-stones in hardness.'[2]

Furthermore, Xenophon says: 'Those horses whose feet are hardened with exercise, will be as superior on rough ground to those which are not habituated to it, as persons who are sound in their limbs to those who are lame.' In the same work, when treating of the duties pertaining to a commander of cavalry, he dwells on the necessity of attending to the horses' feet: 'You must pay attention to their feet, so that they (the horses) may be in a condition to be ridden even on rough ground, knowing

[1] Hipparchicus, p. 611.
[2] *Dumas:* The Horses of the Sahara.

that when they suffer from being ridden they become useless.' He also, in the treatise on horsemanship, speaks of the water used to wash the horses' legs as doing harm to the hoofs by, I suppose, softening them, as the spirit of his teaching was to keep them hard and dry. He makes no mention whatever of any defence for the horses' feet; though he notices the fashion of defending the legs of soldiers by *embattai* or leggings (ἐμβάται), and in passing them under the feet, he says, they might also serve as shoes. These may have been used in cases of emergency for horses, but nothing is said on this point. He specifies horse-armour and its value: 'Since, then, if the horse is disabled, the rider will be in extreme peril, it is necessary to arm the horse also with defences for his head, his breast, and his shoulders. But of all parts of the horse we must take most care to protect his belly, for it is at once a most vital and a most defenceless part; but it is possible to protect it by something connected with the housings. It is necessary, too, that that which covers the horse's back should be put together in such a way that the rider may have a firmer seat (than if he sat on the horse's bare back), and that the back of the horse may not be galled. As to other parts, also, both horse and horseman should be armed with the same precaution (so that the armour may not chafe).' [1]

In a treatise on hunting, ascribed to this author, in speaking of the horse, it is remarked: 'Before the task is accomplished, he falls, the hoofs worn off.' [2] And in another work [3] he incidentally relates that certain people of

---

[1] Hipparchicus, c. xii.   [2] *Sturz*, Lex. Xenoph. Cynegeticon.
[3] De Cyri Min. Expedit., p. 228.

Asia (Armenians ?) whom he saw, were in the habit of tying sandals, or rather, drawing socks over the feet of their horses when the snow lay very thick on the ground, to prevent their sinking too deeply. 'The horses in this country were smaller than those of Persia, but far more spirited. The chief instructed the men to tie little bags (Κυρ Αναβ) round the feet of the horses, and other cattle, when they drove them through the snow, for without such bags they sank up to their bellies.'

This is the only mention made of a garniture for the feet of horses by the renowned author and soldier, and I am not aware of any recent writer mentioning this contrivance in the uplands of Armenia. It may be remarked, however, that in Kamschatka the dogs employed to draw sledges or catch seals wear socks provided with small holes to allow the claws to protrude. These may to some extent not only protect the feet from injury, but also help to guard against sinking in the snow. Arctic travellers have likewise availed themselves of these appliances for their dogs.[1]

The only Greek writer before the Christian era, after Xenophon, who alludes to a defence for the feet of animals is Aristotle (B.C. 340). In describing the camel's foot, he writes : 'The foot is fleshy underneath, like that of a bear; wherefore, when camels are used in war, and become foot-sore, their drivers put them on leather shoes ('ΥΠΟΔΕ-ΟΥΣΙ Καρβατιναις).'[2] They were probably most frequently

---

[1] *See* Beiträge zur Phys. Oekonomie der Russischen Länder. Berlin, 1786. Captain Cook's Last Voyage, and the later Voyages of Arctic Explorers.

[2] Hist. *A*nimal. lib. ii. p. 850.

made of raw hide or coarse cloth (as Ludolphus tells us the Tartars used cow-hide for their horses' feet), passing round the feet and up the legs, like a laced boot.   They will be noticed hereafter as *solea*.

Polydore Vergil (A.D. 1550), in his ' De Inventoribus Rerum,' informs us that the Thessalians were reported to have been the first who protected their horses' hoofs with shoes of iron.   ' Hos quoque (Peletronios, qui Thessaliæ populi sunt) primos equorum ungulas munire ferreis soleis cœpisse ferunt ' [1]   This author, whose Latin was generally more elegant than his descriptions were faithful, does not give his authorities for this statement, which is unsupported by any proof of its correctness.   In all likelihood, as Mr Pegge observes,[2] he has misled himself by referring to Virgil, where that poet asserts that

' The Pelian Lapithæ
Invented bits, and mounted on the back ;
Broke horses to the ring, and made them spring
Under the arm'd, and proudly pace the round.' [3]

Vergil made a mistake, or allowed himself to be deceived, when he described these primitive people of North Greece as the inventors of horse-shoes.

If we turn from the Greek writers who lived previous to our era, to the wonderful productions of the Greek sculptors, those divine works of art—those graceful chisellings portraying groups of men and horses, which are

---

[1] Lib. ii. cap. 12.   [2] Archæologia, 1776.
[3] Georgics, iii. 115 :

' Frena Pelethronii Lapithæ gyrosque dedere
Impositi dorso, atque equitem docuere sub armis
Insultare solo, et gressus glomerare superbos.'

> ' Not yet dead,
> But in old marbles ever beautiful,'

we will find our suspicions as to the inaccuracy of those who assert that this people provided an armour for their horses' feet, more than confirmed.

It must be remembered that the Greeks were the first true interpreters of nature. To this their physical organization, their climate, but, perhaps, most of all their religion, concurred to develop those principles of beauty that induce man to select from nature the forms and combinations which give the highest and most endurable pleasure.

The creations of these people, who, according to Pindar,

> ' Strew'd o'er their walls, their public ways,
> The sculptured life, the breathing stone,'[1]

now that two thousand years have passed away, yet, and will ever, command the admiration of refined taste, speaking, as they do, to our imagination and understanding, while carrying with them the greatest beauty of proportion, the utmost simplicity and truth in design, and blending a harmony with a purity and regard for nature such as has never been surpassed. We recognize in their sculptures of horses that intense and astonishing expression of life, which none but the greatest artists are capable of bestowing on their imitations of nature, when teeming with vitality and action. Theocritus, two thousand years ago, was enraptured with these chisellings:

> ' How true they stand, and move, and quite appear
> Alive, not wrought! What clever things men are l'[2]

[1] Olympic Ode, VII.   [2] Idyll xv. 83.

Such a people must have loved the bold, dauntless courage of the horse, and while seeking to do its un matchable powers justice in their poetry and adoration in their religion, they have testified to all posterity, by the unerring delineations of their chisels, the beauty and the grandeur of his form and disposition. We have an example of this in the Panathenaic frieze, where the horses are not only of exquisite beauty, but full of life and fire. No two out of the hundred and ten which are introduced are in the same attitude, and each is charac- terized by a different expression. Flaxman ever spoke of these horses with enthusiasm, and we cannot wonder at it. ' The horses in the frieze in the Elgin collection,' he said, ' appear to live and move, to roll their eyes, to gallop, prance, and curvet; the veins of their faces and legs seem distended with circulation ; in them are dis- tinguished the hardness and decision of bony forms, from the elasticity of tendons and the softness of flesh. The beholder is concerned with the deer-like lightness and elegance of their make, and although the relief is not above an inch from the background, and they are so much smaller than nature, we can scarcely suffer reason to persuade us they are not alive.'[1]

The horses of Thessaly are there depicted as they exist at the present day, even to the characteristic large heads and thick necks.[2]

To say that they are exactly portrayed in every anatomical detail, is to declare nothing but the simple truth, and is sufficient for our object. And yet the very

[1] Lectures on Science, vol. iv. p. 104.
[2] *Dodwell.* Travels, vol. i. p. 339.

closest scrutiny of the horses' feet in these marbles with a practised—might I add a professional—eye, leads to the unhesitating conclusion that they are exact copies of nature in every respect, but nature never adorned or protected by an iron or bronze furniture. So true do they appear to real life, that we can almost fancy the animals in their spirited movements have chipped their hoofs at the sides (or quarters); and they are of a shape and perfectness which one seldom sees in hoofs that have been shod for any length of time.

These unrivalled relics of antiquity offer additional proofs that metal shoes were not in use. The ancient Greeks were very careful in representing the different costumes worn by the riders of these horses, even to the fashion of their foot covers. Not only this, but they had their marble statues adorned with metals in many instances, which again were not unfrequently gilt. 'For the fragments show that the weapons, the reins of the horses, and other accessories, were in metal, probably gilt.'[1] The horses appeared to have had bits in their mouths, and the holes yet remain at the commissures of the lips wherein they have been fixed; but no evidence is to be found that any metal was attached to the hoofs. In a bas-relief of Castor and Pollux in the Townley gallery of the British Museum, instead of metal bridles for the two horses, red paint appears to have been used. No paint, however, is to be discovered on the feet of any horses to indicate that shoes were worn.

In the Temple collection (case 56) in the British

[1] Description of the Collections of Ancient Marbles in the British Museum. Part IV. page 26. London, 1830.

Museum, among bronze fragments of a statue and sacrificial implements, is a very perfect hind foot and pastern of a horse, from Magna Græcia. This is unshod, and from the shape and general appearance of the hoof, there can be no doubt that the original of this model had never been submitted to this badge of servile subjection, as old Gwillin has been pleased to designate the modern horse-shoe. And among all the relics to be found in this and other museums, nothing can be discerned that the most lively imagination would transform into a horse-shoe, as employed by the ancient Greeks. Weapons there are without number, articles belonging to religious and domestic requirements, armour and spurs for riders, armour and bits for horses, and in the British Museum are also two excellent specimens of muzzles for horses. Xenophon informs us that, in his day, the groom put on the muzzle (κημὸς) when the horse was led from his stable to be groomed or exercised; indeed on every occasion when he had no bridle on his head or bit in his mouth, to prevent his doing any mischief to other horses or to men. While it prevented the horse from biting it did not interfere with his breathing.[1]

A civilized nation which prized the horse so highly, and so largely employed it in war and in the public diversions, could not but display its wisdom in providing everything for its comfort and well-being; but it appears that the Greeks did not understand extending its utility by preventing undue wear of the hoofs and consequent lameness. All the paintings on vases and elsewhere represent the horse with nude feet.

[1] Xenophon, Hipp., chap. v. 3.   Pollux, i. 202.

The climate of Greece, it must not be forgotten, is dry, and favourable to the hardness and durability of horses' hoofs; so that solipedes brought from the north or west, where their journeys would be of a limited character without shoes, may there acquire sufficient strength and cohesiveness in the horny box covering the inferior extremity of the limbs, as to perform a certain amount of labour with no defence.

Paul Louis Courier,[1] who translated Xenophon's treatise on horsemanship, was so pleased with his method of managing the feet of horses, that during the very brief campaign in Calabria in 1807, while with the army corps to which he belonged, he rode horses without shoes, and, as he believed, with advantage. In a note he adds: 'The ancients did not shoe their horses; this is evidenced in all the writings and monuments they have left us, and we cannot be astonished that the people who, in so many different countries, do not know the use of shoes, should not yet have introduced them. The Tonguses, as well as the majority of the Tartars—the best and the most indefatigable horsemen in the world—scarcely work at all in iron; and for that reason it is impossible for them to shoe their steeds. The Dutch at the Cape of Good Hope have little horses which are never shod, according to Sparmann. And M. Thunberg has made the same remark in the island of Java. Another traveller assures us, that at Mogador, and the west coast of Africa, all the horses journey without shoes, and Niebuhr says the same for those of Yemen. Pallas has seen the horses of the Kalmucks, which have small and extremely hard hoofs,

[1] Traite de Xenophon sur l'Equitation. Panthéon Littéraire.

ridden without any shoes, and the Cossacks' on the banks
of the Jaïk, he adds, are never shod.'

Of the evil effects of prolonged marches, and consequent excessive wear of the undefended hoofs in the
Greek armies, we find casual mention now and again in
the early historians. Diodorus Siculus (B.C. 44) in one of
his volumes, when describing the victories of Alexander,
states that 'the hoofs of the horses, through ceaseless
journeying, had been worn away, and the matériel of
war was used up.'[1]

And Cinnamus speaks in the same strain of the war
in Attalia. 'He ordered them to await the rest of the
army in Attalia, and to look after the horses, for a disease
to which they are liable had attacked their hoofs, and had
done serious hurt.'[2]

In the account which Appian gives of the victory
achieved by Lucullus over Mithridates, King of Pontus,
at the siege of Cyzicum (B.C. 73), we find that Mithri
dates sent part of his cavalry back to Bithynia, such as
were useless, feeble from want of forage, and footsore or
lame in consequence of their hoofs being worn out ($\kappa\alpha\grave{\imath}$
$\chi\alpha\lambda\varepsilon\acute{\upsilon}o\nu\tau\alpha\varsigma$ $\grave{\varepsilon}\xi$ $\dot{\upsilon}\pi\sigma\tau\rho\iota\beta\tilde{\eta}\varsigma$).[3]

This description has been differently given by H.
Stephanus (edit. Stephanus, 1592, p. 221), and this has

---

[1] Diod. Siculus, lib. xvii. cap. 94, p. 233. Edit. Weissilingii.
'Equorum ungulæ propter itinera nunquam remissa detritæ et armorum
pleraque absumptæ erant.'

[2] Edit. Tollii Traject. ad Rhenum, 1825. Lib. iv. p. 194. 'Cæteras
copias manere in Attalia et equos curare jussit, nam malam cui est
obnoxium equinum genus plantes pedum acciderat, graviterque effi-
cerat.'

[3] De Bello Mithrid. p. 371. Edit. Tollii.

given rise to a serious mistake. His translation is as follows: 'Equos vero tum inutiles et infirmos ob inediam, claudicantesque solearum inopia, detritis ungulis, aversis ab hoste itineribus, misit in Bithyniam.' No such words as *solearum inopia* occur in the original text; they are an interpolation by the learned translator without the faintest authority, and have led several writers of note to believe that horse-shoes were then in use : whereas the contrary may be inferred, for the horses, it is explicitly mentioned, were lame by the attrition of their hoofs; which implies that horses were not shod. Montfauçon was led astray by this addition to the original account. He writes · 'There are *certain and undoubted proofs* that the ancients shod their horses; thus much Homer and Appian say ;'[1] and Fosbrooke[2] remarks that 'an *iron horse-shoe* is men tioned by Appian ; so that the conclusion from Xenophon's recommendation for hardening the hoof, that the ancients did not shoe beasts of burden, is too rash.'

Subsequent to the Christian era, we find Arrian[3] (A.D. 200) comparing the human body to a pack-ass—ὀνάριον ἐπισεσαγμένον, and speaking of a kind of shoe for that animal: 'Οταν ἐχεῖνο ὀνάριον ᾖ, τἄλλα γίνεται χαλινάρια τοῦ ὀναρίου, σχημάτια, ὑποδημάτια, κριθαί, χόρτος. Some translators have rendered ὑποδημάτια as 'ferreæ calces ;' but Didot, in his new Collection of Classical Greek authors, translates it as *sparteæ calces :* 'Si asselus est corpus, cetera freni erunt aselli, clitellæ, sparteæ calces, hordeum, fœnum.'

Artemidorus, in his Interpretation of Dreams, about

[1] Antiquité Expliquée, vol. iv. p. 50.
[2] Ency. of *A*ntiquities.   London, 1840.
[3] Commentar. in Epictetum, lib. iii.

the same period as Arrian, also speaks of a horse shod with a sock or shoe, ὑπόδημα, which was probably made of spartea, like the above.

I find on a silver coin of Tarentum,[1] now in the British Museum, and struck, it is surmised, about B.C. 300, a curious representation of a horse and two men, which might, at the first glance, be supposed to be connected with our subject (fig. 1).

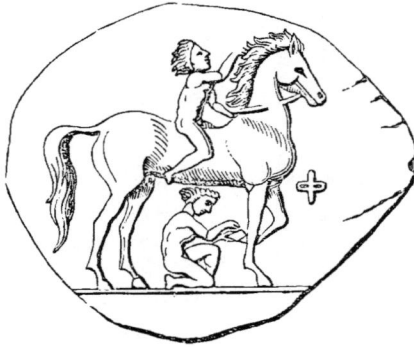

fig 1

The horse is beautifully delineated, and admirably represents the breed then famous in this part of Magna Græcia. A groom or boy, nude as the horse attendants are generally represented on ancient Greek vases and sculpture, is seated on the horse's back, and strokes his

---

[1] Tarentum, the modern Taranto, an ancient town of Italy, in the kingdom of Naples, is built on a small island, in the Gulf of Taranto, near Brindisi. It was founded B.C. 700, as a Greek colony, by Lacedæmonian Parthenii, the descendants of a people noted for their love of horses and excellent horsemanship. This city was one of the most flourishing and powerful of Magna Græcia, and was distinguished for its luxury and splendour, as well as for its encouragement of the fine arts. For a long time it resisted the Romans, but at last submitted to them, B.C. 272. The above drawing is twice the size of the coin.

mane as if to soothe him, while another individual, also nude, holds up one of the fore feet, as if to apply a shoe. The attitude is very striking, and it would be interesting to discover why such a group should be represented on a coinage.

It may be observed, however, that there is no instrument in the hands of the dismounted figure whereby to fasten on the shoe, if such be his vocation, and that his attitude is not a very convenient one. This is, nevertheless, the posture assumed on the continent of Europe, and generally all over the East, by the workman who arms the hoofs, but then there is another person to hold up the limb. In this example he may be only trying on a shoe; though the figure on the horse's back would not add to the facility with which this operation might otherwise be performed. I may mention that I have seen and heard of troop horses which, though otherwise tractable, would scarcely allow themselves to be shod unless a man were seated on their backs, stroking their ears and necks in the manner shown on the Greek coin; and Cæsar Fiaschi,[1] in the fifteenth century, recommends for horses that will not be shod quietly, that 'mots plaisants' be used, and 'faire mettre un cavalier sur le dos.' It has been suggested that a stone is being removed from the sole; but without shoes it is almost, if not quite, impossible that a stone could lodge in the foot. Might he not be fastening on a temporary shoe or sock?

Beyond the illustration this affords, we have no evidence of shoeing among the Greeks; and, after all, this may be only an allegorical representation, or a reference to some mythological subject.

[1] Maréchalerie. 3rd French edit., cap. 29. Paris, 1563.

CHAPTER II.

THE HORSE WITH THE ROMANS. THEIR CAVALRY. PLINY. CAMEL
SHOEING. SILENCE OF ROMAN HIPPIATRISTS IN REGARD TO SHOE-
ING. CATO, VARRO, HORACE, VIRGIL, LUCAN, CLAUDIANUS, FITZ-
STEPHEN. ROMAN ROADS, AND COURIERS. COLUMELLA, JULIUS
POLLUX. DIOCLETIAN'S EDICT. HOOF INSTRUMENTS. APSYRTUS,
PALLADIUS, VEGETIUS RENATUS, RENATUS FLAVIUS. POLYBIUS.
CARBATINAI AND EMBATTAI. SOLEÆ FERREA. CATULLUS, SCALIGER,
SUETONIUS. GOLD AND SILVER SOLEA. EXTRAVAGANCE OF THE
ROMANS. CALIGULA, NERO, POPPÆA, AND COMMODUS. THEOMNES-
TUS. SOLEA SPARTEA, AND THE GLANTE FERREO. HIPPOPODES.
CHARIOT-RACING. OPINIONS AS TO THE EXISTENCE OF SHOEING
WITH THE ANCIENTS. MONTFAUÇON, WINCKELMANN, FABRETTI,
CAMERARIUS, PANCIROLUS, VOSSIUS, PEGGE, SMITH, HEUSINGER,
RICH. SUPPOSED NEGATIVE EVIDENCE OF WRITTEN HISTORY
AND SCULPTURE. TEMPORARY SHOES AND OTHER EXPEDIENTS
TO PRESERVE THE HOOFS IN JAPAN, CHINA, MANILLA, SINGAPORE,
ETC. STRAW SHOES. ICELAND AND CENTRAL ASIA.

THE Romans began to use the horse at a very early
period, but not with much advantage until seven hundred
years after he had been introduced into Greece; so that
the Greeks were well advanced in the management of that
animal, and skilled in its employment long before the
Romans. For this reason it is that we find much in the
writings of the latter that was borrowed from the older
civilization; while their system of equitation and general
care of the horse was altogether Grecian. During a long
time, and even up to a comparatively late date, the army

on which the Romans depended for their conquests was
mainly composed of infantry—they were not an equestrian
nation. But, by degrees, they began to perceive the
advantages of cavalry, and during the period when Rome
was mistress of the world, and even before, many of the
Roman battles were specially planned with a view to the
operations of that arm. We can trace on and on, through
the history of the Empire, a growing regard for, and
dependence on it. Then it played a most important, and
in most cases a decisive, part in their battles, as the number of horses and horsemen began to be increased. 'A
storm of horse' was the language of Antonius, for the
brilliant charge of cavalry against an enemy.[1]

But their country, and particularly their capital, was
in general more humid than Greece, and their horses
more lax in fibre, consequently softer-hoofed. Their
legions, scattered in many regions of the world, were
brought into contact with nations of horsemen, living
and fighting on the backs of small, agile, hard-footed
steeds, inured to incessant fatigue.

Though mounted on stronger animals, the Roman
cavalry could make but little impression against that of
Persia and Arabia. The faculty of moving quickly, and
coming down in a flying cloud of skirmishers, as well as
rapid retreating and rallying, always assured the superiority
of the Numidian and Parthian horse when contending
against the heavy infantry and cavalry masses of the
Romans.

Dureau de la Malle offers the following reasonable remarks with regard to this subject: 'The durability of the

[1] *Tacitus,* lib. iii. cap. 53.

hoof for a cavalry not shod was an indispensable condition. It appears that the Parthian horses, bred in the plains of Mesopotamia, were not provided with shoes, and this fact alone explains why, in the wars with the Romans, the Parthian armies, almost entirely formed of cavalry, and always victorious in their sandy deserts, melted away or suddenly disappeared when they had pursued their adversaries into the mountainous and volcanic regions of Armenia, which are covered with obsidian and sharp stones ; it was simply because the Parthian or Persian horses were not shod.   The absence of a protection to the horn explains why—and I believe that this fact has not yet been remarked or appreciated at its just value—the Ten Thousand Greeks, in their retreat after the battle of Cunaxa, and of Mark Antony and Julian, falling back on Armenia and its mountains after their defeat in the plains, were able to escape from the numerous Persian and Parthian cavalry which incessantly pursued them.' [1]

If the Greeks were unacquainted with the art of attaching a rim of metal or other hard substance to the part of the hoof brought into contact with the ground, it might be expected that the Romans who imitated them so closely in equestrian matters would not, at any rate for some time, be in a position to devise anything of the kind ; and that, as a consequence, the utility of the horse must have been as limited as with the Grecians.   And such would appear to be the fact.   When nearly all the arts had attained a high degree of perfection, the one in question, which would have been of the greatest assist-

---

[1] *Megnin.* Op. cit. p. 9.—*Notice sur les Races Domestiques des Chevaux.*   Moniteur Universel, March 16, 1855.

ance to the conquering armies of Greece and Rome, was yet, it seems, unknown to them. Of this, in their writings, we have apparently ample evidence.

We have similar injunctions and observations with regard to the care and quality of the hoofs, and to their being uncovered, as well as to the injuries sustained in travelling, as we had from the Greek writers. No author mentions metal plates for horses' hoofs fastened on with nails.

Pliny (A.D. 60) is very minute and circumstantial in his history of discoveries, and in other portions of his writings. He tells us that Tychius, the Bœotian, first invented or taught the art of making shoes for the feet of men, and enumerates many other discoverers ; but nothing whatever as to the invention or employment of horse-shoes, though he speaks of the introduction of bridles and saddles by Pelethronius, and the people of Phrygia as being the first to use chariots. With regard to the camel, however, he follows Aristotle closely in his description of that animal's foot, and the way in which it was then protected : 'The camel has pastern bones like those of the ox, but somewhat smaller, the feet being cloven, with a slight line of division, and having a fleshy sole, like that of the bear ; hence it is, that in a long journey the animal becomes fatigued, and the foot cracks, if it is not shod (*calceatu*).' [1]

The term employed by the Roman naturalist to

---

[1] Hist. Naturalis, lib. xi. cap. 106. 'Camelo tali similes bubulis, sed minores paulo. Est enim bisculus discrimine exiguo pes imus, vestigio carnoso, ut ursi ; qua de causa in longiore itinere sine calceatu fatiscunt.' Edit. Gabriels Brotier. London, 1826.

designate shoeing is referred to in a foot-note in the edition of his writings from which this paragraph is extracted: 'Quam ob causam, inquit Philos. loc. cit. in bellicis expeditionibus, carbatinis calceantur, cum ipsis pes dolet. Est autem καρβατίνη vile et rusticum calceamentum, una sappactum solea.' The Mongol Tartars, as I have before noticed, seldom if ever shoe their ponies, chiefly, perhaps, because of the scarcity of iron, their peripatetic mode of life, and the large numbers of these animals they always have to select from; but perhaps also as much from the presence of camels in their droves of animals, and which are their principal beasts of burthen. In consequence of these creatures being able to traverse the dreary steppes of Mongolia without suffering much injury, they are preferred; and in thus economizing the labours of the horse, they diminish the need for shoeing it. According to M. Huc,[1] however, the camel in that distant region is not exempt from some of the evils which are incidental to the unshod feet of horses; and he relates that, after a long journey, when this most useful creature has become footsore, the Tartars make sheepskin shoes for it.

My friend Mr Michie, who has travelled overland from Peking to Siberia, across the desert of Gobi, tells me that whenever a camel's feet have become tender from long journeying, it assumes the recumbent position; and this being observed by the driver, an examination is at once made of the soles, when, if the thick cuticle which covers these pads is found raised and looking white-blistered, as it were, shoeing is determined on. This is

[1] Travels in Tartary, Thibet, and China, in 1844-5-6.

accomplished as follows. Two or three strong Mongols watch their opportunity, and when the creature is still reposing and off its guard, they make a simultaneous rush upon it, throw it on its side, and in a few seconds of time secure it; then with much dexterity a square piece of leather, large enough to cover the bruised place, is applied, and nimbly, yet *firmly stitched with a slightly curvec needle to the foot, through the thick skin of the sole.* After this the beast is able at once to resume its toil.

This is bold treatment, and eminently suggestive of that originality which must have prompted the desperate attempt, when made for the first time, to nail a rim of iron to the horse's foot. The one appears at first sight as hazardous as the other, and were we still ignorant of the art of nail-shoeing, I fear many of us would be incredulous if told that it was practised by other nations.

Roman writers on agriculture and other subjects are silent on that of shoeing, as it is now understood; though from the general minuteness with which they treat all details connected with their studies, had they not been unconscious of it altogether, it must, one cannot help concluding, have received at least some passing allusion. Nearly all, however, speak of the deperdition of the hoofs, and the qualities they should possess to enable them to withstand wear.

Marcus P. Cato, commonly designated the Censor (B.C. 234-149), says nothing in reference to this matter in his 'De Re Rustica.'

Marcus Varro (B.C. 60), in his celebrated work, when advising as to the choice of a horse, says: 'It ought to have upright, straight, and symmetrical limbs, round knees, not too large, nor yet inclining inwards, and *hard hoofs*,'[1] showing that the latter were an essential quality in unshod horses. He also asserts that the hoofs are injured by standing in manure, as the horn thereby becomes softened.[2]

Q. F. Horace (B.C. 30), in one of his famous satires, alludes to the mode of buying horses as practised by a certain class in his day. 'This is the custom with men of fortune; when they buy horses they inspect them covered: that if a beautiful forehand (as very often happens) be supported by a *tender hoof*, it may not take in the buyer, who may be eager for the bargain, because the back is handsome, the head little, and the neck stately. This they do judiciously'[3] And the same author, in one of his admirable Odes, alludes to the sound caused by the horses' unshod feet on the smooth flagstones of their wonderfully paved roads, and in a sense similar to that noticed in the Greek writers already quoted: 'And the horseman will beat the streets of the city with sounding hoofs.'[4]

It is interesting to note, that the poetical epithet of 'sounding foot.' is almost constantly applied to the horse by various writers, at this and a later period. For example:

Virgil (B.C. 20) in the Æneid, exclaims, 'Infatuate!

---

[1] De Re Rustica. 'Cruribus rectis et equalibus, genibus rotundis nec magnis, nec introrsum spectantibus, ungulis duris.' Lib. ii. p. 306. Edit. Gesner.

[2] 'Ne sternis comberat ungulas cavendum.' Lib. ii. cap. 7.

[3] Book ii., Satire 2.

[4]
Et urbem
Eques sonante verberabit ungula.

who, with brazen car, and the prancing of his *horn-hoofed* steeds, would needs counterfeit the storms and inimitable thunder.'[1] And again: 'Their acclamations rise; and, a squadron formed, the *hoof* beats with trampling din the mouldering plain.'[2] In another place he also alludes to the favourite epithet by which this animal was popularly known to the Roman—that of *Sonipes.* 'On its sounding hoofs the horse stands, and impatient champs the foaming bit.'[3]

In the Georgics, when he wishes to point out in a particular manner, one of the most cherished qualities in the noble animal he so beautifully describes in that poem —the density and shape of the external covering of the foot,—he eloquently says of the war-horse: 'With his hoof of solid and deeply-resounding horn, he hollows out the earth.'[4] Or as Sotheby more poetically expresses it

> ' earth around
> Rings to the solid hoof that wear the ground.'

Virgil mentions the wheels shod with iron as *ferati orbes,* but makes not the most distant allusion to a like garniture on hoofs.

And M. A. Lucan (A.D. 60) in his poem 'Pharsalia,' frequently mentions the nature of the horse's feet. For instance, when speaking of the horses belonging to Curio's

---

[1] Book v. 592-4.   [2] Book viii. 596-8.

[3] Book iv. 135. ' Stat *sonipes,* ac frena ferox spumantia mandit.' Another example is found in the same poem : ' Quo *sonipes* ictu furit arduus altaque jactat.'

[4] Book iii. 88,—

> ' Cavatque
> Tellurem, et solidus graviter sonat ungula cornu.'

detachment, which had fallen into an ambuscade when attacking the Numidians, he says : 'Not there did the charger, moved by the clanging of trumpets, shake the rocks with the beating of *his hoof.* .... Nor avails it any one to have cut short the delay of his *horny-hoofed* steed, for they have neither space nor force for the onset.'[1] And referring to an incident in the campaign which culminated in that important engagement, it is written : 'Pompey care deters, by reason of the land being exhausted for affording fodder, which the horseman in his course has trodden down, and with quickened steps the *horny-hoof* has beaten down the shooting field.' [2]

The poet Claudianus, three centuries later, addressing the Emperor Honorius, in one of his epigrams exclaims,

'O felix *sonipes* cui tanti fræna mereri
    Numinis.'

Even so late as the 12th century, Fitz-Stephens, when describing London, and the excellent quality of the horses, remarks, 'Cum talium *sonipedem* cursus imminet,' etc. The expression was, doubtless, borrowed from Virgil, or some of the old Latin poets.   And yet later, the characteristic designation is alluded to, for Ludwig Carrio, in commenting on Leutprand's Chronicle, quotes an old verse, a line of which runs : 'His parvus *sonipes*, nec marti notus.'

Though the appellation may be traced to the Greeks, yet it has been surmised that it had its origin with the Romans, from the circumstance that in consequence of their not knowing how to protect their horses' feet in a substantial manner, they were compelled to construct their roads to accommodate the unarmed hoof; thus were formed

[1] Book iv. 749-67.   [2] Book vi.

those mighty works which surpassed all the other monuments of this people. Made at immense labour and expense, they extended, it may be said, from the Pillars of Hercules, through Spain and Gaul, to the Euphrates and the most southern parts of Egypt. Everything was sacrificed in their construction ; hills were sometimes perforated, and mountains and great rocks were deeply cut for their passage, as at Terracina. Those of Italy, if we are to judge by their remains, were the best made ; the Appian Way is perhaps the most solid. These admirably formed highways were elaborately and curiously built. The centre, being subjected to the greatest amount of wear, was higher than the sides, and consisted of strata of sand, gravel, and excellent cement, overlaid by the pavement, in the form of not very large flat stones, laid close together and firmly bound by the cement, thus making a hard smooth causeway. Near Rome the flags were of granite. From their very even surface, and their passing between banks, mounds, and through valleys, the hard hollow hoofs of prancing steeds would sound loud enough, when compared with the noise made by other quadrupeds. Hence the epithet of ' sounding feet' was very appropriate, and naturally suggested itself, according to Bracy Clark.

Montfauçon says the surface was very smooth, like glass, a circumstance which must have made the horses in wet weather slide about very much ; even in the best weather, travelling must have been uncommonly slow, had horses worn iron shoes, because of their slipperiness. Besides, they would not have lasted nearly so long, and so far as I can ascertain there are no traces of horse-shoe wear to be discovered on their surface—a fact worthy of notice. The Romans travelled very fast on them, so well adapted were they, all things considered, for the preservation of the horses' hoofs.

Towards the Christian era, Augustus introduced couriers (*publici Cursores,* or *Veredarii*) to forward the public despatches, and along these roads government post-houses (*mutationes*) were erected at intervals of five or six miles, and each was constantly furnished with forty horses. By means of these very frequent relays, no doubt necessary where the hoofs were exposed to damaging attrition, it was possible to travel a hundred miles a day.

About a century before our era, Cicero received at Rome, on the 28th September, a letter dated in Britain the first day of the same month. Considering the passage by sea, and crossing the Alps, or making a wide *détour* to avoid this troublesome mountain range, the twenty-six days appear a remarkably short space of time to travel this distance in. And three hundred years later, during the reign of the Emperor Theodosius, Cæsarius, an important magistrate, travelled from Antioch to Constantinople, a distance of 725 Roman (665 English) miles, in six days.

At Terracina, where a stony ridge is cut through to a depth of 26 feet to form the public way, the glassy surface of this rocky thoroughfare is grooved (*sillonné*) transversely, so that the horses might have foot-hold.

It may here be noticed that at Tempe, by the side of the Peneus, the highway is excavated in the rock, but is so steep and rugged, that possibly to save their horses' hoofs, as well as to prevent their tumbling into the river, the Greeks scooped out resting-places or wide steps to diminish the risks attending a descent.[1]

We will return again to the Roman authors.

L. J. M. Columella of Cadiz (A.D. 40), a writer well acquainted with the science of his day, and a scholar, gives us an admirable outline of veterinary medicine as it was then known to the Romans ; and his influence on the development of this department of the healing art has been very great. In one of the twelve books of the ' De Re Rustica,' still in existence, he alludes to the stable management of a country villa in the following terms : ' The master should frequently go into his stable, and should be particular in observing that the floor of the stalls is sufficiently high in the centre, and not made of soft wood, as ignorance or negligence often makes it. The floor should be made of hard oak-plank closely laid ; for this kind of wood *hardens the hoofs of horses and makes them like stones.*' [2]

It is somewhat remarkable that, as already observed, in Java, where horses are unshod, they are kept standing on hard-wood floors without any straw or other soft substance between the boards and their hoofs ; and at Singapore and Manilla—places I visited in 1860—all the

---

[1] *See* Montfauçon, ' *A*ntiquité Expliquée,' vol. iv. pt. 2, p. 177 ; Bergier, ' Hist. des *G*rands Chemins de l'Empire Romaine,' livre ii. chap. i.; Procopius, ' Hist. *A*rcana,' cap. 30 ; Libanius, ' Orationes,' 22, and ' Itineraria,' pp. 572-81.

[2] Lib. i. p. 73 ; edit. Manheim. ' Diligens itaque dominus stabulum frequenter intrabit, et primum dabit operam, ut stratus pontilis emineat, ipsumque sit non ex mollibus lignis, sicut frequenter per imperitiam vel negligentiam evenit, sed roboris vivacis duritia et soliditate compactum ; nam hoc genus ligni equorum ungulas ad saxorum instar obdurat.'

horses are made to stand on planks raised above the ground, in order, I suppose, that the undefended hoofs may be kept dry and hard.

In selecting horses, Columella recommends that they should have '*hard*, upright hoofs, hollow in the sole, and round, with medium-sized coronets.' [1] Elsewhere he advises that the foal should be taken from its dam when a year old, and pastured among the mountains and in other exposed or inhospitable places, 'so that the hoofs may be hardened to resist wear, and then become fitted for long journeys.' [2]

And Pliny, about this period, observes, in speaking of mules, 'They are produced by an union between the mare and the domestic ass; they are swift, and have *extremely hard feet.*' [3]

Julius Pollux, a Greek, and the favourite and preceptor of the Emperor Commodus, in whose reign he died (A.D. 238), has left us, in one of his works,[4] some excellent maxims concerning horses. Indicating the particulars in which a good horse differed from a bad one he maintains that it is more especially in the nature of their feet. 'A corpore quidem ungulæ cavæ, ut scilicet quam vocant testudinem, elata sit, ne in solum impingens, molestetur: hujusmodi enim ungula (ut Xenophon inquit)

---

[1] Lib. vi. p. 50. 'Duris ungulis et altis, et concavis rotundisque, quibus coronæ mediocres superpositæ sunt.'

[2] Ibid. p. 63. 'Ut ungulas duret sitque postea longis itineribus habilis.'

[3] Hist. Natural. 'Generantur ex equâ et onagris mansuefactis mulæ velocis in cursu, duritiâ eximiâ pedum.'

[4] Onomasticon, lib. i. cap. 11; De Corpore et Animo Equi Boni et Mali.

cymbali instar ad solum resonat.' A bad horse was known
by the inferior quality of its hoofs and their softness,
' mollis ungulas;' while a good one should have them
' carneæ pleneæ.' It will be observed that he refers to
Xenophon ; he also follows him in recommending a stable
paved with large round stones to harden the feet. In this
work, he mentions every article of horse-furniture then in
use, but is silent with regard to that for the hoofs.

In 1827, an edict of the Emperor Diocletian, supposed
to have been promulgated about A.D. 300, was discovered.
It fixes the maximum rate of wages and price of provisions,
and two passages in it give us an idea, not only of the
functions and emoluments of the individual who minis-
tered to the requirements of sick animals, but also affords
another proof that the hoofs of solipedes were not shod.
The mulomedicus who clipped the hair and trimmed
the hoofs, was to receive for each animal six denarii ;
and for currying and cleansing the head, twenty denarii.[1]
Had shoeing been known or practised, it must have
been mentioned in such an edict as this. And here
we may notice, in connection with this hoof-paring
among the Romans, that Bonanni has given drawings
of two iron objects found at Rome, near the Castra
Peregrina, which Montfauçon[2] reproduces as ancient
Roman instruments of farriery. One, he notes, is like
the present *boutoir* or *boutavan* of the French *maréchal*

---

[1] *Martin Leake.* Transactions of the Royal Society of Literature,
vol. i. p. 196. ' Mulomedicus tonsuræ et aptaturæ pedum.' ' Eidem
deplecoræ et purgaturæ capitis.'

[2] Vol. iii. lib. v. cap. 5, pt. 5. Plate 197.

ferrant, and the other has been intended to remove the horn and incise it in cases of disease (fig. 2).

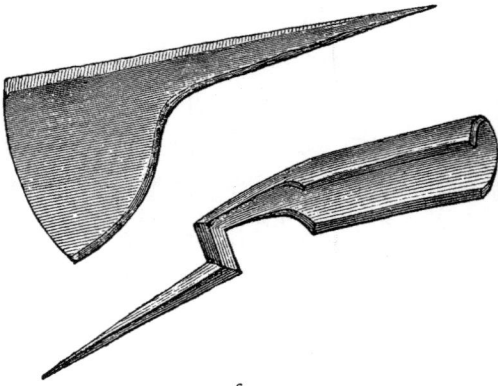

fig 2

These are the only relics of Roman farriery I have been able to trace; and their having been found at the capital of that empire, would show that the hoofs required paring and dressing, and that this was of frequent occurrence, since the mulomedicus was bound to be satisfied with a fixed price for performing that duty. Vegetius recommends the employment of such instruments.

Apsyrtus (A.D. 330—340), a Greek of the Byzantine empire, and one of the most renowned veterinarians of this period, who was employed in the army of Constantine the Great, says that those horses which have a small frog are swift of foot and valuable ;[1] and those which have their frogs growing close and small were best for work.[2] Leading us to infer that those horses which had wide flat soles and prominent frogs, being unshod were liable to become lame from bruises to these parts.

Palladius Rutilius Taurus Æmilianus (A.D. 300—400) advises that strong oaken planks be laid down as a flooring for stables, and that straw be laid over them at night

---

[1] Apsyrtus, Scrip. Græc. Vet. p. 252. Χελιδόνα δὲ μικρὰν ἔχοντες εὔποδες καὶ ἀγαθοί.

[2] Ibid. Οἱ συμφυεῖς κάτωθεν καὶ χελιδόνας μικρὰς ἔχοντες.

only, so that it might be soft for the horses when resting, and hard for their hoofs when standing.[1]

Publius Vegetius Renatus (A.D. 450—510?)[2], a veterinarian, has left us the most complete treatise on veterinary medicine of any ancient writer. He describes more fully than any other Roman hippiatrist the maladies and accidents to which horses were liable in his day; and though he speaks of contracted tendons, horses and mules walking on the fronts of their hoofs, and the casualties these animals are exposed to, as well as the method of curing them, yet he says nothing of shoeing (in a modern sense), either as producing disease or injuries, or as a means of remedying these.

When treating of the hoofs and the feet generally, however, it is plainly intimated that such a practice as nailing on iron plates was not available in his age. He

[1] Scrip. Rer. Rustic., edit. Schneider, vol. iii.

[2] There is much uncertainty with regard to the period in which Vegetius lived. Nothing whatever is known of him, and his writings alone offer evidence as to the date about which they were composed. Eichenfeld thinks he lived in the second century, and Sprengel, in his History of Medicine, carries him forward to the twelfth century, while others have placed him at various periods between these two extremes. A recent writer, M. Megnin (Recueil de Méd. Vétérinaire, 1867, p. 803), gives what is termed a *mathematical* demonstration that Vegetius knew the art of horse-shoeing, and that he lived and composed his work in A.D. 945. He partly founds his demonstration on Lebeau's 'Histoire du Bas-Empire,' in the chapter in which reference to Constantine VII. is made. According to M. Megnin, the reason why Vegetius did not speak of shoeing, was because he did not wish to do so (c'est qu'il n'a pas voulus et qu'il la connaissait parfaitement). For lack of better evidence than is here adduced, I think it will be preferable to follow Heusinger, and retain the date I have given above. Niebuhr (Merobaudes, p. 12) found at St Gallen some short fragments of a very old codex (palimpseste) which were ascribed to Vegetius, and supposed to

says: ' By the ruggedness of roads, and long journeys, the hoofs of animals are worn out, and hinder their walking. *(Animalium ungulæ asperitate ac longitudine itinerum deteruntur et impediunt incessum*, etc.) From a twisting or contusion also, if horses or mules be forced to gallop or run on a rugged or stony road, bruises and chafings arise; lastly, though no cause has preceded, when they stand idle in the stables, they begin to halt and go lame. . . . . . You shall foment the feet that are bruised and worn underneath with warm water.'[1] After a journey, it is recommended that the horses' feet ' be carefully washed and examined, lest any clay or mud remain about their joints and soles. They must also be rubbed with ointment, that their hoofs may be nourished, and that what horn the journey has worn away may, through the virtue of the medicament, grow up again.' He then gives various prescriptions for applications which nourish the hoofs and make them firm. These were to be rubbed in around the coronets and over the feet. At the wane of the moon ' the soles and hoofs of the animals must be trimmed with a paring iron, which allows the heat to escape, cools and refreshes them, and makes their hoofs the stronger.'[2] ' It is a more prudent counsel to preserve the soundness of horses' feet, than to cure any disorder in them; but

have been written in the seventh or eighth century. The codex of Corbey belongs to the ninth century. From the quotations afforded above, it will be seen that he could not have known anything regarding shoeing with nails, otherwise he could not avoid mentioning it. As will be noticed hereafter, this art was practised at Constantinople before 945.

[1] *Vegetii Renati. Artis* Veterinariæ. Lib. ii. cap. 55. Basil, 1528.
[2] Lib. i. cap. 56.

their hoofs are strengthened if the horses or mules stand in a very clean stable, without dung or moisture, and if their stalls are floored or laid with oaken planks. . . . . . You must remember that the hoofs are renewed by growing, and therefore after a certain number of days, or every month, such care ought not to be wanting, by which the weakness of nature is assisted and amended.' In another place, speaking of the stable and stalls, he closely follows Columella. 'A careful master must go frequently into the stable. In the first instance, take care that the place where they stand and lie be raised higher than the other parts of the floor, and that it be compactly made—not of soft wood, as frequently happens through unskilfulness or negligence, but of solid, hard, lasting oak, well put together; for this kind of wood hardens the horses' hoofs like rocks. Moreover, the trench which is to receive the urine ought to have a sink or drain under the ground to convey it away, lest the urine overflowing touch the horses feet.'[1]

'The hoofs of animals that are too small, grow larger, or such as are worn, are repaired if you take,' etc. *(Animalibus exiguæ crescunt, vel attritæ reparantur,* etc.) Numerous recipes are given to harden soft hoofs, especially the soles. Frequent mention is made of suffusion in the feet, and casting the hoofs, doubtless through injuries sustained from the want of shoeing. 'If perchance, from the fatigue of a journey, a suffusion or defluxion shall happen in his feet,'[2] etc. 'If a horse or mule has cast his hoof the cure is difficult.'[3] 'But such horses or mules whose hoofs have become diseased by suffusion or spread

[1] Lib. i. cap. 56.   [2] Lib. i. cap. 38.   [3] Lib. ii. cap. 57.

ing of matter, or by some voluntary act of your own, or by the under part having been injured by some obstacle in the way, and have been a long time lame, this is the cure.'[1] The principal remedy proposed for these hoof-worn animals consisted essentially of pitch and rosin melted, and applied to the sole and the part coming in contact with the ground. It may be well to note here, that in the East Indies, melted pitch is largely applied to the feet of elephants when they become lame from journeying, or are about to travel over rocky ground.

Perhaps a stronger proof than any that horses were not accustomed to be shod at this time, lies in the fact, that in the many directions given with great detail as to the management of the feet, and the performance of various operations in and on the sole, not a word is said as to removing the shoe previously, or replacing it afterwards. Besides, Renatus mentions every malady to which the un-shod foot is liable ; had nailed shoes been in vogue he must have spoken of the accidents arising from their use, such as pricks from the nails, which give rise to great lameness and often dangerous consequences now-a-days ; and he could scarcely omit noticing wounds and fractures caused by kicks from shod hoofs. Mention is made, however, of horses and mules being squeezed or bruised with the stroke of a wheel or an axle-tree.

Vegetius appears to have been no stranger to the manners and customs of other and oftentimes distant countries, and to have been perfectly acquainted with the breeds of horses in them. For instance, in treating of the characteristics of horses, by which their native country

[1] Lib. i. cap. 26.

could be ascertained, he writes : ' In exchanging or selling horses, a lying story with regard to their native country is used, to introduce the greatest fraud. For men being desirous of selling them at the dearest rate, they falsely pretend that they are of the best breed; which circumstance has induced us, who, by travelling frequently into so many different and distant foreign countries, are perfectly well acquainted with all kinds of horses, and have often kept them in our own stables, to explain the characters and real merit and qualifications of every nation. For not to mention the meaner services they are employed in, it is manifest that horses are chiefly necessary for three uses—for war, for the circus, and for the saddle. The horses of the Hunni are by far the most useful for war, by reason of their endurance of fatigue, cold, and hunger. Next to them, those of Thuringia and Burgundy withstand fatigue and bad usage the best. The Phrygian or Friesland horses are reckoned invincible, both with respect to swiftness and perseverance in running. Next, those of Epirus, Sarmatia, and Dalmatia, although they are obstinate and refractory to the bridle, yet are reckoned very fit for war. The noble disposition of the Cappadocian breed for chariots is much renowned; equally, or next to these, the glory of the prize in the circus is reckoned due to the Spanish horses ; nor is Sicily much behind in affording for the circus such as are not inferior to them, although Africa is accustomed to furnish the Spanish breed with the swiftest of any. Persia, in all its provinces, furnishes better horses for the saddle, and they are reckoned as a great part of their patrimonial estate; being very gentle and easy to ride upon, tractable and submissive, and of exceeding great value for the nobleness of their breed and pedigree. The Armenian and Sophenian follow next; nor in this respect must you despise the Sicilian horses, nor those of Epirus, if their manners, or good temper and behaviour, and beauty do not forsake them. Those of the Hunni have a great crooked head, projecting eyes, small nostrils, broad jaws and cheek-bones, a strong and stiff neck, manes hanging down to their knees, large ribs, crooked spine, strong bushy tail, strong legs, the lower part of their feet small, and *full, spreading hoofs;* their flanks hollow, and bodies angular; no roundness in their quarters, or brawny development of their muscles; their stature is rather in length than height; the bones are large, there is a graceful leanness, and their very deformity constitutes their beauty. Their temper and disposition is moderate and prudent, and they are patient of wounds.

'The Persian horses do not differ very much in their stature and build from other kinds of horses, but they are known and distinguished from them only by a certain gracefulness in their gait and manner of walking. Their step is short and frequent, and such as delights and elevates the rider; nor is it taught by art, but freely bestowed upon them by Nature,—for their action is a mean between 'pacers' and those commonly called 'gallopers;' and whereas they are like neither of them, they are thought to have something common to both. These, as has been proved, have more gracefulness in a short journey, but in a long journey their endurance is but small. They have a proud spirit, and unless it be subdued with continual labour, they are stubborn and contumacious with their riders. Nevertheless, they are prudent, and, what is wonderful with so much fire and spirit, with the greatest care do they maintain their graceful carriage, the neck being bent into a bow, so that the chin appears to lean upon the breast.'[1]

A writer who thus carefully describes the varieties of foreign horses, and enters into such details with each, would surely have mentioned the practice of preserving the feet of these useful creatures had it been known to him; but nowhere in his writings does he allude to it.

Vegetius Renatus Flavius, who flourished towards the end of the fourth century, in the reign of the Emperor Valentine, has often been confounded with the preceding writer, and his 'De Re Militari' has been, by Bracy Clark and many others. ascribed to Publius Vegetius. In this much-valued and classical military treatise, there is a particular enumeration of everything pertaining to an army forge; yet there is no mention made of workmen to shoe horses, nor yet of any implement or article intended for such a purpose.

For examples of the losses sustained during war through horses' feet being unprotected, we are not so well supplied as in Greek history. One marked instance, however, would appear to be shown in Polybius, when that writer informs us that the horses of Hannibal's army (B.C. 216) lost their hoofs in the marshes of Etruria: 'Equorum etiam multis, ob longum per paludes iter, ungulæ exciderunt.'

That a defence for the feet of some of the larger domestic animals was in use, there can be no doubt. Aristotle for the Greeks, and Pliny for the Romans, state

---

[1] Lib. iv. cap. 6.

that the feet of camels were in time of war, or on long journeys, shod. And we infer that the Καρβατιναι mentioned by them were formed of a pliable leather sock covering the foot, stouter perhaps on the sole than elsewhere, and which, passing up the leg, was there fastened by thongs or bandages.

A friend who was for a long period surveying in Africa, and whose duties carried him as far as the Soudan, informed me that horses are but seldom shod on the immense alluvial surface of the Sahara, where, for enormous distances, not a stone the size of a pebble is to be seen. In the rocky or stony regions, however, all are shod, and on long journeys the retention of the shoes and protection of the hoofs is a matter of much concern to the horsemen. To guard against the evil consequences that would follow the loss of one or two shoes by a horse when others could not be readily supplied, the conductors or followers of caravans, as well as the horsemen, are careful always to carry with them a sufficient quantity of leather to make socks to wrap the exposed hoof in. On the death of a camel—an event of frequent occurrence— a piece of the thickest part of the hide is removed ; and when this begins to dry, it is subjected to long-continued and almost incessant manipulation, to make it soft and pliable, so as to fit closely to the hoof when required. The Arabs are often observed on the march pulling, rubbing, twisting, and stretching the lately-stripped camel-skin, solely with the intention of using it as a sock for the horses or camels when they become foot-sore.

In Japan, in 1860, the large black bulls used as pack animals, were often seen wearing foot-covers of this description, to enable them to traverse the roads with their heavy burthens.

There is nothing, however, to show that the 'Embattai' of Xenophon, or the 'Carbatinai' of Aristotle and Pliny, were employed for solipedes. Nevertheless, now and again a curious passage occurs in the writings of some of the authorities we have just quoted, and in historical descriptions, which acquaints us that on certain occasions, contrivances, which would appear to have been only of a temporary character, were put on the feet of horses, mules, or oxen, to prevent injury to the horn, or to assist in remedying disease. As with the camel, the foot-defences of these creatures seems to have been suggested by that worn by man himself, and improvement in material, according to the ingenuity or wealth of individuals, would, of course, from time to time appear. But there is no description of these improved defences, and their form and means of attachment to the limb have given rise to endless surmises and disputes.

Catullus (B.C. 50) speaks of some kind of shoe, when he is desirous of throwing one of his too solid townsmen off a bridge into the river, so that he might shake him out of his lethargy, as a mule leaves its shoe in a stiff bog · 'And leave your sluggish mind sunk in thick mire, as the mule his iron shoe in a tenacious bog.' [1]

Joseph Scaliger,[2] in a note on this passage from

---

[1] Carm. xvii. 20.

> Nunc eum volo de tuo ponte mittere pronum,
> Si pote stolidum repente excitare veternum,
> Et supinum animum in gravi derelinquere cœno,
> *Ferream* ut *soleam* tenaci in voragine mula.'

[2] Encyclopédie Methodique, vol. ii. p. 651. *Art.* Antiquités.

Catullus, is of opinion that this solea was drawn over the hoof, and not fastened with nails, and in this opinion he is perhaps justified. An ordinary leather sock, such as would prove serviceable for the wear of a camel, would soon be found to be but little adapted to the rough usage of a horse or mule ; the sharp unyielding margin of the hoof-wall must in a very brief space, and particularly on paved roads or rocky ground, have cut through any envelope of hide or other soft material ; so borrowing the idea from their own caliga or calceus, or the wheel—the *ferati orbes* of Virgil, they shod this covering with stronger materials, such as brass, iron, or even silver, or gold, but most frequently iron. Like their shoes, these *soleæ*, or horse-sandals, were in all probability fastened round the legs with loops and straps, or fillets. It may be observed here that the name given to their own shoe or sandal— *calceus* or *calceamentum*—was never given to this appliance for horses and mules, which is always designated *solea ;* the act of shoeing, however, is found expressed by the verb *calceo,* and is alike employed for man and beast.

The fastening with thongs or straps must of course have been a very insecure one, as modern experience has taught us, and the leathern sole covering the ground surface of the foot would still further tend to weaken it, particularly in marshy or clayey soil. Even now, with our incalculably firmer-attached armature, it is well known that in the hunting-field, when crossing heavy ground, a leather sole acts like a sucker, and is almost certain to cause the shoe which covers it to be left in the mire. Such must have been a frequent occurrence with

the solea ; so that Catullus only referred to it in a figurative but popular sense.

To show that the soleæ were probably fastened to the
extremity in this manner, the example afforded by Suetonius (A.D. 120), may be quoted. In that historian's
' Lives of the Twelve Emperors,' when treating of Vespasian (A.D. 60), he casually intimates that this good
Emperor was in the habit of preserving the feet of his
mules when travelling. Suspecting once during a journey
that his mule-driver had alighted to shoe his mules, in
order to have an opportunity for allowing a person they
met, and who was engaged in a law-suit, to speak to him,
he (Vespasian) asked him how much he got for shoeing
the mules, and insisted on having a share of the profits.[1]

The Commentator of Suetonius, under the Life of
Vespasian, has made the same blunder in introducing
words into the text which do not belong to it as
Stephanus ; and this, as Bracy Clark has pointed out, has
induced Schœffer, the author of ' De Re Vehiculari
Veterum,' to perpetuate the error. He writes : ' Ut testa-
tur Suetonius in Vespasiano, qui frequenter solebat lectica
deferri in villam suam Catiliam, sed a mulis quoniam
quadraginta milliarum intervallo abesset Roma : Hinc
qui lecticam ejus deferebat, solicitatoris cujusdam donis
corruptus, è mulis retentus fingeret se aptaturum *soleam
ferream* pedi unius ex mulis, tempus dabat supplici ad
porrigendum Imperatori libellum.' It is seen that there
is nó authority for this ' soleam ferream ' in the text.

[1] *Suetonius*, Vita Imp. Vespasian de Facetis, Lib. xxiii. p. 120.
' Mulionem in itinere quodam suspicatus ad calciandas mulas desilisse,
ut adeunti litigatori spatium moramque præberet : interrogavit, quanti
calciasset : pactusque est lucri partem.'

As Mr Clark has remarked, the circumstance of the emperor's muleteer dismounting and fastening on the shoes of the mules, in order to detain the car while the solicitor who had bribed him presented his petition, would show that they were not attached by nails; for nailed shoes are not so readily put on in the highway, and coachmen would not be likely to carry tools and other requisites for this purpose. The passage in Suetonius is against such an inference. The muleteer doubtless dismounted to reädjust, or make more secure, the fastenings of some of the soleæ, which were supposed to have broken loose.

And Ribauld de la Chapelle,[1] in the last century, was also of opinion that the ancient Romans did not put the modern-shaped shoe on their horses or mules, but enveloped them in a sock (*sabot*), an act indicated by the words, 'Jumentis soleas inducere.' He alludes to this instance in the Life of Vespasian, where the muleteer could change the coverings of the mules' feet when they were worn out.

Suetonius, in commenting on the great extravagance of Nero (A.D. 60), asserts that he never travelled with less than a thousand four-wheeled chariots, drawn by mules whose feet were shod with silver; and the drivers of which were dressed in scarlet jackets of the finest Canusian cloth.[2] And the elder Pliny, speaking of the instances o luxury in silver plate among the Romans, amongst others relates the following: 'We find the orator Calvus com-

[1] Dissertation sur l'Origine des Francs, etc., p. 199.
[2] De Nerone ipso Tranquillas, cap. xxx. ' Nunquam carrucis minus mille fecisse iter traditur, *soleis* mularum argenteis.'

plaining that the saucepans are made of silver ; but it has been left for us to invent a plan of covering our very carriages with chased silver, and it was in our own age that Poppæa, the wife of the Emperor Nero, ordered her favourite mules to be shod even with gold.'[1] This reference to shoeing has troubled many commentators. Vossius[2] notes from Xiphilinus, that Poppæa's mules were many of them furnished in their feet with shoes made of broom twisted and gilt. He calls their golden shoes επιχρυσια ΣΠΑΡΤΙΑ. In Dion Cassius' History of Rome, it is mentioned that this Sabina had her mules shod with gold, and that the milk of 50 she-asses was devoted to her lavatory.[3] In the same work, we learn that the barbarous Emperor Commodus (A.D. 190), caused his horses' hoofs to be gilt or covered with gold. 'When the horses became too old for the race-course, they were sent away to the country, Commodus replacing them by others, and introducing these into the circus with their hoofs gilt, and their backs covered with a cloth of gold. When they were suddenly brought before the people

---

[1] Hist. Nat., Lib. xxxiii. cap. 49. 'Nostraque ætate Poppæa, conjux Neronis principis, delicatioribus jumentis suis soleas ex auro quoque induere.' 'Poppæa, the empresse, wife to Nero, the emperour, was known to cause her *ferrers* ordinarily to shoe her coach-horses, and other palfries for her saddle (such especially as shee set store by, and counted more dainty than the rest), with cleane gold.'—Holland's Plinie.

[2] Ad Catullus.

[3] *Historiæ Romanæ*, Lib. lxii. 'Sabina vero hæc adeo delicate vixit (nam ex paucis quibusdam cætera intelligentur omnia) ut mulas, quibus agebatur, haberet *auresis soleis calceatas ;* et ut quingentæ asinæ, quæ recens peperissent, quotidie mulgerentur, quo ipsa lacte earum lavaretur.'

loud shouts arose from every one, " Behold, Pertinax is here ! " [1]

The allusion made by Pliny to the garniture of Poppæa's mules, Mr Pegge remarks, would seem to imply that the solea was pulled on like an ordinary sock ; but, as previously mentioned, Vossius doubts this : ' Verum qua ratione absque clavis id fieri possit, non satis liquet ; ' and then he makes the assertion before alluded to, to prove that even the Greeks put on the hoof-armature with nails : 'in vetusto exemplari Hippiatricorum Græcorum, quod habeo, cui etiam picturæ accedunt, clavorum quibus trajiciantur ungulæ signa et vestigia manifeste apparent.' And yet, Pegge maintains, the σπαϱτία επίχρυσα mentioned above could not well be nailed, but must have been drawn on and fastened in a different manner, perhaps by being tied round the leg, like the snow-bags Xenophon saw, and as ὑποδήματα used for the soleæ or shoes of mules seems to imply.   Scaliger,[2] from attentive examination of all the passages referring to this subject, certainly was of opinion that the shoes of horses and mules, whatever may have been their materials, were not fastened

---

[1] Ibid. Lib. lxxxiii.   ' Post hæc equum eundem, quum ob senectutem dimissus esset a cursu, et ruri ageret, Commodus arcessiverat, et introduxerat in circum, *inauratis ungulis,* ac inaurata pelle in dorso ornatum : qui ubi de improviso comparuit, rursum conclamatum est ab omnibus, " Ecce Pertinax adest.

Stephanus thinks that Poppæa's mule-shoes were merely the soleæ spartea gilt, and he adds (though we must not forget the mistake he previously makes) : ' Equi bellatores apud Romanos non habebant munimenta pedum seu soleas, sed sole jumenta, ut ostendit Fabrettas (Col. Traj.) . . . . . . Pertinacis tamen equi παρηβηχότος ungulas inaurabat Commodus, τάς ὁπλας χαταχρυσώσας.

   [2] Pitisc. ad Suet. Nero, cap. 30.

on with nails, particularly in Suetonius' and Nero's time.

Aldrovandus[1] remarks, that Suetonius, in his Life of Caligula (A.D. 40), expressly notices the iron shoe, with eight or more nails; and Colonel Smith,[2] who quotes this naturalist, appears to think him correct. 'We read concerning Caligula, in Suetonius, that the day previous to the races in the circus, he ordered the soldiers to maintain strict silence in the neighbourhood, lest his horse should be disturbed. He remembered when a journey was to be undertaken, if the country to be traversed was mountainous or rough, that, instead of eight, fourteen nails were to be affixed; because such ground wore away the nails rapidly.' I have carefully read two editions of Suetonius (one of them the 'Bibliotheca Classica Latina' of C. B. Hase; Paris, 1828), but do not find the most distant allusion to horse-shoes in the 'Life of Caligula.' The reference is not trustworthy.

For reasons which will be hereafter given, it might be concluded, that when shoes for horses or mules are mentioned by any of the Roman or Greek writers immediately preceding or following the commencement of our era, that the modern method of applying a shoe to these animals' feet is not meant, and that there is no proof that it was known. But as additional evidence that the solea was a temporary

---

[1] De Quadrupedibus, p. 50. Francofurti, 1623. 'De Caligula itaque legimus apud Suetonium pridie quam Circensis fierent, viciniæ silentium per milites indixisse ne eques suus incitatus inquietaretur. Cum iter faciendum est, meminerit, per quæ loca fiet eundem nam si per montes vel quævis asperiora loca fuerit agitandus, loco octo clavorum, quatuordecim invenio affigendos, quod plurimum illic atterantur clavi.'

[2] Naturalists' Library, vol. xii. Edinburgh, 1841.

contrivance, secured round the pastern or fetlock with straps or thongs, we may refer to the writings of Roman and Greek hippiatrists, who testify to their nature and uses in several instances, and in a more or less explicit manner.

Columella, the agricultural writer already noticed, and who lived near the time of Augustus, prescribes a shoe or sandal of broom, or wicker-work, for lame oxen, though not for ordinary wear, but only as a surgical appliance, under the designation of *solea spartea*. Speaking of cattle that had become crippled in the limbs, he says that if it be low down, or in the hoofs, ' you should make a small opening between the digits with a knife, and after wards apply soft bandages steeped in salt and vinegar; then have the foot covered with a shoe of spartea, let there be great caution exercised to avoid wet, and keep the stable very dry.' [1]

Theomnestus, a Greek veterinarian of the Byzantine empire, of whom extremely little is known, save what is to be casually gleaned from his vivacious writings, but who is supposed to have lived in the 6th century, speaks about excessive abrasion of the hoofs, and the application of this rush or wicker slipper. ' *If a horse is much worn in the hoofs by travelling*, and is then neglected, he becomes feverish, and is soon destroyed by the fever if not attended to. To prevent this, you must use warm water in which the roots of althæa or wild mallows have been boiled, and

---

[1] De Re Rust. lib. ii. p. 27. 'At si jam in ungulis est, inter duos ungues cultello leviter aperies, postea linamenta sale atque aceto imbuta applicantur, ac *solea spartea* pes induitur, maximeque datur opera ne in aquam pedem mittat, et siccè stabuletur.'

foment the feet with it till they become clean and soft.
Then the loose parts must be removed from the hoofs
and all bruises be laid bare in the water; and then you
are to have in immediate readiness *slender twigs of broom*,
or twine cords, and rough cloths, tow and other coarse
stuffing, with garlic (αλλιον) and axle-grease—one by
one, so as to have them ready to fix by ties (or bands)
round the hoofs. If they (the feet) should inflame, let
blood be abstracted from the coronets, and cause the horse
to remain in a warm place where there is sunshine, or let
a fire be kindled if it be winter-time, and make him a bed
of dry dung, that he may not stand on what is hard. The
feet may suffer in this way without being much inflamed.
Let him be attended for eight days, and stand in-doors on
dung; also have his water brought to him, that his hoofs
by walking be not torn asunder, but may grow, being
nourished by what comes from the dung.'[1]

As Bracy Clark has noted, the twigs of the 'spartium'
are here recommended to be simply employed as cords to
maintain the soft dressing to the tender feet, enclosing the
hoofs like a net.

The word *spartum*, as used by the Greeks and Romans,
was meant by them to indicate several species of plants
which, like hemp or flax, could be easily manufactured
into various articles of utility. But the former people,
more particularly, applied this term to a shrub, the *Spartium Junceum*, or Spanish broom, which is found in a
wild state on the dry lands of the Levant and the southern
parts of Europe, and the slender branches of which were
woven into baskets, while the shoots were prepared and

[1] *Ruellis.* Scriptores Græci Veterinarii, p. 254.

put to the same uses as hemp. At the present day, the people of Lower Languedoc, towards Lodeve, manufacture it into various household textures, such as table cloths, shirts, and other things, employing the bark as fuel. It is the species called by Pliny (Book xxxix. cap. 9) *genista*, but which he seems, though wrongly, to consider as another variety—the *Stipa* (*macrochloa*) *tenacissima*. This last variety certainly grows in Spain and Africa, and is there designated *sparto* or *esparto*. As described by him (Book xix. cap. 2), it is still in great request for the manufacture of baskets, mattresses, *ship-cables* and *cordage*, and when treated as hemp, is converted into more delicate articles. The Spaniards make of it a kind of shoes called *alpergates*, which form a large export commodity, being in popular demand in the Indies, where these sandals are more suitable than anything else. It is also an essential material for the fabrication of coverings for rooms, balconies, and chairs; and makes, besides, excellent panniers for mules. It is most likely that the Greeks employed the *spartium* and the Romans the *stipa*, in making shoes for their beasts of burthen.

In more modern times, however, sandals for horses have been made from *spartum*, as appears from J. Leonis.[1] It is also now largely employed in the manufacture of paper.

We have already examined what Vegetius had to say about horses' feet, and their injuries from non-shoeing. We will now consider what he relates with regard to some portions of their treatment, as a supplement to his mention of ' detritus pedibus,' ' subtritus pedibus.' etc. He

[1] Africæ Descriptio.   Lib. iii. p. 120.

several times alludes to the *soleæ spartæa*, or shoes of Spanish broom, particularly for the ox when foot-sore, or when disease was present; and to show that this animal sometimes wore this, or something analogous, when travelling or at work, he writes: 'If the sock has hurt his pastern or hoof, wrap up hard pitch and hog's lard,' etc   'But if the sock has entered into it, the sea-lettuce, which the Greeks call Tithymallos, mixed with salt, is put upon it. Also when his feet are worn and bruised underneath, they are washed with ox's urine made warm ; then he is forced to tread upon the burning-hot embers of vine twigs, and his hoofs are anointed with tar, together with oil and hog's lard.   Nevertheless, they do not go so lame if, when they are unyoked from their work, their hoofs be washed with cold water, and their pasterns and coronets, as well as the cleft of the hoof itself, be rubbed with old hog's lard.' 'If he has trodden upon a nail, or pierced his hoof with a sharp tile or stone . . . . Then having a shoe of Spanish broom put upon it for the space of three days,'[1] etc.

With regard to the horse, we often find the words 'animal calciabis,' 'calciatis pedibus per multos dies;' and when describing the treatment for a horse that has bruised or inflamed his foot, he finishes by adding, 'you shall take care to put a shoe of Spanish broom upon it, that, after the evacuation of the humours, the hoof may be repaired.'[2] *(Sparcia calciare curabis, ut post egestione humore ungula reparetur.)*

From this veterinarian, then, we might be led to think that the Romans did not generally shoe their horses, mules, or oxen ; and that when they were impelled to do so from

---

[1] Lib. iii. cap. 1.   [2] Lib. i. cap. 26.

motives of pride and display, or from urgent necessity, the shoeing was of the most simple kind, and much as they were accustomed to cover their own feet in a sock of leather or pelt by enveloping the whole surface. It is not improbable that the portion covering the front of the hoof may, when display was wanted, have been gilded, or covered with gold or silver, and the under portion also strengthened by gold, silver, bronze, or iron plates. That this was the case we find amply illustrated elsewhere in Vegetius' writings, where he speaks of *lemnisci*, which were doubtless intended to strengthen the *solea*, and may have been of strong leather, or even iron; a circumstance of some importance to remember. In the following passage this is found more particularly noticed: 'Pedes quos sanos habet *glante ferreo* vel si defuerit, spartea calceabis, *cui lemniscos subjicies*, et addita fasciola diligentissime colligabis, et suppositicum facies parti illi quæ misera est, ut planas ungulas possit ponere.'[1]

The *glante ferreo* is found for the first and only time here, and Bracy Clark thinks that it may have been only an insertion into, or corruption of, the text with which, by frequent transcription, the work abounds. He adds ⋅ 'There is, however, something very singular about it, for *glans* signifies an acorn, the fruit of the oak, and the figure which this fruit presents projecting from its cup, would, if divided by a longitudinal section, not badly represent the figure of the modern horse-shoe, or a section of its cup would do the same; but as nothing is said of nails for fastening it on, it cannot properly be considered, without other collateral evidence, to mean any such thing.

[1] Lib. iii. cap. 18.

It may have been possibly a piece of iron turned round to the figure of the horse's hoof, and which was then fastened on by rivets or otherwise to the *lemnisci*, or leather soles, and this, it is not at all impossible, might, under the pressure of necessity, have been applied directly to the foot itself, and given birth to the modern horse-shoe. It is therefore probable that these metal plates, or acorns of iron, used to strengthen their *soleæ*, or shoes, were distinguished by the name of *glantes ferrei*, and the passage tells us if these were not to be had they were to be contented with the *lemnisci*, and if not these, with the *sparteum opus*, which was rarely honoured with the title of *solea.*'[1]

The English edition of Vegetius, published in 1748, thus translates the above passage, which relates to the treatment for disease in the hip: 'You shall shoe his feet that are sound with an *iron patten*, or sandal, or if this be lacking, with a shoe made of broom, and you shall put bandages upon it, and bind it up most carefully, and so make it able to support that part which is in misery, that the animal may be able to set down his hoofs flat and full upon the ground.'[2]

At the present day, in this country, what are called poultice-bags or boots, and which are made of leather, fastening with a strap round the pastern, are very frequently shod with an iron shoe to guard them from wear. The Roman *soleæ* may have resembled these, and it is possible that on other, though rarer, occasions they may

[1] Op. cit. p. 25.
[2] *Vegetius Renatus.* Of the Distempers of Horses, &c., p. 275.

have been entirely of iron, suspended to the hoof by a bandage, or strap and buckle.

It is satisfactory that Vegetius has so particularly described the mode of attaching this garniture to the limb: ' et addita fasciola diligentissime colligabis;' because it elucidates what might have otherwise been an obscure reference in Apsyrtus, a Greek veterinarian who lived more than a century before Vegetius.   In chapter 107 of that writer's work, in the Hippiatrica, is found the heading: ' Apsyrtus on the injuries from foot defences or fastenings of the same.'   And the chapter goes on to relate: ' It happens that the legs ($\mu\epsilon\sigma\omicron\varkappa\acute{\upsilon}\nu\iota\alpha$, the parts from the knees to the hoofs) of the horse, from the foot defences or shackles ($\acute{\iota}\pi\pi\omicron\pi\acute{\epsilon}\delta\eta\varsigma$), or its fastenings by the thong or cord, become injured, so that the skin is torn off or destroyed, and the tendons of the fetlock are laid bare. There is danger of this accident proving fatal if it happen to both joints. It is proper, therefore, in the first instance, to apply wine, vinegar, or brine and vinegar; next, to use the lipara and soft applications of white plasters ; and, to complete the cure, of ceruss one part, of ammoniacum one half, of myrtle-berries a sufficient quantity—then triturating the ammoniacum, mixed with the ceruss, pour upon them the myrtle, and use it.'[1]

---

[1] Ruellii (Hippiatr. lib. ii. p. 100) renders this passage from the *Greek* as follows: ' APSYRTUS IIS QUI COMPEDIBUS AUT VINCULIS COLLISI VITIANTUR. Usu venit ut suffragines, quas *mesocynia* vocant, tricis, pedicis, vinculisque quibusdam loro vel fune districtis plerunque lacessantur, quibus corium procidit, sic ut nervuli hujusce partis aperiantur, ac nudi pateant: id quod vitæ discrimen adfert, præsertim si in utroque flexu articulorum evenerit,' etc.

This passage, and the term 'hippopodes,' here used for the first and only time in the ancient veterinary writers, obviously refers to the sandal or solea worn by horses or mules on rare occasions, and to the way in which it was maintained on the extremities by the *corrigiæ,* or rather the *fasciolæ,* mentioned by Vegetius. That this was really the case, a very fine terra-cotta or baked clay (the kind named 'typi' by Pliny), now in the British Museum (2nd vase Room, and marked T 337), has been brought forward by Bracy Clark as a proof (fig. 3). The example is cer-

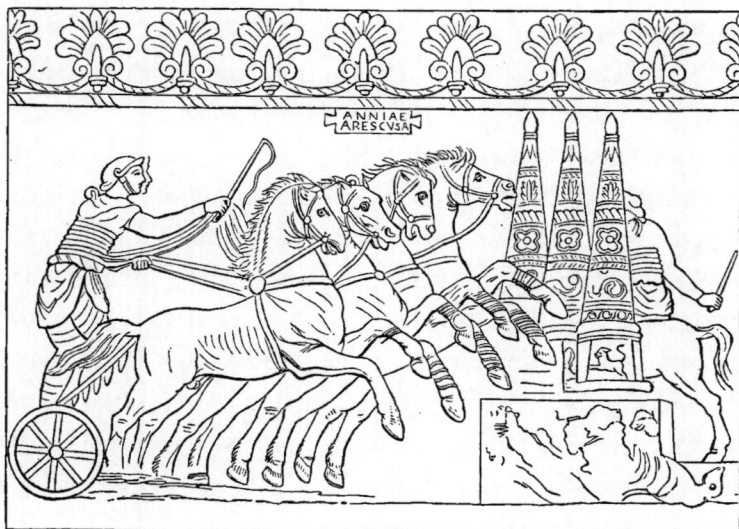

fig. 3

tainly, so far as I can ascertain, unique; but taken in connection with what the ancient authors have said in regard to this matter, it would appear to afford conclusive evidence. The age of the tablet is, unfortunately, unknown; but it belongs to a number which were found about the year 1765, in a dry well, near the Porta Latina, at Rome ; and which were sometime afterwards added to Mr Townley's collection. The bas-relief exhibits a chariot-race, having something of the Greek character in design. The charioteer, wearing a helmet and what Suetonius calls the 'quadrigarian' dress,[1] stands in a two-wheeled curriculus or car, drawn by four horses, which are galloping towards the *metæ* or pillars, round which the competitors were obliged to turn in these contests of the circus. The upper part of his body appears to be swathed in his robe, and the reins, four in number, two in the left and two in the right hand, according to the fashion of the times, encircle his waist.[2]

The bits are the simple snaffle, and not the curb, which we know the Romans introduced ; and Combe,[3] who has made these terra-cottas his particular study, says the instructions of Nestor,[4] that in turning round the goal, the right-hand horse should be urged on with a loose rein, are exactly followed in this instance. The reverse, however, appears to be the case. At the base of the metæ, there may have happened an accident; but this part is rather disfigured; while turning the goal the back of a horseman is seen, with what seems to be reins round his body, and who may only be keeping the course clear. On

---

[1] *Suetonius,* Vita Calig. cap. 19. ' Per hunc pontem ultro citroque commeavit, biduo continenti. Primo dei phalerato equo—Postridie quadrigario habitu, curriculoque bijugi famosorum equorum, præ se ferens Darium puerum ex Parthorum obsidibus; comitante prætorianorum agmine, et in essedis cohorte amicorum.

Lampridius (Vit. Commodi, cap. 2) has also ' *A*urigæ habitu currus rexit.'

[2] *Statius,* Theb., lib. vi. 104.

[3] Description of the *A*ncient Terra-cottas in the British Museum.

[4] Iliad, 335—341.

the upper part of the tablet, which is in size one foot four inches by one foot, is an inscription, ANNIAE ARESCUSA, who may have been the winner of the race, or the artist of the terra-cotta. Most important of all, however, for our present purpose, is the representation of what look like bandages on the fore limbs of all the horses—a little rubbed on the nearest, but certainly most distinct on the middle and left-hand horses. There is nothing of the kind on the hind limbs, and this may easily be accounted for. Admitting that these are the bands of the hippopodes, it is well known to all horsemen that the fore feet are more liable to suffer from attrition, when unshod, than the hind ones, simply because they have to support more weight and strain. In India, for instance, cavalry and other horses are frequently only shod on the fore feet, as they require this defence; while the hinder ones can be submitted to a great deal of wear without suffering at all to the same degree.

The *fasciolæ* cover the limb apparently from the knee downwards, and though nothing of the sandal itself can be distinguished, yet it is to be observed that the hoofs of the fore extremities are much larger, and altogether look clumsier than those behind, which have no bandages above them; a circumstance that leads to the inference that the hippopodes enveloped the hoofs as closely as they could be made to do.

In the same collection of terra-cottas are some very fine bas-reliefs in which horses are admirably represented, but none have their limbs swathed liked these, which had probably been subjected to an extra amount of racing, being noted horses, and had consequently become foot-sore.

It is very probable that an ancient seal, reported by
Bracy Clark and others to be in the British Museum, but
which I have been unable to trace, is also intended to
convey the idea of the hippopodes being used for cavalry.
From the attitude of a warrior, who kneels down in front
of a horse, and with his right hand seizes its right leg,
while another soldier is aiding him by holding up the left
one as high as the elbow, it has been conjectured that this
boot is being attached to the animal's foot.

The Abbé Winckelmann has described this paste, and
also made some interesting remarks on shoeing; so, in
consequence of my inability to discover its whereabouts
in the Museum, if it ever was there, I reproduce what he
says : 'Pâte Antiq.   Un homme avec un bonnet, qui tient
levé avec force le pied droit d'un cheval, tandis qu'un
soldat armé qui est à genoux devant le cheval, paroit lui
lier des bandages au dessus du sabot.   Il seroit, sans doute,
hardi d'avancer, que ce soldat soit là pour mettre des fers à
son cheval.   Il ne veux pas repeter ici, que les mulets des
Anciens étoient ferrés, et je sais bien qu'on ne trouve des
chevaux ferrés sur aucune ancien monument.   Je soutiens
de plus que le pied ferré d'un cheval qui est sur un bas
relief du Palais Mattei à Rome, représentant une chasse
de l'Empereur Galien, où Fabretti a cru trouver l'époque
des chevaux ferrés, je soutiens, dis-je, que cette jambe *est
une restauration moderne.*   Je ne disconviens pas pourtant
qu'on ne sache que les Anciens, et en particulier les peuples
de l'Asie, firent des fers à leurs chevaux, comme on voit
dans ce qui dit Appian dans l'Histoire de la guerre de
Mithridate.   Scaliger se fondant sur la parole *solea*, le fer
de mulets dans Catulle, et sur celle ὑπόδημον, le fer des

chevaux dans Appian, est un sentiment qu'on leur lioit les fers.'[1]

But even these defences must have been rarely resorted to, as the above are the only two instances in which there is any attempt to represent them. It may also be observed, that in the Greek or Latin languages there are no words corresponding to those we employ to designate a horse-shoe, or the artisan who applies it, and there is nothing to prove in a logical manner, in ancient history or the writings of veterinarians, that hoofs were furnished, as now-a-days, with a defence attached by nails.

As before observed, this subject has given rise to much dispute and research for very many years. Montfauçon[2] asserts: 'The custom of shoeing horses is very ancient, although there are certain proofs that it was not general among the Romans. Fabretti says, that among the great number of horses which occur in ancient monuments, he never saw more than one which was shod, though he made it his business to examine them all, both upon columns and other marbles. As to the mules, both male and female, they are often said by writers to have been shod. There are, nevertheless, certain and undoubted proofs that the ancients shod their horses; thus much Homer and Appian say (?); though it does not appear, indeed, that the custom was general.' In another place, he writes: 'The horses' feet (on an Etruscan tomb) have iron shoes, a particular rarely seen on ancient monuments. Fabretti says, that of all the horses he saw

[1] Description des Pierres Gravées du Feu Baron de Stosch. Florence, 1760, p. 169.

[2] Antiquité Expliq., vol. iv. p. 50.

on monuments, he never observed but one with four shoes.'[1]

Fabretti's remarks are valuable in many respects, but with regard to shoeing it can scarcely be doubted that he has allowed himself to be deceived. (See above for Winckelmann's notice.) He writes: 'I am certain that the shoeing of draught animals was introduced before the time of Trajan (A.D. 98); but in this country we cannot recognize shoes on the statues, though many other details are found. For neither in the marble nor old brass statues, as it would seem, is a single thing else excepted. It would be by no means vain to assert that the Romans at this time did not shoe their war-horses, for lack of which they were not a little lightened in their work, and were less liable to receive injury from each other when at large.' After referring to the writings of Xenophon, Suetonius, Catullus, Pliny, and to Poppæa's mules, which, he acknowledges, had foot defences attached by golden bands, he adds that there was seen a statue on the fourth landing of the staircase of the temple dedicated to the memory of Cyriacus Matthæius, in the Cælian Garden, with shoes on the horses' feet fixed by nails. 'But this statue has nothing to do with Trajan; because it was either destroyed by Severus, 120 years from Trajan's time, or it refers to something which took place in the last days of the Cæsars. This conclusion only do we arrive at, that those authors are ignorant of this matter who suppose that the application of iron shoes to the hoofs of horses was first made at the time of P. Theophilum Raynaudum in Tabulâ Chronologicâ, year DCCIC., by

[1] Op. cit., vol. vii. p. 558.

Lascus Polonus. Nearer to the time of Trajan we find the equestrian statue of Marcus Aurelius, and another marble one on the first platform of the orator's staircase, *nudas ferro ungulas habent ;* at the bottom, also, two statues of Trajan himself on each side of the Arch of Constantine. But lest it should be asserted that details were not intended to be shown on these statues, it so happens that the artist has designed the soles of the shoes worn by the soldiers with iron nails, which Festus and Isidorus in their Orig. xix. cap. ult. termed "*clauta*," and to which kind of shoes and sharp nails Josephus in " De Bell. Judaic." frequently refers.'[1]

Joachim Camerarius asserts that the ancients were not accustomed to shoe their horses.[2]

Guido Pancirolus observes, that some are of this opinion, because such shoes are not seen in the equestrian statues; the reason for which was not known to him.[3] He, however, cites Nicetas for an equestrian statue shod with iron shoes; but as that Byzantine historian lived in the 13th century, when shoeing was well known, it is extremely likely that the statue was either a very recent one, or the horses' feet were armed in the same fashion as Eustathius caused Homer's horses to be.

Isaac Casaubon [4] was of opinion that shoeing was not known very anciently.

---

[1] *Raphaelis Fabretti.* De Col. Trajani, cap. vii. p. 224. Romæ, 1683.

[2] Thesaur. Græc. Antiq., vol. xi. p. 822. De Curandis Equis. *' Prisci solea ungulis assigere non consuevere.*

[3] Nova Reperta, Tit. 16. *Sunt etiam qui velint ne calceatos quidem olim fuisse equos: eo quod in equestribus statuis ferrea ista calceamenta non conspiciantur ; cujus rei causam sanè haud scio.*

[4] Aristoph. Equit., 549. *Vetustissimos homines hoc ignorâsse certum est.*

Vossius shows from Palladius [1] that mules were usually shod with *spartum*, for by ' animalia,' the word Palladius uses, Vossius thinks mules and asses were intended.

Pegge [2] asserts that there is no clear, express, or positive proof that the Greeks shod their horses *very anciently*, or even customarily, in later times. ' I think it not improbable they might begin to do it occasionally, and in some certain places, a little before the age of Mithridates; a conjecture grounded upon the practice of the Romans, with whom shoeing prevailed so soon after.' By shoeing, this antiquarian perhaps meant the use of the *solea*—not the modern shoe. He adds : ' But why, it may be asked, should mules and asses be more commonly shod than horses ? I answer, these animals were much used in ancient times, more so than horses, for riding in Judæa, and for draught almost everywhere ; besides, they are usually more tractable and patient, asses especially, and shoeing, consequently, was much more easily performed upon them.'

This is scarcely correct. The use of the horse for draught and riding purposes was very limited, principally because shoeing, as now practised, was, if written testimony be accepted, unknown to the Romans. Mules and asses were probably preferred, because their hoofs are far more strong and durable than those of horses. These animals are also much less tractable, and, as a rule, are more diffi cult to shoe, from their obstinate and often vicious tempers.

Colonel Smith says : ' With regard to horse-shoeing, Bishop Lowth and Bracy Clark were mistaken in believ_

[1] Lib. l., cap. 24.   [2] Archæologia, 1776.

ing that the Roman horses' or mules' shoes were fastened on without nails driven through the horny parts of the hoof as at present. A contrary conclusion may be inferred from several passages in the poets; and the figure of a horse in the Pompeii battle-mosaic leaves little doubt on the question.' [1]

As this writer, however, does not quote the passages from the poets which lead to the inference that shoes were applied by means of nails, and as the authenticity of the details in the Pompeii battle-mosaic, which represents the defeat of Darius by Alexander, rests entirely on the authority of a *coloured engraving*, the horse-shoe supposed to be seen on the foot of a Satrap's charger is, we can scarcely doubt, of the same age as the copyist—a very modern affair, and as likely to prove the antiquity of the present method of shoeing as the presence of shoes with immense calkins on the feet of St Paul's horse in the painting by Lebrun, now in the Louvre; or the *virtuoso* in Dr Johnson's 'Rambler,' who possessed 'a horse-shoe broken on the Flaminian Way.' It must not be forgotten that another artist, in a print of Aristotle, carefully put a modern pen into the fingers of the illustrious Greek writer. When the engraving of the Pompeii mosaic was drawn and published, shoeing had been long known in Italy. Some years ago, while workmen were excavating on the site of that buried town, the ruins of an inn were reached, and in it were found the bodies of cars, with iron rings for fastening horses to the wall; bones of horses in the stables were also discovered, but *no shoes*.[2]

[1] Kitto's Cyclopædia of Biblical Literature.
Having placed myself in communication with Her Majesty's Con-

Heusinger,[1] whose profound acquaintance with ancient literature, particularly with that pertaining to the early Greek and Roman hippiatrists, few will dispute, declares that shoeing was not known to the Romans; that the writings of the ancient veterinarians are full of remedies for preventing and remedying undue wear of the horn; and that old authors were well acquainted with the use of shoes for diseased feet, but never make mention of the modern iron shoes in the treatment of such.

Mr Rich[2] asserts of the soleæ ferreæ, that 'they were a protection for the feet of mules employed in draught, intended to answer the same object as the modern horse shoe, though differing materially in its quality and manner of fixing; for the concurrent testimony of antiquity, both

sul-General at Naples, in order to ascertain if the recent investigations at Pompeii had afforded any additional evidence as to the absence of horse-shoes, that gentleman writes to the following effect, on the 24th January, 1869 : ' I have been informed by the Director of the Museum at Naples and of the excavations at Pompeii, that two pieces of bronze have recently been found which may have been used as shoes for a horse, but no other indications of horse-shoes having been in use have been met with. On the other hand, pieces, or rather small plates, of iron have been found, which are believed to be tips or half-shoes, as used at present, as a protection to the hoofs of oxen.

I have caused further inquiry to be made, and have also applied for drawings of these objects. Should anything satisfactory arrive before the publication of this work, it will be inserted as an appendix.

[1] Recherches de Pathologie Comparée, vol. i. p. 9. 'On ne trouve aucun indice de la ferrure chez les anciens Romains.' 'Les ouvrages des anciens vétérinaires sont remplis de remèdes pour prévenir et guérir l'nsure de cornes ; mais les suites de la ferrure sont seulement mentionnées dans les ouvrages modernes. Les anciens auteurs connoissent bien des sabots pour les pieds malades (soleas sparteas, etc.), mais jamais ils ne font mention des fers dans la cure des pieds malades.'

[2] Companion to the Latin Dictionary and Greek Lexicon, p. 608.

written, sculptured, and painted, bears undeniable evidence to the fact that neither the Greeks nor the Romans were in the habit of shoeing their animals by nailing a piece of iron on the hoofs as we now do. The contrivance they employed was probably a sock made of leather or some such material, and similar in form and general character to the solea spartea : being passed under and over the foot, and bound round the pastern joints and shanks of the animal by thongs of leather, like the *carbatinæ* of the peasantry. This sock was not permanently worn, but was put on by the driver during the journey in places or upon occasions when the state of the roads required, and taken off again when no longer necessary. Both the nature of the contrivance, showing that it was a close shoe covering the entire foot, and the practice of putting it on and removing it occasionally, is sufficiently testified by the particular terms employed to designate the object itself and the manner of applying it—*mulas calceare, mulis soleas induere.* When the underneath part of the sock was strengthened by a plate of iron, it was termed *solea ferrea.*' This writer describes the *solea spartea,* and compares it to the sandal used by the Japanese, which, he says, is 'a small basket, made to the shape of the animal's foot, on to which it is bound by a strap round the fetlock.' I have seen nothing in or from Japan answering to this description, nor at all like the drawing he gives.

The 'Nouveau Dictionnaire des Origines, Inventions, et Découvertes,' also maintains that the Greeks and Romans were ignorant of this art, and that they were content to attach the coverings they used by means of straps, in the same manner as men's shoes.

A like conclusion was recently arrived at by M. Nickard,[1] a careful investigator, who has examined all the accessible ancient records and monuments, in order to satisfy himself with regard to this subject ; though, as an archæologist, he has ignored this modern science.

So much for the written history of this art in the ages preceding the Christian era, and for some centuries sub sequently. Notwithstanding the various assumptions put forward by modern writers, founded on obscurely written or incorrectly rendered passages, that nail-shoeing was in use, the balance of evidence, it will be seen, is of a negative character. The frequent allusion to the injuries caused by travelling ; the mention of losses incurred in war-time by the horses breaking down from over-worn hoofs ; the repeated occurrence of words implying that the feet were unprotected ; the studied and judicious manner in which strong hoofs are spoken of and commended by the Greek and Roman horsemen ; the limited use made of the horse, with its comparatively easily damaged hoofs, and the extensive employment of the mule and ass, inferior animals, but whose feet are so much better protected by horn ;—all would go to prove that no effective armature for this vulnerable part of the horse's body was then known.

But we have noticed that a special device, though far inferior to that now employed, was had recourse to in the form of a sandal, which, though of a very inconvenient shape, and usually made of unthrifty materials, yet doubtless served for short journeys, and by being often renewed, answered to some extent for a longer space of time when a horse's feet had become tender from prolonged walking

[1] Mem. de la Soc. des *A*ntiq. de France, 1866.

on broken or stony ground; as well as assisted in re-taining healing applications to the soles when these were injured. At any rate, there would be no difficulty in em-ploying it; as a rider or driver, when apprehending injury to his horse or mule, could easily apply the *solea*, whether of broom, leather, or other materials; though he would always have to guard against the evil results incidental to the too prolonged use, or the constriction of the bands which bound it to the limb.

From such inquiries, and from the knowledge that a large portion of their stable management was devoted to making the horn of the foot tough, and the edges of the crust round and smooth, so as to obviate splitting and chipping, together with the known fact that no horses in any part of the world will bear severe and continuous labour without shoes,[1] we appear to be justified in con-

[1] Major Rickard, speaking of the district of San Juan, near the Cor-dillera, in Peru, describes it as very stony. ' For such districts the mules ought to be shod, as otherwise they will soon become foot-sore, and consequently worthless. I mention this because it is not usual to shoe horses or mules in the ordinary transitable districts of South *America*; and I would strongly recommend the traveller to *insist* upon *his own* mule, at least, being shod, irrespective of place or distance.'—*A Mining Journey Across the Great Andes*, p. 144.

And Tschudi, describing the village of San *Geronimo de Surco*, in the valley of Lima, says that the horses are shod, and that shoeing must be extremely valuable, if we may judge from its price. ' In this village there is an old Spaniard who keeps a tambo, and at the same time exercises the calling of a farrier. One of my horse's shoes being loose, I got him to fasten it on. For hammering in eight nails he made me pay half a gold ounce, and at first he demanded twelve dollars. Shortly after my arrival in the Sierra, I got myself initiated in the art of horse-shoeing, and constantly carried about with me a supply of horse-shoes and nails, a plan which I found was generally adopted by travellers in these parts. It is only in the larger Indian

cluding that the art of arming the ground surface of the
hoof with a metal plate and nails was unknown to the
antique civilization of the Greeks and Romans. Had
such a handicraft been in existence among them, without
a doubt it would have obtained particular notice in more
ways than one, but especially by the veterinary writers.
And so proud were the Romans of everything relating to
the horse, that shoes on his hoofs, making him a still more
perfect animal, and adding to his appearance, would have
been portrayed by the chisels of their sculptors, who,
faithful to their art in every respect, never omitted the
most apparently trivial or minute detail from the subjects
they have immortalized. We find them, for example,
giving an exact representation of the shoes worn by the
soldiers, with the nails that oftentimes studded the soles;
and even in the carriage-wheels depicted by them, we can
see the nails or rivets which bound the iron hoops to their
circumference. Yet neither in the remains of ancient
sculpture, among the ruins of Persepolis, on Trajan's
column, or those of Antoninus, Marcus Aurelius, and
others, nor yet on the equestrian statues which still remain
to us, is such a trophy of man's skill to be found.

As another instance, however, of the wonderful identity
and universality of purpose and instinct which impels
mankind in the most widely separated regions of the globe
to adopt certain measures and particular objects for the
requirements of their existence, the soleæ of the Roman
writers, and the desire for hard hoofs, are not without
interest to the ethnologist.

villages that farriers are to be met with, that is to say, in places fifty or
sixty leagues distant from each other.'—*Travels in Peru*, p. 266.

In Eastern countries at the present day, as has been already briefly remarked, the greatest importance is attached to the toughness and durability of the hoofs, even where horses are shod with iron plates. Among the Afghan tribes, for instance, not satisfied with the natural qualities of the horn, even when best developed, the native shoers adopt the following means for increasing its resisting powers. After removing the old shoe, and cutting away enough of the superfluous growth of horn, the lower margin of the wall and the sole are pretty freely charred by a red-hot iron, and while these parts are yet in a state of partial fusion, the whole foot is dipped into a strong solution of alum.

In some of the islands of the Eastern Sea—Java, Manilla, and Singapore—where shoeing is not practised, and the small horses have no defence to their feet, the stable floors are constructed exactly as Xenophon, Varro, Columella, Palladius, or Vegetius recommends, with the object of making the horn hard and keeping it dry.

Travelling to the North Pacific Ocean, there is the remarkable island-empire of Japan, so long isolated from other countries that it is indeed wonderful to find its inhabitants, so far as the arts and sciences are concerned, a highly cultivated and ingenious people. From time immemorial they have been skilful workers in metals; with the properties and many of the uses of iron they have for ages been familiar; and for centuries they have employed horses on a large scale, not only in their traffic, but in their feudal armies, of which a large proportion is cavalry. And yet they are in exactly the same condition as we suppose the Greeks and Romans were as regards

shoeing, and as evidenced in the quotations just referred
to.   The art of fastening metal plates on their horses' feet
is unpractised, and was probably unknown until a few
years ago ; so that strong hoofs with them is a matter of
much importance, and from year to year these are untouched by any instrument ; indeed, they become injuriously over-grown when the animal is not allowed
sufficient exercise ; and at all times they are permitted to
grow crooked and mis-shapen, just as wear or disease may
allow.   On unpaved roads, cases of lameness are not rare,
and where long journeys have to be performed over rocky
mountains and along stony paths, the hoofs must suffer
very much.   To obviate this inconvenience, the ingenious
Japanese have been compelled to resort to sandals which
are identical in principle, and not far removed from them
as regards material, with the *soleæ sparteæ* of Vegetius
and Columella.   The invention of these is probably coëval
with the introduction of their beautiful hardy little horses,
as the people themselves wear shoes of a similar construction.   Though made of rice-straw for ordinary wear
on the horses of the humbler classes, and of silk or cotton
stuff for those of *grandees*, yet their use is universal; and
if the large number worn out in a day's journey by one
horse be any criterion of what will be expended in a busy
commercial town, the manufacture of these slippers must
give employment to very many people (fig. 4).   Riding
horses do not always wear them, and when they do they are
generally fastened only on the fore feet, as on these the
weight chiefly falls ; but the pack-horses—which form,
with bulls, the only means of conveying m erchandise by
land, carriages not being in use—nearly always have sandals

on. The arrangement of these is very simple. Rice-

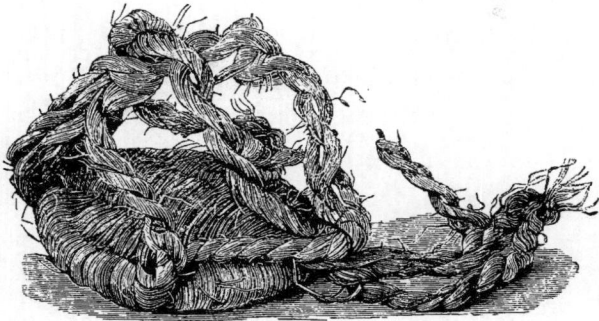

fig 4

straw is plaited into close ropes or bands, which are interwoven to form a thick circular pad, intended to cover the
whole of the sole. Around the border of this cushion
are loops of the same material; and at the front part
a stronger loop, the main fastening, and through which
run two narrow bands from the heels, the *corrigiæ*, made
to secure the whole apparatus firmly to the pastern.

Kæmpfer, the veracious historian of this curious empire, notices these contrivances. 'Shoes for the servants
and for the horses. Those of the latter are made of straw,
and are fastened with ropes of the same to the feet of the
horses, instead of iron shoes, such as ours in Europe,
which are not used in this country. As the roads are
slippery and full of stones, these shoes are soon worn out,
so that it is often necessary to change them. For this
purpose, those who have the care of the horses always
carry with them a sufficient quantity, which they affix to
the portmanteaus. They may, however, be found in all
the villages, and poor children who beg on the road even
offer them for sale, so that it may be said that there are

more farriers in this country than in any other; though, to speak properly, there are none at all.'[1]

Captain Sherard Osborne, describing the equipment his steed carried on a journey, amongst many other articles notes 'a string of the copper coin of the country, far too cumbrous for the pocket; a clothes-brush and fly-flap; a paper waterproof coat; a broad-brimmed tile for heavy rain or strong sunlight; *and lastly, a bundle of spare straw shoes for the horse.*' A noble's horse is thus painted: 'It is, indeed, a gorgeous creature; its headstall richly ornamented with beautiful specimens of Japan skill and taste in casting, chasing, and inlaying in copper and bronze, the leather perfectly covered with these ornaments. The frontlet has a golden or gilt horn projecting. The mane is carefully plaited, and worked in with gold and silver, as well as silken threads. The saddle, which is a Japanese imitation in leather, lacquer, and inlaid bronze, of those in use amongst the Portuguese and Spaniards in the days of Albuquerque, is a perfect work of art, and only excelled in workmanship, weight, and value by the huge stirrups. The reins are of silk; a rich scarlet net of the same material hangs over the animal's shoulders and crupper. The saddle-cloth is a leopard's skin; and lastly, as a perfect finish, the long switch tail is encased in a blue-silk bag reaching nearly to the ground; *whilst, instead of the shoes being of ordinary straw, they are made of cotton and silk interwoven.*'[2]

And Sir Rutherford Alcock writes: 'Refreshed by our breakfast, we began to turn inland to the screen of hills

[1] Histoire du Japan. *A*msterdam, 1732.
[2] Japanese Fragments, p. 97.

which skirt the bay, and soon came upon some roads as bad as any "Camincha real" in Spain. My horse's straw shoes, having already been half shuffled off, were tripping him up at every step, and compelled me to dismount in order to get rid of them altogether. An Englishman riding with the fore-feet of his horse muffled in straw slippers, might furnish a subject for "Punch." I am happy to say that at both the legations this absurdity has been got rid of, and means found of teaching the Japanese to shoe our horses properly with iron ; and more than one of the Daimios, I was told, had followed the good example.'[1]

High, black, and small hoofs are with the Japanese, as with the Greeks and Romans, in most favour, and for the same reasons.

The massive, powerful black bulls of Japan, which carry immense loads on their backs, often have their feet encased in strong, half-tanned buskins, which lace round the leg; probably these resemble the hippopodes of Apsyrtus.

Captain Blakiston informs us, that near Chung-King, province of Sz'chuan, on the upper waters of the Great Yang-tsze, the cattle wore straw shoes to prevent their slipping on the wet ground.[2]

In the far north of China, as we will have occasion to notice hereafter, horses and cattle are shod with iron shoes and nails.

Colonel Smith[3] mentions, that in Iceland horses are occasionally shod by the peasants with sheep's horn ; cer-

---

[1] The Capital of the Tycoon. London, 1863.
[2] Five Months on the Yang-tsze, p. 214. London, 1862.
[3] Naturalists' Library, vol. xii. p. 129.

tainly a step in advance of the sandal. In the valley of
the Upper Oxus, towards Budukshan, the people shoe
their horses with stag-horn. 'I heard of a singular practice,' says Burnes,[1] 'among the people of these districts,
who shoe their horses with the antlers of the mountain
deer. They form the horn into a suitable shape, fix it on
the hoof with horn pins, and never renew it till fairly worn
out. It is said the custom is borrowed from the Kirghizzes.'

Speaking of the Kirghiz, Wood writes : 'What flesh
they consume is obtained by their matchlocks ; and the
number of horns that strew Pamir bear evidence to the
havoc they make among the wild flocks of the mountain.
These horns being of a remarkably large size, supply shoes
for the horses' feet, and are also a good substitute for
stirrup-irons. The shoes are nothing more than a semicircular piece of horn placed on the fore part of the hoof.
When the horse is in constant work, it requires renewal at
least once a week.'[2]

---

[1] *Travels into Bokhara,* vol. iii. p. 180.
[2] *Journey to the Source of the River Oxus,* p. 340.

CHAPTER III.

OVERTHROW OF THE ROMAN EMPIRE BY THE BARBARIANS. THE 'DARK AGES.' THE EMPEROR LEO, AND HIS 'TACTICA.' FERREA LUNATICA. THE EMPEROR CONSTANTINE, AND 'SELENAIA. ARCHÆOLOGY. ANCIENT CUSTOMS OF EUROPE. CHIFFLET'S DESCRIPTION OF KING CHILDERIC'S TOMB. DOUGLAS AND THE ABBÉ COCHET. DISCOVERY OF ANTIQUE HORSE-SHOES. BURIAL WITH HORSES. THE ANCIENT GERMANS, AND OTHER RACES; THEIR SUPERSTITIONS. THE GAULS AND BRITONS. RARITY OF HORSE-SHOES IN GRAVES. THE CELTS SHOD THEIR HORSES; THEIR HISTORY. THE GAULS AS A NATION: WARRIORS AND AGRICULTURISTS. THE DRUIDS. GALLIC NAMES. AN EQUES-TRIAN NATION. HORSES, WAGGONS, AND ROADS. ALESIA AND ITS TOMBS. PRIMITIVE FARRIERY. THE DRUID'S WORKSHOP AND ALTAR. THE PONTIFF BLACKSMITH. THE GAULISH CAVALRY. DEFEAT OF VERCINGETORIX. NAPOLEON III. AND HIS 'VIE DE CÆSAR.' BESANÇON AND ITS RELICS. SMALL-SIZED HORSE-SHOES. GALLO-ROMAN SHOES; THEIR PECULIARITIES. SPECI-MENS FOUND WITH ROMAN REMAINS. VAISON AND ITS TESTI-MONY. CRECY. SUPPRESSION OF DRUIDISM IN GAUL. INVASION OF THE FRANKS, AND EFFEMINACY OF THE GAULISH NOBLES. THE FRANKS NOT AN EQUESTRIAN PEOPLE. LEVIES OF COWS IN-STEAD OF HORSES. ABSENCE OF HORSE-SHOES FROM MEROVIN-GIAN GRAVES. THE CARLOVINGIAN DYNASTY. ADVANTAGES OF CAVALRY. CHARLEMAGNE AND REVIVAL OF EQUESTRIANISM. TRADITIONS. SHOEING IN FRANCE IN THE NINTH AND SUBSE-QUENT CENTURIES. THE COMTE DE L'ETABLE, AND ECUYER. ORIGIN OF CHIVALRY AND ITS CONSTITUTION. DUTIES OF THE KNIGHTS. THE MARESCHAL.

WE have now reached a comparatively modern date in the history of the domestication of the horse, without discovering any incontrovertible evidence as to those who employed it having extended its usefulness by a durable armature to its vulnerable hoofs. All the authorities worthy of acceptance have been examined, and their testimony, taken as a whole, would lead to the belief that plates of iron or other metal, securely attached to the feet by nails, were not in use during the period of time over which our inquiry has extended; these authorities have been historians, agricultural and veterinary writers, and sculptors, who would, we may be almost certain, have left us ample testimony in this respect, had they been cognizant of the art. But we appear to have evidence that a very temporary and clumsy defence was resorted to, and which was more or less firmly fixed to the extremity by thongs and bands, or straps and buckles.

Unfortunately, further inquiry is rendered all but nugatory on account of the dearth of historical or other records by which one might be enabled to pursue an uninterrupted investigation towards the period when *iron shoes* were attached by *iron nails* to the feet of horses, and that such an artisan as the *faber ferrarius* was needed to garnish the hoofs with these now indispensable appendages. The third century saw the Roman Empire rapidly declining; successive hordes of barbarians issuing from what are designated 'the frozen loins of the north,' began to disturb the equilibrium of the western world, and to spread confusion and destruction everywhere. The Huns, originally of Tatar or Scythian origin, first made their presence felt in Europe about the middle of the 4th century, and about a hundred years later ravaged the continent far and near, under the leadership of their king,

Attila, the 'Scourge of God.' With an immense army, the greater portion of which was cavalry, he invaded and laid under tribute the Roman empire, but not before devastating many of its provinces. After his death, this wandering people, who appear to have been largely composed of Kalmuck or Mongol Tatars, were without a leader, and, being broken up, formed themselves into a number of petty states, which continued to maintain their independence until the close of the eighth century, when they were subdued by Charlemagne. During these and subsequent centuries, well termed the 'Dark Ages,' learning was at a low ebb, because of the disturbed condition of the civilized world, and the overthrow of kings and dynasties by the irruptions of these strange and less than semi-barbarous nations, who swept away or destroyed in their progress nearly everything valuable to future ages, leaving only the more salient and remarkable historical facts to be imperfectly described by a few monks or refugees. These were, for the most part, buried in cloisters or secluded spots, and had but few opportunities, even if they possessed the inclination or ability, to note the various changes which befell many of the arts, or chronicle those which appeared for the first time. So that it is not to be wondered at that the annalists of those days should be silent with regard to these foot defences, and that the first intimation of their existence should only be given at so late a date as the ninth century.

The change of designation which was formerly employed to indicate the coverings for the feet, χαρβατιναι, εκβαται, *soleæ*, and ἱπποπεδης, was that which first led investigators to the conclusion that our present method of shoeing was practised in the ninth century. From the ancient terms being much less frequently met with, it was surmised that the old-fashioned *solea* had gone out of use, and that the new armature, if it was adopted, must have a particular designation of another kind to distinguish it. In the 'Tactica' of the Eastern Emperor Leo VI. surnamed the Philosopher (A.D. 886—911), there is a list of everything necessary for the equipment of a cavalry soldier, and amongst other articles are included 'lunar or crescent-shaped iron shoes and their nails.'[1]

In the 'Tactica' of the Emperor Constantine Porphyrogenitus, son of the former, the same passage also occurs,[2] and in a book by this monarch on court ceremonies,[3] iron horse-shoes are mentioned on two occasions: first, when in speaking of the horses to be provided for the imperial stables, he directs that they are to be furnished with everything requisite, and to have σελητναῖα—*selenaia*; and, secondly, where it is ordered that a certain weight of iron is to be issued from the imperial magazines for the purpose of making these iron shoes, and other articles of horse necessaries.

These are, so far as is known, the first instances that occur in history of horse-shoes, with their nails; and it is somewhat remarkable, that about this period they are also noticed in the writings of Italian, French, English, and

---

[1] Tactica Imperatoris Leonis, vol. v. cap. 4, p. 51.　Leyden, 1612. 'πέδικλα σεληναῖα σιδηρά μετὰ καρφίων—Ferra lunatico cum clavis eorum.'

[2] 'Calceos lnnatos ferreos cum ipsis corphiis, id est, clavis.'　Maffei, who translated an edition of this work, attributed it to Constantine, son of the Emperor Romanus Lecapenus.

[3] De Ceremoniis *Aulæ* Byzantinæ.　Leipzig, 1754.

other authors. We will refer to these at another time ; at present it is necessary to observe, that this mode of preserving horses' feet must have been in vogue long ages before it is casually alluded to by the Byzantine Emperors ; and in all likelihood was even practised by the Romans in the early centuries of our era, though their writers are silent with regard to it.

For some years, the study of the ancient languages and of old monuments has assumed the dignity and position of a science, and has gradually introduced great modifications in the opinions held in regard to the primary phases of humanity ; while discoveries, conveniently and reasonably discussed, have brought into view other horizons, and given a novel direction to ethnologic research. This new science, which investigates the unwritten history of our race, and illustrates, in a most unequivocal manner, that which has been written, has been styled ' Ethnological Archæology ;' to it the discourse of our subject is already much indebted, as we will see presently.

The researches of archæologists and ethnologists have, in this and other countries, thrown much light on the manners and customs of the ancient inhabitants of Europe, and thus largely compensated for the absence of written documents ; and the result has been to carry back the probable date of the introduction of modern shoeing to a generation much beyond that supposed by inquirers, who relied solely on the evidence of Greek and Roman authors, and the creations of the sculptor's chisel.

In the year 1655, Jean Jacques Chifflet published a description of what he supposed to be the tomb of Childeric, father of Clovis, discovered at Tournay, in

7 *

Belgium, in 1623.[1]   This king, who lived in the fifth
century, was the founder of the French monarchy; and in
the grave, with human bones, those of a horse, ornaments
and equipments of various kinds, was also found what
Chifflet believed to be the remains of an iron horse-shoe.
This article was in a state of extreme oxidation, and from
the small fragment that could be preserved the author
contrived to delineate an ordinary horse-shoe of the seven-
teenth century.   Chifflet, two years after the discovery,
published his account of it, in which he says: ' The remains of his (Childeric's) horse were found: the bones of
the head, the teeth, cheek-bones, and an *iron shoe ;* but
the latter was so eaten away by rust, that while I was
trying to cleanse the nail holes—of which there were four
on each side—with a small spike, the rotten iron broke in
pieces, and could only be imperfectly restored.'[2]   This
restored shoe has given rise to much dispute.   Bracy
Clark thought from its shape and size that it must have
belonged to a mule; forgetting that the use of such an
animal for riding purposes in the age of the Merovingian
kings, and by a king, was possibly as great a degradation
as it is now-a-days to the Indians, or to the Bedouins, who
sing—

> Honourable is the riding of a horse to the rider,
> But the mule is a dishonour, and the ass a disgrace.[3]

---

[1] *Anastasis Childerici.   Auctore J. S. Chiffletio.   Antwerp,* 1655.

[2] Op. cit. ' Inventæ sunt ejus equi reliquiæ, capitis ossa, dentes,
maxillæ et ferrea solea, sed ita rubigine absumpta, ut dum veruculo
clavorum foramina (quæ utrinque quaterna erant) purgare leviter
tentarem, ferrum putre in fragmenta dissiluerit, et ex parte duntaxat
hic representari patuerit.'   Page 223.

[3] Froissart, however, would appear to indicate that in Spain, in the

Douglas, in his ' Nenia Britannica,' throws great discredit on Chifflet's description, because of his not being present when the tomb was opened, and also because of the condition the various objects were in. When Douglas visited France in 1787, the shoe and some other articles were not to be found, which caused him to look with yet greater distrust on the whole account.

The Abbé Cochet, an accomplished antiquarian, is also suspicious of this fragment of iron, which was so oxidized that it fell into powder on the slightest touch, and has entirely disappeared, being the remains of a horse-shoe ; he is more inclined to think it must have been a portion of the iron-mounting of a box, although the skeleton of a horse was found in the tomb. He bases his doubts on the fact, that in no Frankish grave has anything been discovered at all resembling an iron nailed shoe, and he is of opinion that the Franks did not shoe their small and coarse-bred horses.[1]

middle ages, it was not derogatory even for a king to ride a mule. Immediately before the battle of Navarette, he mentions King Henry ' mounted on a handsome and strong mule, according to the custom of his country,' riding through the ranks, paying his compliments to the lords and knights, and entreating them to exert themselves in defending his honour.—*Chronicles of England, France, and Spain,* vol. iii. p. 302. London, 1806.

[1] Jusqu'ici, rien ne s'est montré plus rare dans les sépultures franques que les sabots ou les fers de chevaux. En effet, sur les trois ou quatre chevaux que nous avons trouvés à Envermeu, nous n'avons jamais rencontré de fers et pourtant les jambes ne manquaient pas. En revanche, nous avons trouvé des boucles et des mors bien caractérisés. M. Lindenschmit, à Selsen, a rencontré un squelette de cheval, mais sans fer. Il en a été de même à Sinsheim, à Ascherade, à Langweid, à Nordendorf ; dans cette dernière localité, on a trouvé trois squelettes avec brides, mais toujours sans fers. MM. Durrich et Menzel, dans la fouille si in-

Montfauçon, however, believed it to be really a horse-shoe, and adds, ' the shoe is small; whence it is conjectured the animal it belonged to was of a diminutive size.'   And in reply to the objection that the Franks did not shoe their horses, he replies : ' Perhaps only the greatest persons had their horses shod in those times ; and afterwards, probably when the practice of shoeing was more general, the Franks only shod their cavalry *occasionally*, as in frost, for example, in the ninth century.'

In the accompanying copy of this restored, but doubtful, shoe (fig. 5), it will be seen that there was but a slender instalment to base such an outline upon. Mont fauçon says, in explanation of the drawing: ' The horse-shoe of Childeric has been here represented entire, although only a portion of it

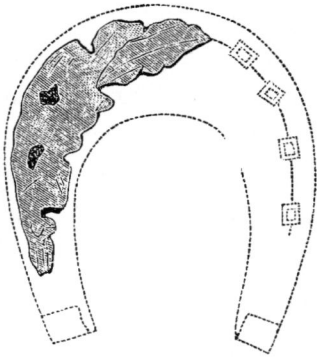

fig 5

téressante d'Oberflacht, ont rencontré un équipement complet de cheval sans fer. . . . . . Le fer de Childeric Ier, ainsi que les squelettes de chevaux francs trouvés en Allemagne, prouve que cette race était petite, ce qui est confirmé par Tacite :

Equi (eorum) non formâ conspicui.

.   .   .   .

Namur, rapporteur des fouilles de Dalheim, dit : ' Il paraît établi que les chevaux gaulois des premiers siècles de l'ère chrétienne étaient de petits chevaux de selle, demi-sauvages, à petits sabots durs et rétrécis, comme le sont encore aujourd'hui les chevaux demi-sauvages élèves dans l'Ukraine et dans les steppes qui avoisinent la mer Caspienne.'—*Le Tombeau de Childeric Ier*.   Paris, 1852.

has been found; but by this piece it is easy (?) to judge of the size of the whole. The horse was a small one.'[1]

Since Chifflet's publication appeared, relics of races whose history has never been written, and whose story has never been told, have been found in various parts of Europe and in our own country; and among these not unfrequently have appeared horse-shoes of a primitive, peculiar, and somewhat marked form, which plainly indicates that they are of high antiquity. The researches of archæologists, carefully and skilfully conducted, have, in many instances, led us to form an estimate of their age; but in other cases we are left much in doubt, from their not accompanying any remains which can be traced to any race or epoch, and also from their often occurring with relics which mark no particularly definite period.

One source from whence these memorials of an age long passed have been derived, has been the graves, cromlechs, tumuli, barrows, kists, or cairns, as the last resting places of primitive peoples have been variously named; and their presence there has been due to the prevalence of

---

[1] Op. Cit. ' Solea ferrea equi regii hic tota repræsentatur, etsi pars ejus tantum reperta sit; sed ex illa parte totius formam excipere haud difficile fuit. Modicæ magnitudinis equus erat, ut jam diximus.

Elsewhere he says : ' Parmi les pièces que nous venons de décrire se trouverent aussi le crâne, la mâchoire et les dens du cheval de Childeric *avec une partie du fer d'un pied,* qui faisoit juger que ce cheval étoit assez petit. On voit souvent des chevaux de médiocre taille, qui pour la vigueur, la forme et la gentillesse, passent les plus grands. On y mit apparemment celui que Childeric aimoit le plus. La coutume de ces anciens peuples étoit d'enterrer avec les hommes les chevaux et les autres animaux qui étoient à leur usage, et qu'ils aimoient le plus.'—*Les Monumens de la Monarchie Françoise,* p. 235.

a custom which shows that the early inhabitants of many
parts of Europe were horse-loving nations, from whom
the noble creature could not be separated, even by death.
I allude to the interment of horses with the mighty dead,
the fame of whose deeds was not allowed to pass to our
time, and whose bones, fragments of weapons, or adorn
ment, and the silent evidence of their friendship for the
horse, alone remain to denote their having once upon a
time existed.   To a certain extent, the horse-shoes found
in graves are trustworthy testimony to the antiquity of
nail-shoeing, and the degree to which it prevailed.

The practice of burying the horse with his master is
extremely ancient, and general to a most wonderful extent.
With the Greeks, as with ourselves, horses served to
heighten the solemnity of death.   Homer tells us, that
when the Greeks were mourning for Patroclus,

> Thrice round the dead they drove their sleek-skinn'd steeds,
> Mourning !

and the body of that warrior being consigned to the
flames,

> round the edges of the pyre,
> Horses and men commix'd.

In the funeral feasts of his people, which are represented
on funeral monuments the image of a horse's head was
usually placed in one corner, as an emblem that death was
a journey.

Among the ancient Germans, the body of the dead
warrior was consumed in the flames of a particular kind of

wood, and only the arms of the deceased, with his horse, were given to the flames with him; then a mound of earth was heaped up over all.[1] Cæsar speaks of Celtic tribes as burying with the dead their most valuable possessions, and sacrificing human beings, probably, also, the horse.

In Celtic, Slavonic, and German graves or cairns, horses' bones are expected to be found. At Mecklenburg the presence of horse-remains is not unfrequent. In a barrow on the Baltic coast, the skeleton of a very tall man was discovered eight feet below the surface or summit of the mound; and beside the skull, on the left side, lay bones of a horse's head, and several flint knives at the top and bottom. More than a dozen human skeletons lay around in a circle, the skulls inwards towards the principal one, and a number of stone weapons. At another place a stone cairn was opened in which were two graves; in both were arms, stone implements and weapons, amber ornaments, and the remains of unburnt horses' bones. Similar remains were found in other stone cairns. At Calbe, near the former place, Wagner discovered the skeleton of a horse, surrounded by at least twenty urns, in a grave marked on the surface by three large stones. Wilhelm mentions a grave in which the skull of a skeleton rested on the cranium of a horse, and the other bones of the animal lay around the grave. In tombs supposed to belong to the Alemannic tribes, this antiquarian discovered similar remains.

At Selzen, on the Rhine, Lindenschmidt found a

[1] *Tacitus.* Chap. 27.

horse's skull in the resting-place of a primitive warrior (fig. 6).[1]

In the vicinity of Hamburg, graves which were supposed to belong to what is termed the 'iron period' were opened, and horses' bones were found. At Nienburg, horse and human bones were met with, mingled together, in a cairn belonging to the same period.

The Slavonians sacrificed horses on their graves; for the Arabian traveller, Ibn Fozlan, was a witness to this practice in the 10th century, at the funeral of a Russian prince. The Lithuanians and Samogitians did the same; and the Finn and other Mongolian

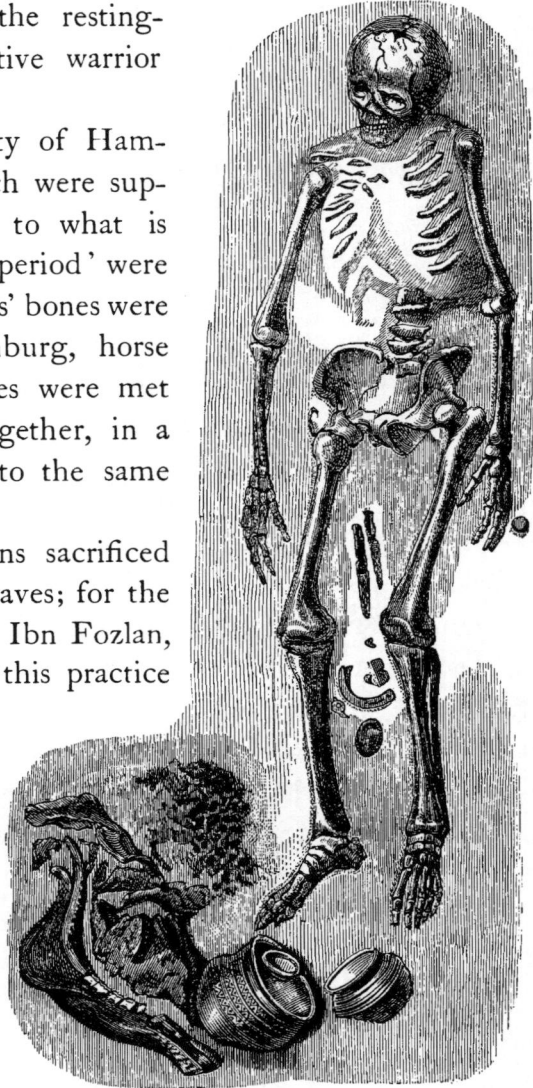

fig. 6

races, among which may be reckoned the Tschuds, generally buried their horses with the dead. The remains of horses are very often found in the graves of

[1] *Das Germanische Todtenlager Bei Selzen.* Plate 8. Mainz, 1848.

the tribes who formerly tenanted Liefland. Marco Polo, in alluding to the custom of interring the bodies of the chiefs of the race of Ghengis Khan at a certain lofty mountain, no matter where they may have died, adds. 'It is likewise the custom, during the progress of removing the bodies of these princes, for those who form the escort to sacrifice such persons as they may chance to meet on the road, saying to them, "Depart for the next world, and there attend upon your deceased master," being impressed with the belief that all whom they thus slay do actually become his servants in the next life. They do the same also with respect to horses, killing the best of the stud, in order that he may have the use of them.' This was in the 13th century.

Tumuli containing the remains of horses and men are met with in Central Asia and Siberia. The vast plains of these regions have ever been nurseries for horse-loving nations. This sacrifice and burial of horses was particularly practised by the early northern nations, but especially by the Scandinavians. When a hero or chief fell gloriously in battle, his funeral obsequies were honoured with all possible magnificence. His arms, his gold and silver, his war-horse, and whatever else he held most dear, were placed with him on the pile. His dependents and friends frequently made it a point of honour to die with their leader, in order to attend on his shade in the palace of Odin; for nothing seemed to them more grand and noble than to enter Valhalla with a numerous retinue, all in their finest armour and richest apparel. The princes and nobles never failed of such attendants. The warrior and his horse were to salute the god in the regions of ever lasting war and feasting. They believed, because Odin himself had assured them, that whatever was buried or consumed with the dead, accompanied them to his palace. And another reason why the horse was buried with them was, that they durst not approach the palace of Odin on foot.' Probably this was a wise feature introduced into their religion, to impress upon them the value of cavalry, and a high regard for the services of the horse. At the funerals of Harold Hildetand and Skalagrim, horses were sacrificed to accompany these doughty warriors.

Balder, the beautiful and youthful god of eloquence and just decision, the innocent who appears brilliant as the lily, and in honour of whom the whitest flower received the name of Baldrian, was slain with a spear of the misletoe by the blind god Hoder, whose violent deeds the gods never forget, but whose name they never hear pronounced. The Prose Edda thus refers to his funeral : ' Balder's body was then borne to the funeral pile on board the ship, and this ceremony had such an effect on Nana, the daughter of Nep, that her heart broke with grief, and her body was burnt on the same pile as her husband's. . . . . Balder's horse was led to the pile fully caparisoned, and consumed in the same flames with the body of his master.' Longfellow has beautifully described this scene:

> ' They laid him in his ship
> With horse and harness,
> As on a funeral pyre.
> Odin placed
> A ring upon his finger,
> And whisper'd in his ear.

' *Mallet.* Northern Antiquities. 1847.

They launch'd the burning ship,
It floated far away
O'er the misty sea,
Till like the moon it seem'd,
Sinking beneath the waves.
Balder returned no more!'

It is curious to note, that among the Sea Dyaks of Borneo, the dead chief is placed in his canoe with his favourite weapons and principal property, and is then turned adrift.

In the Scandinavian barrows, great quantities of horses' bones are found with human skeletons. The only pleasure and business of life with these old turbulent spirits, was war; and their political, domestic, and religious institutions were all founded on this characteristic. A warrior, therefore, could not but fight well when the pleasures after death were, as his religion taught him, those which he most relished during life. 'The heroes who are received into the palace of Odin,' says the Edda, 'have every day the pleasure of arming themselves, of passing in review, of ranging themselves in order of battle, and of cutting one another in pieces; but as soon as the hour of repast approaches, they return on horseback all safe and sound to the hall of Odin, and fall to eating and drinking.'

With the Danes the age of tumuli or hillocks was styled Hoigold and Hoielse-tüde. The corpse was buried with all the arms he had wielded or worn during life, and all his ornaments; and his horse was killed and laid beside him.

The Patagonians, to whom the horse is, comparatively speaking, a novelty, also inter it in their burial-places, and the stories about the immense size of these people probably originated from the circumstance that this animal's bones were mistaken for those of the Patagonians. And the Red Indian desires the company of his steed, when the Great Spirit calls him to the hunting-grounds beyond the setting sun. Longfellow has celebrated the burial of the Minnisink, an Indian chief, in some of his happiest verses.

> ' Behind, the long procession came
> Of hoary men and chiefs of fame,
> With heavy hearts, and eyes of grief,
> Leading the war-horse of their chief.
>
> Stripp'd of his proud and martial dress,
> Uncurb'd, unrein'd, and riderless,
> With darting eye, and nostril spread,
> And heavy and impatient tread,
> He came; and oft that eye so proud
> Ask'd for his master in the crowd.
>
> They buried the dark chief; they freed
> Beside the grave his battle steed;
> And swift an arrow cleaved its way
> To his stern heart! One piercing neigh
> *A*rose—and, on the dead man's plain,
> The rider grasps his steed again.'

In Central Africa, for lack of horses, other creatures accompany the deceased, if he be a wealthy individual.[1]

In France, as we have already mentioned, and as will be again referred to, this mode of sepulture was common

---

[1] ' When a Wanyamwezi dies in a strange country, and his comrades take the trouble to inter him, they turn the face of the corpse towards the mother's village, a proceeding which shows more sentiment than might be expected from them. The body is buried standing, or tightly bound in a heap, or placed in a sitting position with the arms clasping the knees; if the deceased be a great man, a sheep and a bullock are slaughtered for a funeral feast, the skin is placed over his face, and the hide is bound to his back.

among the ancient Gauls, and horses and other creatures were sacrificed. 'When they have conquered,' writes Cæsar, 'they sacrifice whatever captured animals may have survived the conflict.' 'Their funerals, considering the state of civilization among the Gauls, are magnificent and costly; and they cast into the fire all things, including living creatures, which they suppose to have been dear to them when alive; and a little before this period, slaves and dependents who were ascertained to have been beloved by them, were, after the regular funeral rites were completed, burnt together with them.'[1]

With regard to Britain, Sir John Lubbock[2] remarks, that the very frequent presence of the bones of animals in tumuli appears to show that, with prehistoric man, sepulchral feasts were generally held in honour of the dead; and the numerous cases in which interments were accompanied by burnt human bones, tend to prove the prevalence of still more dreadful customs, and that not only horses and dogs, but slaves also, were frequently sacrificed at their masters' graves.

All the remains of horses found in prehistoric barrows

'The chiefs of Unyamwezi generally are interred by a large assemblage of their subjects with cruel rites. A deep pit is sunk, with a kind of vault or recess projecting from it; in this the corpse, clothed with skin and hide, and holding a bow in the right hand, is placed sitting, with a pot of pombe, upon a dwarf stool, while sometimes one, but more generally three female slaves, one on each side and the third in front, are buried alive to preserve their lord from the horrors of solitude.' —*Burton.* The Lake Regions of Central Africa, vol. ii.

According to Crantz, the Esquimaux lay a dog's head by the grave of a child, for the soul of a dog, say they, can find its way everywhere, and will show the ignorant babe the way to the land of souls.

[1] Bell. Gallic., lib. vi. cap. 17, 19. [2] Prehistoric Times, p. 115.

are probably those belonging to a domesticated race. The antiquity of the horse in England is yet doubtful; and if we are to place any reliance on the results of researches in these barrows, we might conclude that horses were very rare, if not altogether unknown, during that period styled the stone age; but during the metallic period his remains are frequently met with.

Mr Bateman[1] concludes, from his researches among the most ancient burial-places, that he does not know in what light the primitive inhabitants of our country may have looked upon the horse, viewed as a creature of sufficient importance to be necessary for their use and happiness in a future state, but certain it is, that however rude and degraded this belief in another world may have been, the teeth, if not some of the bones, of horses have been found in primitive British tumuli, particularly those of Derbyshire; and which have no history but their strange contents.

Two Celtic graves opened in Yorkshire contained skeletons of horses; and in graves of the Anglo-Saxon period they have also been found.[2]   The Hon. C. Neville, describing the remains found in a cemetery near Little Wilbraham, Cambridgeshire, in 1851, remarks: 'Mention should here be made of an instance similar to one described by Sir Henry Dryden (Archæologia, vol. xxxiii.), viz.: the entire body of a horse, interred by the side of his rider, with a perfect iron bit still remaining on its head, and some small stud nails, with fragments of a leather headstall.'[3]

[1] Ten Years' Diggings.   [2] *Knowles.*   Horæ Ferales, p. 65.
[3] Saxon Obsequies, p. 9.

With the Celts, it appears that it was not unfrequently the custom to place in the warrior's tomb, besides his horse, one or two wheels of the chariot, and sometimes the whole carriage and harness. At Alaise, in France, and among the tombs of Anet, Switzerland, this has been noticed.[1]

If my memory serves me right, the remains of a chariot found in a tomb are now in the York Museum.

Unfortunately, as Mr Knowles observes, these remains of horses in graves do not constitute any distinguishing mark of time or race, as the slaughter and burial of horses appear to have belonged to almost all nations and all ages; the custom extending from the Tschuds of the Altai and the Crim Tartars to the Franks and Saxons; even in the sarcophagi of Christian knights, buried in churches during the Middle Ages, besides their own weapons and bones, the less perishable parts of their steeds are there. So late as the eighteenth century the custom was in vogue, for a martial and Christian order of knighthood, in 1781, laid Frederick Casimir in his grave with his slaughtered horse beside him. In 1866, Her Majesty Queen Victoria's huntsman died; his old and favourite horse was destroyed, and the animal's ears were deposited on his late master's coffin before the earth had shut him out from the world.

And still more unfortunately for our subject, these remains of the gentle soliped do but seldom testify to the existence of nail-pierced hoofs and a metallic mounting. From shoes being nearly always manufactured of iron, that metal oxidizes so rapidly, that in the presence

[1] *Troyon.* Habitations Lacustres, p. 334. Lausanne, 1860.

of moisture a thin plate would not be long in rusting to powder. And those who have had the superintendence of these disinterments have not, it is to be feared, been always careful enough to direct their attention to such an insignificant matter as the condition of the hoofs, when these were yet intact.

From their situation, and the remains accompanying the horse-shoes found in certain regions, as well as from their later history, there is every reason to believe that the Celts or Celtæ, and their chief branch, the Gauls or Gaël, were cognizant of the art of shoeing with metal and nails at a very remote period, and before they were conquered by the Romans under Cæsar.

The early history of this great nation is lost in the thick haze of antiquity. Originally a section of the Aryan family, at some very distant period they left Asia and spread themselves over various parts of Europe in their descent from the Caucasus and along the south side of the Danube. Several Celtic tribes took possession of different countries under various names; others settled on the shores of the Adriatic, along the banks of the Danube, and in the southern part of Germany; while the principal branch of the nation located itself between the Pyrenees and the Alps, the ocean and the Rhine, in the country which received its name from them; from thence they passed into Albion and Ierne (Great Britain and Ireland). Everything relating to their history at this time is so obscure, that we have sometimes little but conjecture to aid us in tracing their migrations. It would appear, nevertheless, that the eastern Gauls or Celts who passed along the Danube occasioned the migrations of whole nations, and that about B.C. 300 they had already absorbed a part of the German race named the Cimri, or Cimbri. Defeated, however, in Greece, at an attack on the temple of Apollo at Delphi, destruction awaited them, and with the exception of several tribes who passed into Asia Minor, and assumed the name of Galatians, we hear little or nothing of the Celts on the Danube or the south of Germany. Tribes of German origin occupied the whole country as far as the Rhine, and even beyond that river. But the Cimbri, a mixed race of Gauls and Germans, whom the Gauls themselves designated Belgæ, occupied the whole northern part of Gaul, from the Seine and Marne to the British Channel, from whence they passed over into Britain. Here they drove back those Gauls who had made themselves masters of the country at an earlier period, to North Britain (Scotland), where the latter afterwards appear under the name of Caledonians or Highland Gaels, and still later as the Picts and Scots.[1] These Belgæ or Gallo-Cimbri are, in fact, the ancient Britons, the inhabitants of the land of the Cymry.

The Emperor Napoleon[2] concisely sums up their history in the following words: 'There are peoples whose existence in the past only reveals itself by certain brilliant apparitions, unequivocal proofs of an energy which had been previously unknown. During the interval their history is involved in obscurity, and they resemble those long silent volcanoes, which we should take to be extinct but for the eruptions which, at periods far apart, occur and expose to view the fire which smoulders in their bosom. Such had been the Gauls. The accounts of

---

[1] Popular Encyclopædia, pt. 5.   [2] Vié de Cæsar, vol. ii. p. 1.

8 *

their ancient expeditions bear witness to an organization already powerful, and to an ardent spirit of enterprise. Not to speak of migrations which date back perhaps nine or ten centuries before our era, we see at the moment when Rome was beginning to aim at greatness, the Celts spreading themselves beyond their frontiers. In the time of Tarquin the Elder (Years of Rome, 138 to 176), two expeditions started from Celtic Gaul: one proceeded across the Rhine and Southern Germany, to descend upon Illyria and Pannonia (now *Western Hungary);* the other, scaling the Alps, established itself in Italy, in the country lying between those mountains and the Po. The invaders soon transferred themselves to the right bank of that river, and nearly the whole of the territory comprised between the Alps and the Apennines took the name of *Cisalpine Gaul.* More than two centuries afterwards, the descendants of those Gauls marched upon Rome and burnt it all but the Capitol. Still a century later (475), we see new bands issuing from Gaul, reaching Thrace by the valley of the Danube, ravaging Northern Greece, and bringing back to Toulouse the gold plundered from the Temple of Delphi. Others, arriving at Byzantium, pass into Asia, establish their dominions over the whole region on this side Mount Taurus, since called *Gallo-Græcia,* or Galatia, and maintain in it a sort of military feudalism until the time of the war of Antiochus.

'These facts, obscure as they may be in history, prove the spirit of adventure and the warlike genius of the Gaulish race, which thus, in fact, inspired a general terror. During nearly two centuries, from 364 to 531, Rome struggled against the Cisalpine Gauls, and more than once the defeat of her armies placed her existence in danger.'

Cicero says: 'From the beginning of our Republic, all our wise men have looked upon Gaul as the most redoubtable enemy of Rome.

'The Romans,' says Sallust, 'held then, as in our days, the opinion that all other peoples must yield to their courage; but that with the Gauls it was no longer for glory, but for safety, that they had to fight.'

When the nations we term classical first became acquainted with the northern races, German and Celt had long been in possession of iron, and formed all their warlike weapons of that metal. Indeed, they were far from being the barbarians historians have often represented them. M. Fournet remarks: 'The Gauls were no more savages than the Germans; the Romans found with these people arts hitherto unknown to them, and the barbarism only existed with the sworn calumniators of other nations.'[1]

Among the Gauls, in the north, the breeding of cattle was the principal occupation,[2] and the pastures of Belgic Gaul produced a race of excellent horses.[3] In the centre and in the south the richness of the soil was augmented by productive mines of gold, silver, copper, iron, and lead.[4] The country was, without doubt, intersected by carriage roads, since the Gauls possessed a great number of all sorts of waggons,[5] since there still remain traces of Celtic

---

[1] Le Mineur. Lyons, 1863.   [2] Strabo, p. 163; edit. Didot.
[3] De Bello Gallico, lib. iv. 2.   [4] Strabo, pp. 121, 155, 170.
[5] ' Carpenta Gallorum.' (Florus, i. 13.)—' Plurima Gallica (verba) valuerunt, ut reda petorritum.' (Quintilian, *De Institutione Oratoria*, lib. i. cap. v. 57.)—' Petorritum enim est non ex Græcia dimidiatum, sed totum transalpibus, nam est vox Gallica. Id scriptum est in libro

roads, and since Cæsar makes known the existence of bridges on the Aisne, the Rhine, the Loire, the Allier, and the Seine.

Their skill in agriculture appears to have astonished the Romans. While the latter were using a most primitive plough, Pliny writes of the Gauls: 'There has been invented, at a comparatively recent period, in that part of Gaul known as Rhætia (Gallia Togata), a plough with the addition of two small wheels, and known by the name of " plaumorati " (supposed to be derived from the Belgic *ploum*, a plough, and *rat* or *radt*, a wheel). The Gauls have invented a method of carrying their plough on small wheels. Their ploughshare, which is flat like a shovel, ploughs very well through the soil. A pair of oxen suffice. After sowing the seed, they harrow with a kind of iron hurdle with spikes or teeth, and which is dragged over the ground.' From the various notices of Gaulish agriculture given by ancient writers, we are led to believe that this people were the most skilled in tilling the soil of all the Western nations.

They were naturally agriculturists, and we may suppose that the institution of private property existed among them, because, on the one hand, all the citizens paid the tax, except the Druids, and, on the other, the latter were

M. Varronis quarto decimo *Rerum Divinarum;* quo in loco Varro, quum de petorrito dixisset, esse id verbum Gallicum dixit' (Aulus Gellius, xv. 30.)—'Petoritum et Gallicum vehiculum est, et nomen ejus dictum esse existimant a numero quatuor rotarum. *A*lii Osce, quod hic quoque *petora* quatuor vocent. *A*lii Græce sed αἰολικῶς dictum.' (Festus, voc. Petoritum, p. 206, edit. Müller.)—'Belgica esseda, Gallicana vehiculæ. Nam Belga civitas est Galliæ in qua hujusmodi vehiculi repertus est usus.' (Servius, Commentaries on the Georgics of Virgil, lib. iii. v. 204.)

judges of questions of boundaries. They were not un-acquainted with certain manufactures. In some countries they fabricated serges, which were in great repute, and cloths or felts; in others they worked the mines with skill, and employed themselves in the fabrication of metals. The Bituriges worked in iron, and were acquainted with the art of tinning. The artificers of Alesia plated copper with silver leaf to ornament horses' bits and trappings.[1]

They were also excellent workers in gold, of which they made bracelets, leg-rings, collars, and even breast-plates.[2]

In the time of Cæsar, the greater part of the peoples of Gaul were armed with long iron swords, two-edged (σπάθη), sheathed in scabbards similarly of iron, suspended to the side by chains. These swords were generally made to strike with the edge rather than to stab. The Gauls had also spears, the iron of which, very long and very broad, presented sometimes an undulated form (*materis, σαύνιον*). Their helmets were of metal, more or less precious, ornamented with the horns of animals, and with a crest representing some figures of birds or savage beasts. They carried a great buckler, a breast-plate of iron or bronze, or a coat of mail—the latter a Gaulish invention.

Diodorus Siculus[3] says that the Gauls had iron coats of mail. He adds: 'Instead of glaive (ξίφος), they have long swords (σπάθη), which they carry suspended to their right side by chains of iron or bronze. Some bind their

---

[1] Pliny, xxxiv. 17. Deinde et argentum incoquere simili modo cœpere, equorum maxime ornamentis, jumentorumque ac jugorum, in *A*lesia oppido.

[2] Diodorus Siculus, v. 27.   [3] Ibid. v. 30.

tunics with gilt or silvered girdles. They have spears
(λόγχη or λογχίς) having an iron blade a cubit long, and
sometimes more.   The breadth is almost two palms, for
the blade of these *saunions* (the Gaulish dart) is not less
than that of our glaive, and it is a little longer.   Of these
blades, some are forged straight, others present undulated
curves, so that they not only cut in striking, but in addition they tear the wound when they are drawn out.'[1]

Polybius informs us, that in the battle in which the
Gauls were defeated by the Consul Æmilius, when the
Romans used swords of bronze, those of the Gauls were
long, but so badly tempered that they bent when the
Gallic warriors struck a hard blow against the Roman
armour.   It would appear from this observation that the
Gaulish swords were made of iron, but that the art of
tempering them was unknown.

The priests of the Celts were the learned men and
philosophers of these people.   Besides their other important functions, and attending to their mysterious rites,
they alone afforded instruction in religious matters and all
other kinds of knowledge, the art of war excepted.   There
can scarcely be any doubt as to their possessing an extensive
knowledge of metallurgy, particularly with regard to iron,
the more valuable secrets being closely retained by these
priests. 'The Druids,' says M. Eckstein, 'forged a double
kind of sword and lance, the religious arms—the glaive of
honour, and the deadly weapons—the sword and lance of
combat.'[2]

As before mentioned, the Romans were not an eques-

---

[1] Vié de Cæsar, vol. ii. pp. 36, 39.
[2] *Eckstein.*   *Anciennes Poésies des Gaëls*, p. 152.

trian people, and for a long period had but few cavalry; indeed, not until Numidia and Gaul had become Roman provinces had they a respectable cavalry force. The Gauls were fond of the horse, and were good horsemen; their cavalry was much superior to their infantry, being composed of nobles, followed by their own people.[1] The cavalry was styled 'Trimarkisiæ' *(tri-march-kesec,* Celtic for three horses combined), in consequence of each soldier having the attendance of three horses. Pausanias, mentioning that every Celtic horseman was followed to battle by two attendants, says that this custom was in their language called 'Trimarkisian,' because the name of a horse among them is *markan.*[2] *Mark* or *march* is also a horse, *tri* is three. and *trimarkwys* is literally three horsemen in the ancient British and present Welsh.

The same writer, speaking of those who had reached Delphi, says that 'each of the horsemen had with him two esquires, who were also mounted on horses; when the cavalry was engaged in combat, these esquires were posted behind the main body of the army, either to replace the horsemen who were killed, or to give their horse to their companion if he lost his own, or to take his place in case he were wounded, while the other esquire carried him out of the battle.'

These equestrian habits of the Celtic Gauls are confirmed by a large number of proofs, historic and archæo logic. Not only does the Celtic name for the horse, 'march,' form the root of a long list of districts, towns, nations, and individuals, but also all the terms employed in cavalry or the *manége,* and even those hippiatric

[1] Strabo, iv. p. 163.　　　　[2] Phocid. x. 545.

expressions employed by the Greeks and Romans, were Celtic.[1]

All the Gaulish medals bear the figure of a horse, often accompanied by that of a boar. The sacrifice of a white horse was the greatest oblation that could be offered to the gods of these people; and the many statuettes of horses found in various places would tend to prove that a mysterious importance was attached to this noble creature. The Gauls, as before noticed, buried their chiefs and warriors with their weapons, their dogs, and their war-horses, for on their steeds they were to ride when they entered the abode of everlasting felicity.

The numerous cairns, or Celtic tombs, which abound in Brittany and Franche-Comté, show that this custom widely prevailed.

'The Gauls,' Cæsar writes, 'were so fond of their horses, and valued them so highly, that the German allies could not procure them for their service.'[2]

[1] *Megnin.* Op. cit. p. 14. As illustrative of this fact, we may give the following examples. Names of countries: *Denmark;* of people: *Marsi, Marcomanni;* names of places: *Penmark, Markhausen, Kœnigsmark, Mark of Brandenburg, Marca, Marca Trevisana, Kurmark, Mittlemark, Neumark, Altmark, Vormark, Ukermark,* and *Stiermark.* Marches, or frontiers, such as the Welsh and Scotch marches, the *Marche de Limousin* in France, and *Marchfield* in Austria; the places where the standards of the northern people were arrested, and represented by a horse. The term also signifies a market for horses, and the German *jahr-marckt,* or annual fair, always denoted one where horses were sold. Individuals: French *Marquis,* German *Markgraf.* Cavalry terms: *Polemark,* commander of a body of troops; *maréchal* (qui equorum gerit curam, qui proest stabulo); *merchant, marchand,* horse-dealer. For the Celtic etymology of terms used by the hippiatrists, *see* Recueil de Médecine Vétérinaire, 1858.

[2] *Megnin.* At the great battle before Alesia, the Roman cavalry was composed exclusively of German allies.—*Cæsar,* Commentaries.

The horses of Trèves and the country of the Soutiates (Bigorre) were the most renowned in the time of Cæsar, and those also of Franche-Comté bore a high reputation. 'Under the Romans,' says Clerc,[1] 'Sequani, the most fertile part of Gaul, according to Cæsar, had large fine towns noted for their commerce and wealth. In the country, although covered in great part by forests, there were, chiefly along the rivers' banks and public roads, villages, hamlets, and cottages, the robust and industrious inhabitants of which grew barley, reared flocks of sheep and droves of pigs, and especially fine horses, the best in Gaul. . . . . In the midst of the Roman customs and institutions, I do not know if, in Sequani, anything more national predominated than the ever-ruling passion of the people for horses, which figure on all their medals, and their horsemanship, from which the town of Mandeure (now a little village on the Doubs near Besançon; it was destroyed in the tenth century by the Hungarians) took its name, "Epomanduodurum," signifying the town where they managed horses well, Epona being the Celtic goddess of horses.'

It is, then, very evident that when the Romans came in contact with the Gauls, the horse was largely and widely employed in that country for riding and draught purposes. The 'petoritum' (Celtic *petoar*, four, and *rot*, wheel) was evidently a native vehicle, but the 'esseda' was the chariot most used in warfare, immense numbers always figuring in every Celtic army; and these armies dragged after them a multitude of waggons and

[1] Essai sur l'Histoire de la Franche-Comté.

other conveyances, even in the less important expeditions.[1]

From the extensive employment of chariots, roads must necessarily have existed in Gaul,—and, as we have seen, this was the case; only these roads, instead of being like those of the Romans, which were substantial works of masonry, were formed, it would appear, by the never-ceasing passage of carriages over the same track. The traces of these, however, only exist in rocky situations, which have preserved the imprint of wheels, and even of *horses' feet.* These impressions are sometimes so deep, in consequence of the long and oft-repeated action of the carriages during centuries, that, in certain places, the road is literally channeled or trenched; and on the stony sides of these passes, marks can be plainly seen which have been caused by the axletrees scraping them in passing through. These marks testify to the height of the nave, and consequently of the wheels.

MM. Delacroix and Castan, with Captain Bial of the French artillery, have lately discovered good specimens of these Celtic roads in the Jura, at Trochatay, Moutier-Granval, and Alaise. 'At the latter place the road is most characteristic, where it leads from the valley to the summit of a hill on which stood this old Gallic city. How can the extraordinary effects produced on the living rock by horses' feet be explained, if we do not admit that from remote antiquity iron shoes were in use?' So asks M. Megnin, and apparently with good cause. We have before remarked, that not the faintest trace of wear which could be attributed to horses' feet has been found on any of the Roman roads,

[1] *Cæsar.* De Bello Gallica, viii. 14.

and probably for the simple reason that horn is softer than stone. Never, M. Megnin adds, could the horn of the hoofs alone of ever so many generations of horses, passing and repassing, produce any notable furrowing on the rock, and particularly as seen in the imprints at the staircase-like *Languetine* of Alaise. ' To wear the rock in such a manner iron horse-shoes were necessary.'[1] In a country so rocky and mountainous as Brittany or Franche-Comté, the employment of the horse on anything like a large scale was simply impossible without efficient shoeing, and this attrition of the living rock goes a long way to prove that the Celtic Gauls of this region armed the hoofs of their horses with metal. But the exertions of French archæologists have afforded us additional and incontestable evidence of this fact in their researches in the Celtic graves, particularly those which abound in the vicinity of Alesia.[2] This large hill, covered with the ruins of the

[1] *Megnin.* Op. cit. p. 17. *Bial.* Chemins, Habitations, et Oppidum de la *G*aule au Temps de Cæsar. Paris, 1864.

[2] *A*lesia, now perhaps Alise-Sainte-Reine, in the department Côte-d'-Or, was the capital of the Mandubii, a *G*allic people, who dwelt in what is now Burgundy. Much discussion has lately taken place as to which *A*lesia—for there are several—Cæsar refers. Smith (Classical Dictionary) gives it as an ancient town of the Mandubii in Gallia Lugdunensis, said to have been founded by Hercules, and situated on a high hill (now *Auxois*), which was washed by the two rivers Lutosa (*Oze*) and Osera (*Ozerain*). It was an important fortress, the siege and capture of which was, undoubtedly, the greatest military achievement of Cæsar. All Gaul had risen against the Romans, even the Ædui, the old allies of the oppressors ; but Cæsar conquered them under Vercingetorix, and besieged them in Alesia. No less than 80,000 men were shut up in this town or fort ; while Cæsar, with 60,000 troops, lay before it. The Roman General immediately erected a line of contravallation, extending for four leagues, in order to reduce the place by famine, since its situation on a hill, 1500 feet high, and on all

Celtic city, amid which have grown the secular pines, displays on its surface, on the banks of the Lison, and on the neighbouring plateau of Amançay, so large a collection of tombs (more than twenty thousand have been counted), that only an awful slaughter, like that which decided the fate of Gaul, can explain their presence in such numbers. All the graves which the Archæological Society of Besançon has carefully explored since 1858, contain the skeletons of Gaulish warriors (the Romans burned their dead) in variable numbers, who had been buried with their horses, and sometimes even with their chariots, of which no more remain than the iron-work.

M. Castan, who has examined many of them, gives the following account of the contents of one of these resting-places. Above two skeletons (surrounding them were

sides abrupt, between the rivers Ope and Operain, rendered an attack impossible. Vercingetorix, after making several furious but unsuccessful sallies, called all the Gauls to arms, and in a short time 250,000 men appeared before the place. Cæsar had, in the mean time, completed his line of circumvallation, protecting himself against any attack from without by a breast-work, a ditch with palisadoes, and several rows of pit-falls, to keep off the dauntless cavalry. These defences enabled him to repel the desperate attack of 330,000 Gauls against the 60,000 Romans attacked in front and rear. The Gauls were unable to force his lines at any point, and Vercingetorix, reduced to extremity by hunger, was compelled to surrender, without having carried into execution his design of murdering all the people in the town who were unfit for battle. But the whole tribe of the Mandubii, which had been expelled from the city by the Gauls, and were not allowed by the Romans to pass into the open country, died of famine between the two camps.

It must not be forgotten that some time afterwards it attained a flourishing condition, but was finally destroyed in 864, by the Normans.

twelve more), one of which was furnished with a short
iron sword (figure 7) and bronze scab-
bard, and which were probably the remains of the chariot driver and the
warrior, the principal iron-work of an
' essedum ' was found. This consisted
of eight cylindrical iron boxes with
their nails yet adhering, and which had
served as mountings to the ends of the
axletrees ; four iron hoops almost entire,
one of which was found in a perpendicular position in the ground. From
the traces of wood yet remaining on
their entire inner surface, there is reason
to believe that they were fixed on the
massive wooden wheel the ancients called
a *tympanum*, from its resemblance to a
drum-head. The imprints of wheels on
the Celtic roads corresponded exactly
with the appearance presented by the
débris of the chariots exhumed from
these tumuli. Taking the maximum of
the diameter of the wheels, this was supposed to be about 37 inches, minim. 31
inches for the wide wooden ones; the
thickness of the felloes was from 1 to $1\frac{1}{2}$ inches. These
remains of the car showed workmanship not coarse and
heavy, as we might suppose, but fine, light, and very
advanced. Most important, however, was the discovery,
beside the relics of a horse, of two pieces of a *bronze*

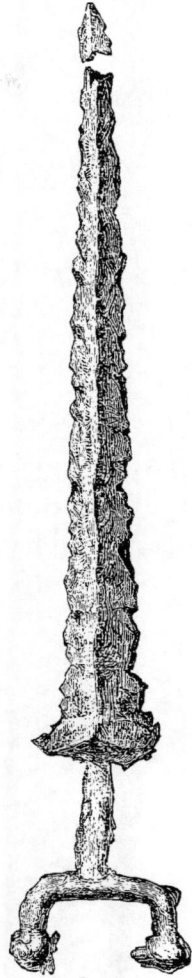

fig 7

horse-shoe which had been worn through at the toe

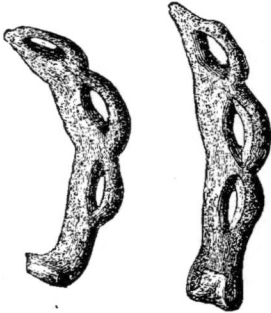

fig. 8

(fig. 8). M. Megnin, a competent judge, and from whose description I have freely translated, saw these fragments at the Besançon Archæological Museum.

Many other tombs have furnished, with the *débris* of arms, cuirasses, girdles, and collars of boars' teeth, various articles similar to the preceding, and among them the characteristic 'kelt' (fig. 9), together with iron nails with a flat head (*clefi de violon*), which had served to attach horseshoes, as in fig. 10, of the same origin, and in which three similar nails are yet fixed.

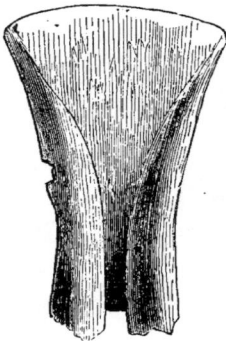

fig. 9

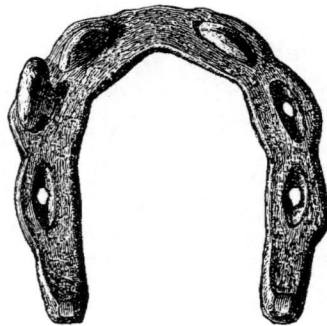

fig. 10

But the most curious discovery made in the tumuli of Alesia was that of a complete Celtic forge, which M. Castan, who presided at the exhumation, thus describes: ' The heights of Alesia terminate towards the north in three

promontories, which are parallel and overhang the Lison.
One of these promontories, situated in the central axis of
the heights, is covered with *tumuli* and ruins. This place
is called the Châteleys, and is an immense tongue of land,
which rests on a gigantic perpendicular basement, 164
yards elevation. On the margin of this region, at a
place called the *Champs-Mottets*, are seen three Celtic
tumuli built of pebbles, and about 33 to 40 feet in
length. Two of these were opened simultaneously, and
were found completely empty. The third contained a
certain number of thick and short bones, which the
osteologists have pronounced to be the remains of a bear
of the largest species. In the same collection was found
the half of a cloven foot belonging to a stag or buck.
These remains of what had no doubt been sacrifices, no
less than the vicinity of the place designated *Ban-du-Prêtre*
(priest's ban), were, in our opinion, indications that we
were touching on sacred soil. Pursuing our exploration, we
reached the extreme point of the promontory of Châteleys,
which was occupied by one of those heaps of stones the
English archæologists term *cairns*. The traditions of
buried treasure, which had always haunted this mound,
had induced a farmer in the neighbourhood to open it.
Quickly deceived in his expectations (he had only taken
away, we were told, the foot of a bronze pot), this gold-
hunter abandoned the spot, leaving the mound pierced
with a large hole at its summit. This opening, which had
been made about sixty years before, and about the origin
of which nearly every one had forgotten, caused the ruin
of the Châteleys to be looked upon as the base of a tower

or circular habitation. In its primitive condition, the cairn or hillock of Châteleys had the figure of a cone with an oval base, and was 98 feet in length, and about 66 feet in width. The neck of land which served for its foundation was naturally in the form of an amphitheatre; and the covering of stones, formed of large pieces, contained absolutely nothing, and appeared to have been constructed solely with a view to protect the bed of *débris* covering the floor of the interior, against the effects of time and the cupidity of mankind. All around the stone which formed the altar, were spread long tracks of cinders mixed with charcoal, fragments of vases, and the calcined bones of men and horses. To one side of these extinguished fires, lay scattered on the ground the maxillary bones of pigs and the skeleton of a bear. In the middle of the hearth, which occupied the north side, were found successively a little triangular file, $2\frac{1}{2}$ inches in length (fig. 11); the fragment of a thick flat file, nearly

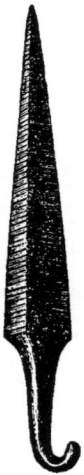

fig 11

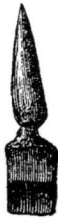

fig 12

an inch in width; a small chisel $1\frac{1}{4}$ inch long, intended to be fixed in a wooden handle (fig. 12); three iron cinders or *scoriæ;* two morsels of bronze castings about $\frac{1}{3}$ inch thick, one of which was ornamented with round points, executed with the graving tool; a large iron hammer weighing 5 pounds, and still retaining six iron wedges which had been used to fix the handle (fig. 13). Not far from this hammer-head, under the heap of cinders that extended to the

north-west, lay an iron buckle, composed of two rings
tied together by a flap, through which passed a tongue
of metal (fig. 14). Then came a fragment of a horse-
shoe (fig. 15), furnished with a flat oblong-headed nail
(fig. 16); afterwards the blade of an iron knife which
had lost its point, and was yet 5 inches long (fig. 17).

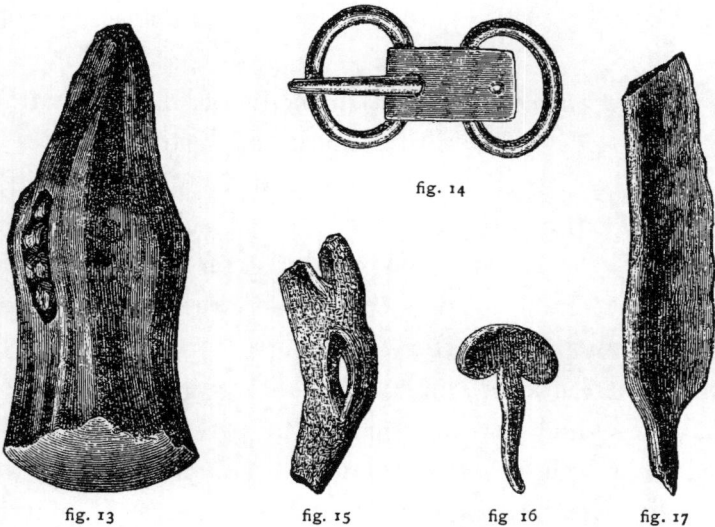

fig. 13   fig. 15   fig 16   fig. 17

fig. 14

The numerous bits of pottery collected from among the
cinders and the charcoal were of grey clay full of silice-
ous particles, but better tempered and more solid than
Celtic pottery in general. Some fragments had acquired,
from prolonged baking, the hardness of stoneware;
others, more friable, were covered with a black varnish
and very salient mouldings. The vases to which these
belonged appeared to have been broken, and their pieces
scattered on the ground designedly, for the scraps
gathered over a wide surface, and which have been put

together, form the neck of a jar (fig. 18). From all this it will be seen that the cairn of Châteleys was not an ordinary tomb. I do not hesitate to assert that it was more than a tomb. This forge-hammer; these imple-ments for working in

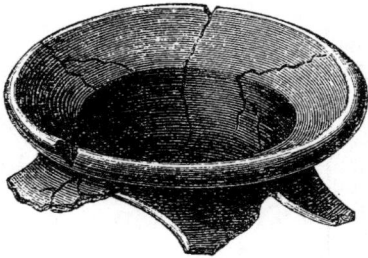

fig 18

iron; these horses and pigs, emblems of Gaulish nation-ality, lying *pêle-mêle* on the sacrificial hearth, beside an altar built by nature—all this composed a page of antique symbolism curious to decipher. The Druidical traditions of Ireland tell us that each of the great regions of the Gallo-Cimbric race had a centre, a sacred rallying-place, to which all parts of the confederate territory resorted.[1] In this centre burned, on an altar of rough stones, a per-petual fire, which was designated the parent flame. The guarding of this sanctuary, and the maintenance of the sacred fire, were entrusted to a school or college of pontiff-artists, commanded or directed by a smith. This Druidi-cal college combined with the exercise of the pontificate, the teaching of mysteries and the industrial arts. ' It forged two kinds of swords and lances:—religious arms—the glaive of honour and death-dealing weapons—the sword and lance for fight.' In this way is the mystery which shrouded the promontory of Alesia cleared up. Instead of being a hill devoted to graves, we have discovered the sanctuary of Alesia, the oppidum which Diodorus termed the primitive metropolis of the Celts. Nothing is wanting to complete

[1] *Henri Martin.* Histoire de France, vol. i. p. 71.

the picture; neither the altar, which the hand of man has not fashioned, nor the insignia of the pontiff-blacksmith, nor the buckle of his magical leather apron, nor yet the sacrificing knife, or the bones of boars, horses, and bears mingled with the remains of human victims consumed by the flames. More able men than ourselves had fanned these embers eighteen centuries ago, and from them had attempted to wring out lamentable secrets. They carry us back to distant ages, and show us the chiefs of Gaul deliberating around this place of worship, and the Druids, the ovates, and the bards seeking to gain, by sacrifices and supplications, the countenance of the tutelary genii of their nation; then, when all hope has disappeared, when the fates have pronounced the fatal decree, the worshipping priests have broken the sacred instruments, and have covered over their holy place to conceal it from the profanation of their vanquishers.'[1]

The publication of this discovery gave rise to much discussion. Col. Coinard denied the accuracy of the conclusions arrived at by the Besançon archæologists, and clung to the written history of the Greeks and Romans. M. Quicherat, however, replied to his attacks in a very direct manner. 'M. de Coinard exults because we admit that the Gaulish horses were shod; he overwhelms us with citations to prove that shoeing was not practised, neither in the Roman cavalry nor yet in that of Mithridates, when we speak of the cavalry of Gaul. Horseshoes are discovered with Gaulish pottery; in two of the tumuli of Alesia they are embedded in the floor of the graves, in the midst of cinders, *under a thick pavement.*

[1] *Castan.* Les Tombelles Celtiques. Besançon, 1858. *Megnin.*

M. Castan has mentioned this discovery in his reports on the tombs of Alesia. *I was present, and I can certify that there was a well-alloyed bed (gisement).* The authority of the compiler Beckmann, quoted by M. de Coinard, cannot prevail against a fact of which Beckmann was ignorant, and of which M. de Coinard cannot speak.'[1]

M. Troyon, the celebrated Swiss archæologist, in noticing these discoveries, and the dispute as to which of the Alesias Cæsar had to contend with, remarks of this one : 'This is not the place to enter into the discussion raised as to whether this Alesia is the place of which Cæsar speaks. Whatever may be the opinion of *savans* on the subject, it cannot be doubted that the majority of the objects discovered in these later years characterize the first age of iron. It is evident that this locality has been the seat of a Gaulish establishment of great importance. The numerous tumuli of Alesia no doubt cover the remains of diverse generations interred in the age of bronze, and during the Roman period. However this may be, the intermediate epoch is largely represented; the majority of the specimens collected belong to the space between these two periods, and give rise to important relations with the Helvetic antiquities.'[2]

Lest it be supposed that this haunt of Druidism was only destroyed in A.D. 864, it may be useful to recollect, that the Druids were banished from Gaul by Tiberius and Claudius in the first half of the first century of our era.

This holy blacksmith, the pontiff of the Druids, will be alluded to hereafter, when we come to speak of the

[1] Moniteur de l'Armée, *A*pril 16, 1864.
[2] Habitations Lacustres, p. 334.

discoveries of horse-shoes in Britain; in the mean time we must not forget to mention, that these researches and speculations on the treasures found in the tumuli surrounding the ruins of the ancient city of Alesia, are supplemented by similar discoveries in the neighbourhood, of articles which may be referred to the same period.

During the war in Gaul, Cæsar had often to encounter the brave and numerous cavalry of Vercingetorix, the Gaulish general. Before the blockade of Alesia, a severe cavalry engagement took place on the Vingeanne, near Longeau, which resulted in the defeat of the Gaulish horse. The Emperor Napoleon thus alludes to the historical proofs of this event:—'The field of battle of the Vingeanne, which M. H. Defay, of Langres, first pointed out, answers perfectly to all the requirements of the Latin narrative, and moreover, material proofs exist which are undeniable evidences of the struggle. We allude to the tumuli which are found, some at Prauthoy, others on the banks of the Vingeanne, at Dardenay, and Cusey, and those which, at Pressant, Rivières-les-Fosses, Chamberceau, and Vesores, mark, as it were, the line of retreat of the Gaulish army, to a distance of twelve kilomètres. Two of these tumuli are situated near each other, between Prauthoy and Montsaugeon. There is one near Dardenay, three to the west of Cusey, one at Rivières-les-Fosses, another at Chamberceau. We will not mention those which have been destroyed by agriculture, but which are still remembered by the inhabitants. Researches lately made in these tumuli have brought to light skeletons, many of which had bronze bracelets round the arms and legs, calcined bones of men and horses, thirty-six bracelets, severa iron circles which were worn round the neck, iron rings, fibulæ, fragments of metal plates, pieces of Celtic pottery, an iron sword, &c. It is a fact worthy of remark, that the objects found in the tumuli at Rivières-les-Fosses and Chamberceau bear so close a resemblance to those of the tumuli on the banks of the Vingeanne, that we might think they had come from the hand of the same workman. Hence there can be no doubt that all these tumuli refer to one and the same incident of war.

'We must add that the agricultural labourers of Montsaugeon, Isomes, and Cusey have found during many years, when they make trenches for drainage, *horse-shoes* buried a foot or two deep under the soil. In 1860, at the dredging of the Vingeanne, hundreds of horse-shoes, the inhabitants say, of excellent metal, were extracted from the gravel of the river, at a depth of two or three feet. They are generally small, and bear a groove all round, in which the heads of the nails were lodged. A great number of these horse-shoes have preserved their nails, which are flat, have a head in the form of a T, and still have their rivet—that is, the point which is folded back over the hoof (the *clench*)—which proves that they are not shoes that have been lost, but shoes of dead horses, the hoofs of which have rotted away in the soil or in the gravel. Thirty-two of these horse-shoes have been collected. One of them is stamped in the middle of the curve with a mark, sometimes found on Celtic objects, and which has a certain analogy with the stamp on a plate of copper found in one of the tumuli of Montsaugeon. When we consider that the action between the

Roman and Gaulish armies was merely a cavalry battle, in which were engaged from 20,000 to 25,000 horses, the facts just stated cannot but appear interesting, although they may possibly belong to a battle of a later date.'[1]

I have not been able to find any more detailed men tion of these grooved shoes than in this brief notice, and it would be important to ascertain if the groove be really continuous in any, or all of them. If the fact be as is stated, then they probably belonged to the horses of the German cavalry which we know Cæsar largely employed to subdue the Gauls. These German shoes we will speak of hereafter. A very careful inspection of the Vingeanne shoes would be most interesting in various ways.

According to M. Mathieu,[2] in the neighbourhood of Alesia, and in the valley of Brenne, the ground can scarcely be dug to the depth of 3 to 6 feet without discovering shoes of small dimensions, and the cover so wide that only a small triangular space is left for the frog. The excavations for the railway between Paris and Lyons, in the valleys of Armançon and Brenne, have exposed thousands even in the brief space separating Ancy-le-Franc from Alesia ; while some have been found below the Roman road leading from Alesia to Agedincum (Sens). This road is supposed to belong to the Augustan era. M. Mathieu considers them to be of two sizes—a very small one, and a larger ; a circumstance which may be accounted for by supposing that the German auxiliaries drew their supply of horses from different parts of Germany. The

---

[1] Vie de Cæsar, vol. ii. p. 362.
[2] Recueil de Med. Vétérinaire. November, 1868.

form of the nail-head in the Vingeanne specimens is that always found with the Gaulish or Celtic shoe.

The museum of Besançon is very rich in specimens of Celtic horse-shoes, as well as those of the Gallo-Roman and middle-age, according to M. Megnin. This may be explained by the importance which always attached to Besançon ; at one time it ranked as the chief town of the Celtic Mandubians (*Man Dubis*=Man of Doubs) ; under the Romans it was the capital of Sequanian Gaul, Visonti uni ; later, it was the principal city of the kingdom of Burgundy ; as Bisanz, it was a part of the German empire ; then it became the metropolis of the Bisontine archbishops, potent individuals in the middle ages ; and lastly, it was the capital of Spanish Franche-Comté

Its sub-soil offers traces of the industry and the arts of each of these epochs. More than a hundred pieces of antique farriery figure in its museum. Twenty of these are from the tumuli of Alesia ; others have been found at variable depths in the sub-soil of the town in digging sewers, or excavating foundations for houses, and often side by side with mutilated marble statues, indicating that they belong to the Gallo-Roman period. Other shoes, apparently belonging to this epoch, have been met with by M. Delacroix in the clayey soil of Beaune and Candar; and some have been found at Montbéliard and Mandeure. At Besançon, but at a less considerable depth, shoes of better workmanship are encountered, but they are much heavier and clumsier than the Gallic and Gallo-Roman shoes, and may be allotted to the middle ages.

M. Delacroix reports in 1863: 'Excavations are

actually in progress in many streets of the town, for the formation of new sewers.   The depth of the cuttings has not been so great as could, in the interests of archæology, have been desired; they have generally penetrated only to the 4th-century layer : that is, to the same level as the *débris* of the first Gallo-Roman villa destroyed by the Emperor Constantine, the veritable barbarian of those days, whose wish it was to raze systematically all the dwellings on the left bank of the Rhine to a distance of forty leagues, and to convert Sequania into a desert. This 4th-century ground is characterized by a layer of *débris* which rests on the admirable paved road so well preserved, and immediately beneath the middle-age strata. From the day of commencing this work, the labourers have been asked to collect carefully all rusty fragments denoting the presence of iron, and to note the level.   As since the Gallo-Roman times, and even the Celtic period, the Grand-Rue of Besançon and the Rue Battant have not ceased to be the lines of thoroughfare, the strata, deposited, it might be said, century after century, have each in their turn rendered testimony to the manner in which animals have been shod during, perhaps, eighteen centuries.   Indeed, in the Rue Battant, the roadway has been cut down to the living rock, which is here found grooved by ruts, and lies at least two mètres[1] beneath the great layer of Roman tiles, cinders, and antique remains by which we at Besançon recognize the ruins of the 4th century.   But everywhere is found, with differences in details only, the horse-shoe as at present known. . . . . . The fol lowing are the most notable characteristics of these shoes :

[1] The mètre is equivalent to nearly 39⅜ inches.

three holes on each side, each hole having a kind of groove, twice as long as it is wide, to receive the similarly elongated head of the nail, and to protect it from wear, at the same time that it permits it to project considerably; the outline of the shoe is wavy (*festonné*), and its contour marks the situation of every hole; each branch terminates in a calkin (*éponge à crampon*), the whole of the projecting nail-heads and the calkins forming a level bearing surface. The wavy outline seems to disappear quickly after the period of the destruction of ancient Besançon; five to six specimens, all having the holes counter-sunk in an oblong manner, resemble more the even margin of modern shoes. One of these pieces, the bed of which was not so accurately determined, terminates by two rapidly tapering branches, on the under surface of which the calkin was represented by a protuberance a little way from the points of the heels. Two very small shoes were pierced by only four holes each. These may have belonged to asses or mules. The metal is extremely ductile, like that of all antique horse-shoes, and very white. Some nails remaining in the holes had been curved round in the hoof, so as to form more than a circle. . .   . The number of shoes collected has been one hundred; many escaped our possession, and yet it was in an excavation of 4 feet wide that so large a quantity of these objects was found. From this numerous collection, an important fact relating to the ancient breed of horses in Sequania was immediately recognized. It is, that towards the 4th century, the size of the shoes indicate excessively small feet; not a shoe exceeds a total width of 4¾ inches. These belonged to the fine breeds of which the various provinces of France boasted in all ages. A superior officer of cavalry, who is much more occupied with the varieties of horses than antiquities, exclaimed, on seeing this lot of shoes, *that they had all belonged to Arab horses.* Their width varies from $3\frac{1}{3}$ to $4\frac{1}{3}$ inches; their length from toe to heels 4 to $4\frac{3}{4}$ inches.' [1]

The Celtic or Gallic, and the Gallo-Roman shoes, as we may then fairly designate them, possess a remarkable identity, and their special features it may be here convenient to notice a little more closely than in the report furnished by M. Delacroix of the interesting and valuable collection made in Besançon, where shoeing appears to have been largely practised at a remote epoch. Their most noteworthy characters are four in number: 1. The general shape of the shoe with regard to size, weight, and width of cover; 2. The shape of the nail-holes; 3. The outer border; 4. The nails. In shape, the Celtic and Romano-Celtic shoes are extremely primitive. 1. Their form is irregular and deficient in outline; the majority of the specimens I have seen give one the idea that the Druid smiths and their immediate successors (if they were really the workmen) did not possess an anvil with a bick-horn, or beak, to fashion them to the proper shape. The width of their surface is irregular, but in no instance have I observed it to be anything like that noted in shoes of the middle ages; and their thickness is inconsiderable. The size varies, but is always small, and such as would suit diminutive round-footed horses, or little horses with long, mule-shaped hoofs. None of the shoes have toe or other clips,

[1] *Delacroix.* Mémoires de la Soc. d'Emulation du Doubs, 1863, p. 205-220.

so far as I am aware, to aid in retaining them on the feet. The great majority of them have calkins or catches at the extremities. 2. The nail-holes are certainly peculiar. They are six in number in all, save very exceptional, instances. For each hole there is a long and wide oval cavity, evidently intended to give partial lodgment to the head of the nail, and through the middle of this socket the opening is made. 3. The disproportionate size of these cavities, and perhaps the absence of a suitable anvil, has left these primitive defences with an irregular bulging or undulating outer margin, and not unfrequently the inner one also, like the undulated 'saunions' these people fought with. 4. The nails are also curious. The head is very large and flat, so that it must have projected much beyond the shoe, even when imbedded in the ovoid groove, and generally approaches the letter T in shape. Their appearance will be more particularly noticed when we speak of individual specimens of shoes.

The shoes of a later date, as will be seen hereafter, are larger, wider across their face, and thicker; they are also more regularly formed, and the holes are *square*, or 'counter-sunk;' their borders are very rarely, if ever, undulated; or they have a continuous groove running along their ground surface into which the nail-heads fit.

The Abbé Cochet[1] reports that, in 1844, a discovery was made which was all the more interesting because it appeared to carry with it a determined date. At Yèbleron, near Yvetot (not far from Rouen), a wooden bucket, mounted with an iron handle and hoops, was found, and inside it were three bronze chandeliers, one of which,

[1] Le Tombeau de Childeric I., p. 161.

borne by a goat, bore the stamp of antiquity; also the coulter of a plough, a hammer, a horse-shoe, and a spur —these latter were of iron. Founding an opinion on the style of the chandeliers, this group of objects was supposed to belong to the Gallo-Roman or Gallo-Frankish period. The shoe (fig. 19) has six nail-holes, and its border is

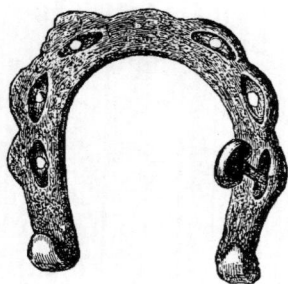
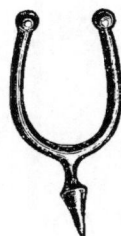

fig. 19   fig 20

markedly undulated; the nail-head is also of the Celtic pattern. The length of the shoe, according to the scale, is about $4\frac{1}{2}$ inches, and the width 3 inches. The spur is undoubtedly very antique (fig. 20).

M. Castan has seen the half of a horse-shoe, which had the sinuous border and the usual number of holes, as well as a calkin, extracted from a Gallo-Roman villa at Egli-series, in the Jura, on the same level from which a coin of Marcus Aurelius (A.D. 161) was gathered. This villa appears to have been destroyed in the second century. Many articles in bronze and iron accompanied it, and all were covered by a thick bed of rubbish, consisting chiefly of tiles and Roman pottery.

In 1842, M. de Widranges met with an iron horse-shoe in the ruins of a Gallo-Roman habitation, in Sauvoy

(Meuse), amongst a heap of tiles with the characteristic border of the period, pottery, cinders, and fuel (fig. 21).

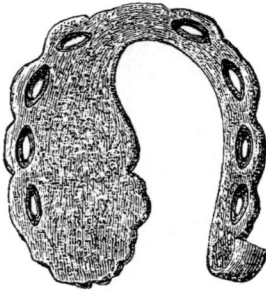

fig 21

This shoe had *eight* holes, the wavy margin, and one of its sides so greatly expanded as to cover one-half the sole. This was no doubt a pathological shoe, intended to cover and protect an injured part of the foot, and perhaps also to retain some healing application. Its length is 5¼ inches, and width 4 inches.

In 1848, a shoe identical with the primitive model was found beside a coin of Trajan, in the foundation of a new hospital at Tonnerre, by M. Dormois, a distinguished archæologist. And the Calvet museum contains a small, wide-covered shoe, with a triangular space between its branches. It was found in clearing away the theatre of Orange, in 1834, on a Roman pavement.

The remains of Celtic farriery have also been found in Switzerland. In the Canton Vaud, at Chavannes, is a mound named the hillock of Chatelard (*motte de Chatelard*), which M. Troyon, a learned Swiss antiquarian, believed to be a place for sacrifices, for on examining it he found nearly five hundred bones of animals. Among the iron articles discovered in this mound, there were spurs, bridle-bits, and horse-shoes. These last, five in number, are of small dimensions and very primitive workmanship. They have no calkins, and the holes, three on each side, have, as with the shoes of Alesia and elsewhere, distorted the sides of the metal. The nails are thicker in the stalks or bodies than those now in use, and have the high, flat head which for a long time would serve the purpose of a calkin (fig. 22).

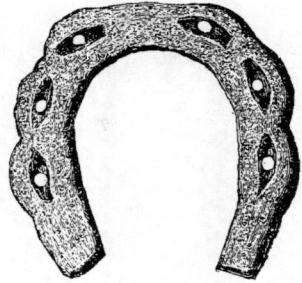

fig 22

The museum of Nantes contains nine shoes with wavy borders. Two of these were found in the river Erdre, near Nantes, in 1827, during the construction of the Orleans bridge ; the others have been extracted from the bed of the Vilaine, in the neighbourhood of Rennes, and from a tumulus near Pousanges.

The museum of Troyes, near Paris, possesses three shoes, two with undulated edges and six nail-holes. The third shoe is evidently more modern, and is very peculiar and fanciful in shape ; being a modification, or rather exaggeration, of our 'bar-shoe.' These shoes were found in cutting the canal, and were described by M. Thiollet at the French Archæological Congress assembled at Troyes in 1853 (fig. 23).

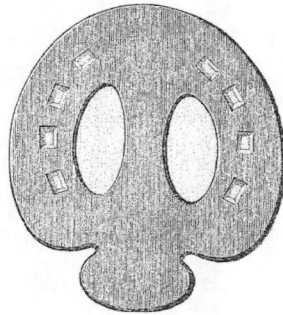

fig. 23

In the museum of Cluny, near Lyons, there is, says M. Megnin,[1] an undulated, very light, and very elegant shoe, which was found at Vassimont,

---

[1] *Megnin,* Op. cit. p. 26. To this veterinary surgeon's able but brief treatise, I am indebted for much of the foregoing description of the contents of several French museums.

at the chateau of the Counts of Champagne (fig. 24).   It
is catalogued as being of the
sixteenth century ; but this
is evidently an error ; it does
not belong to that, nor yet
to very many previous cen
turies.

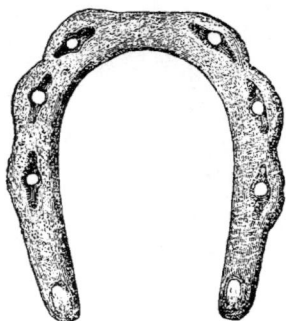

fig. 24

In a French antiquarian
publication,[1] it is mentioned
that when destroying a
Roman bridge to construct
the Canal de Bourgogne
'there was found in the joints of the stones forming the
body of the chaussée, a *horse-shoe.*' Unfortunately no
description is given.

The Abbé Cochet mentions a small shoe with six
nail-holes and uneven border, which was obtained from
the marshes of Dompierre-sur-la-Somme.   It resembled
that found at Chavannes by M. Troyon.   The collection
of M. Houbigant, at Nogent-les-Vierges, contains several
antique shoes, but the Abbé says nothing of their origin,
save that one of them, belonging to a mule (?), and with
six nail-holes, was fished up in the river Oise, in 1842,
not far from Creil, where the same antiquarian had fixed
the Roman station of Litanobriga.   The other shoes were
collected, to the number of one hundred and fifty, not far
from a Roman road at Nogent-les-Vierges.   They had a
fullering or groove around their circumference, and were
so small that it was supposed they were intended rather
for mules than horses.

[1] Mem. des *A*ntiq. de la Soc. de France, vol. xii. p. 47.

M. Traullé, an antiquarian of Abbeville, who died in 1828, stated that he had seen a large number of *mules'* shoes extracted from the battle-field of Saucourt, where Louis III. defeated the Normans in 881 or 882.[1]

M. J. Long, author of a memoir on the Roman antiquities of Vocontia, which appeared in the transactions of the Academie des Inscriptions et Belles Lettres, states :—
'I possess a horse-shoe slightly different from that now in use, and in perfect preservation. It was found in the neighbourhood of Monte-Chalençon, among cinders, with lachrymatories and burnt bones. Its preservation ought to be attributed to the cinders and animal charcoal. The branches of this shoe are very narrow ; the stamping of the nail-holes has produced bulgings. These stampings are elongated apertures ; those of modern shoes are square. The ancient shoe has no *ajusture*, or concave form, which facilitates support. The freshness of the stampings and the state of the toe, leads to the presumption that it has been little worn. It therefore appears that, contrary to the opinion of several authors, horse-shoeing was known to the ancients.' The remains accompanying this article were pronounced to be Gallo Roman.

At Prémeaux, arrondissement of Nuits, a quantity of horse-shoes were exhumed in the vicinity of a road of Roman construction by the pickaxe of a labourer. *Many of them were found buried beneath the strata of the road.* 'This circumstance is worthy of notice, because it has been asserted that the ancients were not in the habit of shoeing their horses. Found in such a bed, these shoes

[1] Le Tombeau de Childeric.

10 *

can belong to no other than the Roman, if not an earlier, period.'[1]

In the Liverpool Museum, two shoes belonging to the Rolfe collection, and said to have been found by M. Boucher de Perthes on the battle-field of Crécy, near Abbeville, in 1851, are of the Gaulish or Roman period in shape. I can scarcely believe that they belong to the age in which the famous battle was fought. All my researches lead me to think that this form of shoe was out of use even long before the tenth century. It must not be forgotten, that the district in which the famous battle was fought, has been the scene of conflicts from the earliest times.

The sub-curator of this museum remarks in his notes to me on these specimens, that they 'are remarkable from the nails used to secure them being oblong throughout the shank, and with oblong and narrow flat heads, as is evidenced by the socketed holes.' The size of the first (fig. 25) is $4\frac{1}{2}$ inches long by 4 inches wide; and the second is the same length, but only $3\frac{1}{2}$ inches wide (fig. 26).

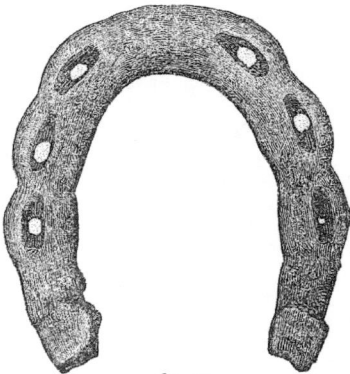 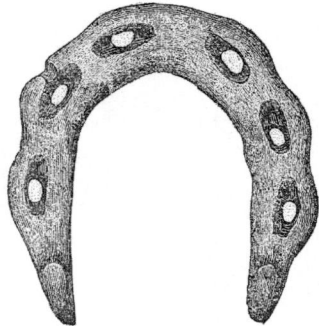

fig 25   fig. 26

[1] *Constitutionnel*, May 31, 1865.

If any other evidence was needed to prove that the ancient people of Gaul shod their horses, beyond that furnished by the discovery of these articles in situations, and accompanied by relics, which cannot leave a doubt as to the fact, it would be supplied in a most conclusive and satisfactory manner by the monument which has been, it may be said, re-discovered in the public museum of Avignon, by that most indefatigable and typical archæologist, Mr C. Roach Smith. This most interesting piece of sculpture was found at Vaison, in the department of Vaucluse, on the Ouvèse, a tributary of the Rhone ; a place retaining almost unchanged the ancient name, Vasio, and described by Pomponius Mela and Ptolemy as one of the wealthiest cities of Gallia Narbonensis. It was the capital of the Vocontii, and the vast quantities of antiquities which have at times been recovered from the ancient site, cover ing, as it did, a large extent of ground, bears witness to its opulence in ancient times. ' All we know of this monu ment is the meagre assertion that it was found at Vaison. The structure, to which the portions about to be described originally belonged, appears to have been of large dimen sions, erected probably upon a quadrilateral basement. The summit is wanting, and two of the sides ; but the two which remain are in fine preservation, and covered with sculptures in a good style of art. The inscription is lost, so that we have no clue whatever to the name or history of the persons to whom such a costly memorial was erected, except so far as the two principal subjects, in the central compartments, may be accepted as referring to the public offices he held, the usual object of such representations. One of those subjects is a travelling scene (plate 2). In a four-wheeled vehicle, drawn by two mules, are no less than four persons, exclusive of the driver. Two of these are seated, face to face, in the inside ; and two, back to back, on the roof. The passengers upon the top of the vehicle are all provided with hoods which fall down upon the back ; and the driver wears the Gaulish *braccæ* or trowsers. The centre figure of the upper group is seated in what resembles, in some degree, the body of the common chariot, or *biga*, while the personage in the rear is seated upon what seems to be a chest, perhaps containing luggage. He carries what appears to be a *securis*, or long-handled axe, which is, unluckily, broken ; but I think may be nevertheless recognized as an axe. The whole gives a striking and interesting picture of the equipment and arrangement of a travelling party in Gaul, not to be found, in all probability, elsewhere ; and it may doubtless be depended upon as a very faithful representation.' Mr Smith believes the carriage to be the *rheda* or *petorritum*, of which Cicero,[1] Ausonius,[2] Isidore,[3] Quintilian,[4] Juvenal, and Martial speak. He then adds : ' The custom of shoeing horses among the ancients has been much discussed *pro* and *con*. If it could remain an unsettled question after the repeated discovery of iron horseshoes themselves, among unquestionable Roman remains, the indications of the nails are so decidedly marked in the feet of the mules in the Vaison monument, as to leave no doubt that the artist intended to show that the mules were shod ; and we may conclude that the shoeing of horses as well as very many more inventions in the useful arts,

---

[1] Oratio pro Milone ; Philippica Secunda ; *A*ttico Epist.
[2] Epist. vii.   [3] Originum, l. XX., c. xii.   [4] Instit. i. 5.

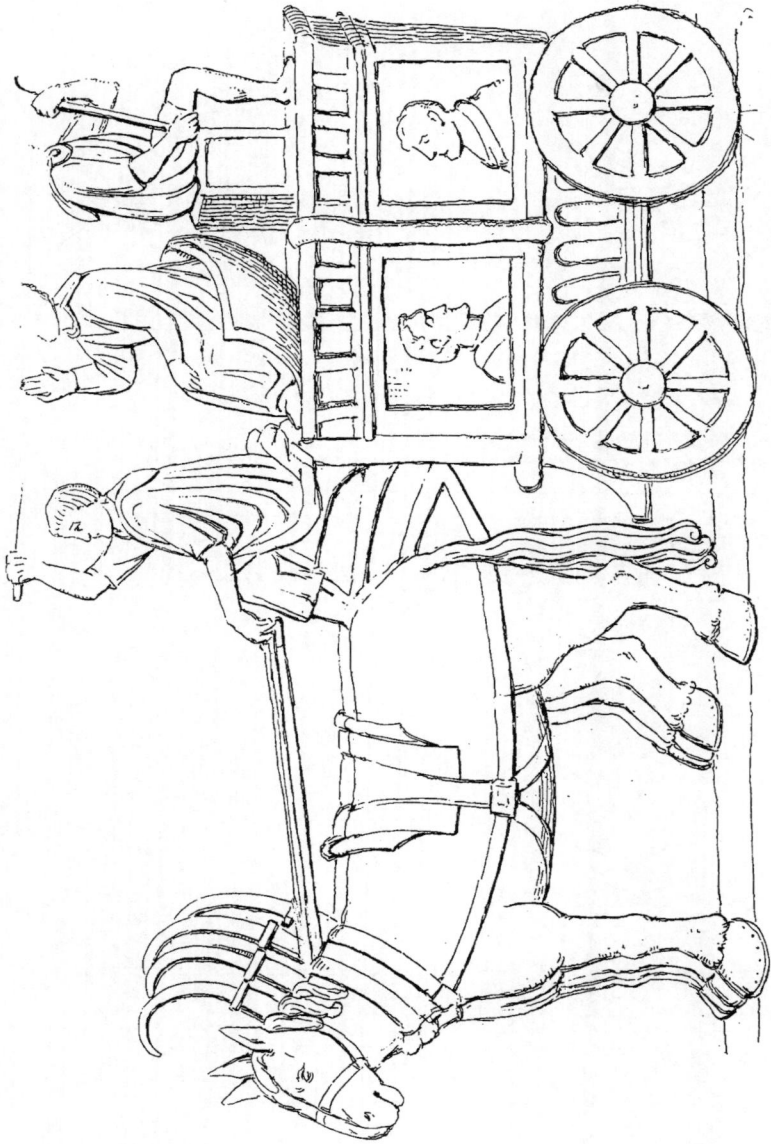

P.S. del.   J.G.W. Sc.

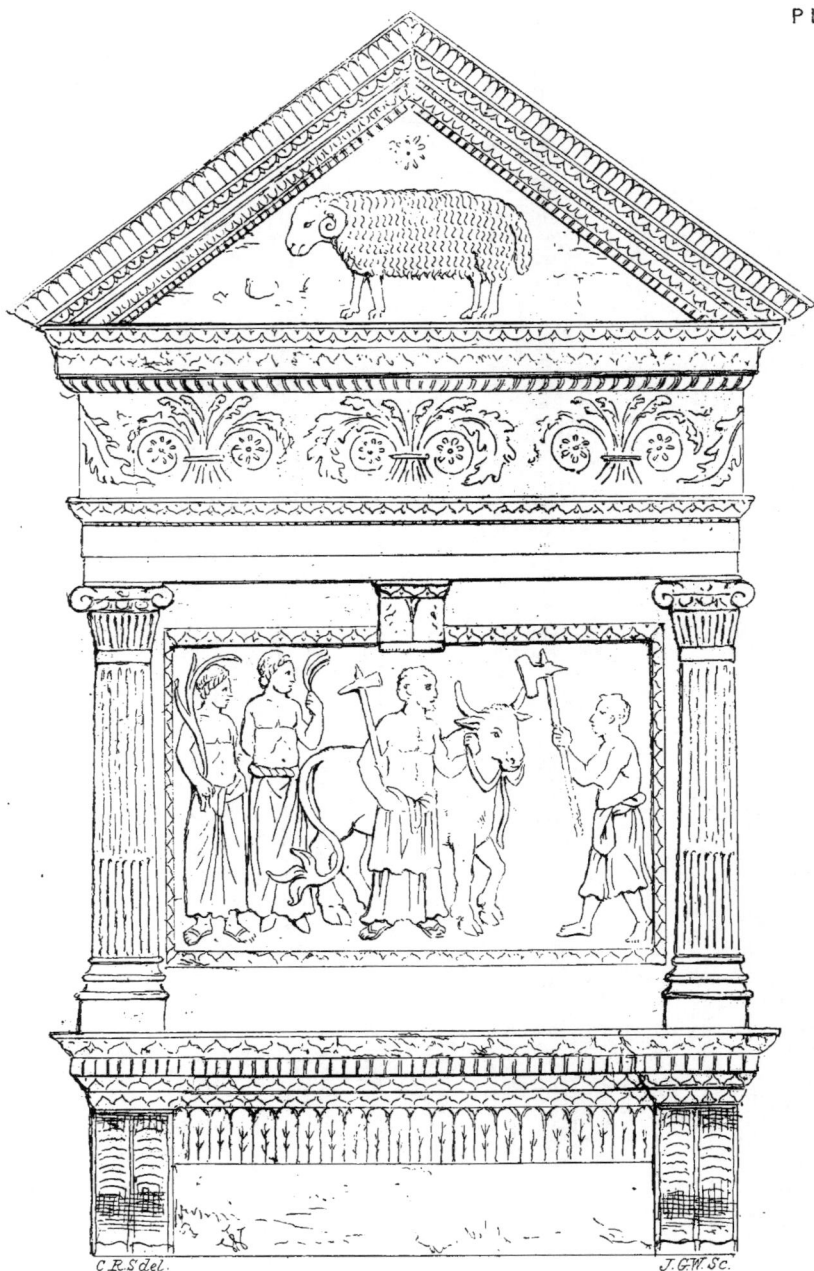

C.R.S del.　　　　　　　　　J.G.W. Sc.

VAISON.

fesses to some doubts as to its real character, however, and says he would rather have seen it on the foot of a horse.[1]

It appears that this Vaison monument was found in the sixteenth century, in building the Château de Marodi, and was kept in that building as an ornament until recently. French archæologists are of opinion, that it has been sculptured towards the second century of our era, at the time of the Roman decadence.

The sacrificial scene (plate 3) on this grand memento of Gallic history lends additional evidence as to its antiquity. 'The chief personage is, I believe, one of the inside passengers in the *rheda,* who, as *flamen,* or chief sacerdotal magistrate of the province, or district, is journeying to superintend some important religious ceremony. The attendant carrying the *securis* is as significant of this office as the eagle, vexillum, or other standard would have been in denoting a military office ; while the whole details of this second scene are so carefully rendered, as to determine a connection between the two, allusive to one of the chief offices which the deceased object of the monument held. Provincial inscriptions prove that distinguished persons commonly held the highest sacerdotal offices in connection with the first civil appointments.'[2]

Shortly after their conquest of Gaul, the Romans appear to have commenced the suppression of Druidism, and the priests shared the fate of the vanquished nation in being doomed to slavery, or at best were permitted to

---

[1] *C. Roach Smith.* Op. cit.   [2] Ibid. p. 22.

enjoy the scanty privileges of freemen.[1]   Many of the most devoted Druids doubtless fled to remote places, and exercised their arts in secret, in order to maintain a precarious living; so that the sound of the anvil in caves and forest fastnesses, would alone denote the dwelling-place of those Druid priests, who had become fugitives to avoid the degradation of slavery.

The Druidical monopoly in the arts was abolished by the Romans, who established large manufactories of arms in eight different parts of Gaul, and in them the slaves fabricated weapons for their conquerors.   When these bondsmen contrived to obtain their liberty, they then worked on their own account, and with the trading class formed a *bourgeoisie* who dwelt in the towns; but they were so heavily taxed and kept under that they never attained any position.[2]   Only the nobles who had given in

---

[1] *Megnin.* 'The freemen were a very numerous class in Gaul, who derived their origin from the various nations against which the Romans had carried their arms.   And the most numerous class at the time of the invasion of the barbarians was that of the slaves. . . . All the Gauls invested with the title of citizen had to renounce Druidism. The edicts of Augustus proscribed it, and the other Celtic notions, together with the language, were consigned to the lower classes. . . . . . The freedmen were in possession of nearly all the arts and handicrafts, and they laboured at them unceasingly; but they enjoyed no consideration or authority, and had to submit to vexatious laws.'—*Sismondi.* Hist. des Français, vol. i. pp. 6, 58, 104.

[2] 'The tradespeople and artisans were responsible for the industrial impost, as the Curials were for the land-tax.   An iron hand stifled free trade and prevented its competing with slave labour, which was devoted to the imperial exchequer.   This oppression gave rise to such a degree of despair, that they abandoned their homes to live in the forests and deserts with the Bagauds and fugitive slaves.'—*H. Martin.* Hist. de France, p. 327.

their adherence to the Roman rule, and in everything, even to their names, had become Roman, became senators, gained a high rank, and in becoming rich became also effeminate, like the Romans themselves. Thus was extinguished the valorous Gallic nation; and, with its decadence, disappeared its love for the horse. During the Gallo-Roman period the cavalry became so scarce, that at the invasion of the barbarous hordes it can scarcely be traced.

That the barbarians who overthrew the Roman empire shod their horses we have no proof whatever ; though it has been maintained by eminent authorities that they introduced this art. The Sarmatians appear not to have known the use of iron, for they had armour of horn plates sewn on cloth and overlapping each other ; and their horses, so extremely hardy, but which were so numerous that every horseman had two or three to select from when the one he rode was fatigued (as with the Mongol Tartars, who do not shoe their horses), were also covered in the same manner.[1]

The confederacy of German tribes who conquered the Lombards, assumed the name of Franks (the Free), and finally obtained possession of Gaul, were not an equestrian people ; their battles were chiefly, if not altogether, fought by infantry.[2] The Franks had no cavalry, and up to the time of Charles Martel, no evidence of it is to be found in their armies. The nobles alone were mounted on horses, and with the descendants of Clovis the

[1] *Amm. Marcell.* Lib. xvii. cap. 23, p. 506.
[2] *H. Martin.* Hist. de France, vol. i. p. 377. *Sismondi.* Hist. de Français, vol. i. p. 340.

Great a most valuable present consisted of a few horses. At the reception of Theodebert by his uncle Childebert, king of Paris, among all the considerable gifts he received, none excited so much admiration as six horses;[1] and when Theodebert entered Italy in 539, with an army of 100,000 combatants, the only mounted men were a few armed with lances who formed his body-guard. All the others were footmen.[2]

The renowned Clovis himself, after defeating the Visigoths at Vouglé, went to the tomb of Saint Martin to return thanks for his victory, and presented the monastery with the horse he rode at the battle. But so scarce were good horses, that in a very short time he repented having bestowed his courser, and offered to buy it again for fifty marks of silver. The monks, however, sent an answer that Saint Martin was very tenacious of the present made to him; so that Clovis was obliged to double the amount in order to overcome the defunct Saint's scruples. This crafty stratagem caused the impious Sicambre to murmur in his beard, ‘Saint Martin does his friends good service, but he sells it somewhat dear.’

When the nobles or their families travelled it was either on foot, or in carriages (*basterne*) drawn by oxen; kings even journeyed in this manner, and the possession of horses did not denote nobility or wealth. Martin, alluding to this period, gives us an example of this undignified mode of progression. ‘Clodowig hastened to send an official ambassador to Gondebald, who, not without hesitation, permitted the deputies to espouse

[1] *Gregor. Turon.* Lib. iii. pp. 24, 198.
[2] *Sismondi.* Op. cit. vol. i. p. 275.

Clotilde in the name of Clodowig, by the *sou d'or* and the *denier d'argent*, according to the Salic custom, and after a *plaid* (court) held at Chalons, between the knights of Burgundy and the French envoys. These last led away Clotilde in a *basterne*, a covered chariot drawn by oxen'' The same author describing the entry of the young chief Sighismer into Lyons when about to marry the daughter of the King of Burgundy, writes: 'His hair resembled the gold of his vestments; his complexion was as dazzling as the scarlet of his dress; his skin equalled in whiteness the silk with which his robes were trimmed. *He came on foot,* surrounded by a troop of chiefs of tribes and a cortège of companions terrible to look upon, even in time of peace. Their feet were covered by velvet boots; their limbs were naked, and their vestments were so short and narrow that they scarcely reached the knee. They wore gowns of green silk bordered with scarlet, and carried glaives suspended from their shoulders by rich baldricks, curved lances, throwing hatchets (*haches de jet*), and double bucklers of iron and copper beautifully polished.'[2]

When the Frankish kings imposed tribute on the Saxons, whom they had vanquished, the impost levied was cows. 'In 632, the Saxon deputies took the oath on their weapons, according to the custom of their nation, to defend the Austrasian frontier until such time as the king (Dagobert) should abolish the tribute imposed upon them and their ancestors by the Frankish kings since the reign of Clotaire I.; then the army would be disbanded.

[1] Hist. de France, vol. i. p. 416.
[2] Hist. de France, p. 406, note.

This annual tribute, which the Saxons considered so onerous, was 500 cows.'[1]

Pepin the Short was the first who sought to substitute the five hundred cows thus levied for three hundred horses. In a campaign against that people, he thoroughly subdued them. 'The battle was very sanguinary, but Pepin gained the victory. He advanced to the Weser, and destroyed the fortresses or *fertés* built by the Saxons. The West Saxons submitted, and were compelled to pay a tribute of 300 horses a year, and to permit the preachers to preach among them in the name of the Lord.'[2] This was also considered a very severe punishment.

This indifference of the Merovingians to horses may have had everything to do with the absence of horseshoes from their graves and other remains, which have been explored in France within the last few years. The Abbé Cochet remarks, in reference to this fact: 'It ought to be mentioned that, up to the present time, nothing has proved more rare in Frankish graves than the shoes of horses. With the three or four horses we discovered at Envermeu no shoes were found, although all the limbs were present. But buckles and bits of a very characteristic shape were there. Lindenschmidt, who found the skeleton of a horse lying beside a warrior, at Selzen, positively asserts that it was without shoes. Of all its harness there was only found a bit and some small bronze rings. This archæologist adds, that it has been the same at Sinsheim, Ascherade, Langweid, and Heidesheim. At Nordendorf three skeletons of horses were discovered, but

---

[1] *Frédégarius.* Cap. lxxiv. p. 441.
[2] Ibid. *Annal.* Metz. ap. Scrip. Rerum Francic. V. 336.

they were also without shoes, and had only their bits.[1]
MM. Durrich and Menzel, in their interesting search
at Oberflacht, found an almost complete equipment of a
horse, but no shoes.[2] . . . . . Thus nothing is more
common than the bridle bit, and nothing so scarce as
shoes.'[3] It was the extreme rarity of these articles that
led the Abbé to doubt Chifflet's reported discovery of
one in the grave of Childeric.

It would also appear that with the second or Carlovingian dynasty, shoeing, and indeed the value of cavalry,
was still held in little esteem. The war with the Moors
began during the reign of Charles Martel, but every
engagement only showed the advantages of cavalry on
the one side, and infantry on the other. This monarch
would have gained a far more decisive battle at Tours,
had the solidity of his infantry been supplemented by
cavalry to crush the defeated and retreating Moors, who
got away undisturbed; and though the world was saved
from Mahommedanism, yet this equestrian people, by
their courage and rapidity of movement, harassed the
Franks long afterwards.

Charlemagne seems to have become aware of the
necessity for mounted troops, and to have organized a
large body of cavalry, to which he owed many of his
victories. His army appears to have been extensively
horsed from Spain, the successes of his lieutenants in that
country, in their contentions with the Moors, giving them
an opportunity for making captures.[4] From this source

---

[1] Das *Germanische* Todtenlager, bei Selzen, pp. 6, 28.
[2] Die Heidengräber am Lupfen, p. 31.
[3] Le Tombeau de Childeric, p. 154.
[4] *Eginhard.* *A*nnales, p. 213.

he was able to present the King of Persia with a number of Spanish horses and mules.[1]

In his expedition against the Avares of Hungary, he had a very strong force of cavalry; but at Ems the horses were attacked with a contagious disorder, which destroyed nearly the whole of them. So great a reliance did he place upon cavalry, and so severe was this infliction, that he preferred waiting for three years, until this arm could be recruited by horses from Spain and elsewhere ; notwithstanding the greatest possible provocations offered him by the enemy in the interval.[2]

An ordinance, or capitulary, published at Aix la Cha pelle in 807 (*De villis imperialibus*), is curiously illustrative of the manners of this time. Among other things it is enacted that the 'Judex,' or steward of each villa, was to provide stallions (C. 13); that care was to be taken of the stud mares, and the colts were to be separated at the proper season; the stables were to be thoroughly prepared; there were to be good artificers, particularly blacksmiths; and at Christmas, in giving an account of their administrations, with many other items, mention was to be made of what profit was derived from the labours of the blacksmith, as well as from colts and fillies. In peace everything was to be prepared for war : ' Our cars for war to be litters well made, covered with hides so closely sewed, that if necessity occurs for swimming rivers, they may pass through (after being lightened of their contents), without water entering.' His cavalry was always kept on a war footing.

---

[1] *The Monk of Saint-Gall.* Hist. des Gaules.
[2] Poet. Saxon. iii., apud Scrip. Rer. Franc. V. 155.

The 'Chroniques de Saint-Denis' recite some wonderful stories of Charlemagne's strength, such as his cleaving a warrior in two with a blow of his sword, and carrying a heavily-armed man by one hand. Shoeing must have been practised in his day, for tradition says of him that he bent, and even broke, with his hands alone, a shoe that had been made by a smith for his horse. He was, however, outdone by the farrier, who, to show his strength, broke in like manner the piece of gold paid him by the Emperor for his shoeing.

The revival of Celtic legends and traditions may have operated largely in infusing into Charlemagne and his successors a love of the horse and equestrian exercises—a revival due, perhaps, to the arrival of St Columbanus and his followers from Ireland.[1] The historian Nitard is particularly careful in informing us how the two kings, Charles and Ludewig, arranged troops of cavalry, consisting of Saxons, Wascons, Austrasians, and Bretons, and manœuvred them against each other, causing them to gallop their horses fiercely, and brandish their arms.

Shoeing would therefore appear to have been practised, though perhaps only occasionally; indeed, there is some ground for believing that the Celts, Gauls, and Franks (when the latter began to avail themselves of this defence for their horses' feet), only resorted to iron plates for the hoofs of their steeds when the horn had been considerably worn way. No implements have been discovered which one might infer were employed to remove the superfluous growth consequent on the wearing of shoes, and it is not at all unlikely that the

[1] *Martin.* Hist. de France, vol. ii. p. 114.

11

hoofs were allowed to be worn down to their natural size when they had attained an undue length, instead of being shortened by instruments as at present. Shoes would, of course, be more particularly required during wet and frosty weather; and such is indicated in the description given by Père Daniel,[1] when speaking of the difficulties surrounding Louis I., the *Debonnaire* (832) · 'La gelée qui avoit suivi (les pluyes de l'automne) avoit gasté les pieds de la plupart des chevaux, *qu'on ne pouvoit faire ferrer* dans un pais devenu tout d'un coup ennemi, lorsq'on y pensoit le moins.' From this passage we might conclude that horses were but seldom shod, though the art of shoeing was known and practised; and that it was only on particular occasions that the hoofs were so protected, as in winter, when ice and frozen roads damaged them, or during war. In some parts of Germany at the present day, agricultural horses are only shod in winter.

Towards the termination of the Carlovingian reign, and the beginning of the Capet dynasty, shoeing became more general. Lobineau, in his History of Brittany, gives many copies of seals of the tenth, eleventh, and twelfth centuries, on which are depicted knights whose horses are shod with iron shoes fastened by nails.

Those who had the care and management of horses became men of high rank, and the *Comte de l'Étable* soon became the commander of armies.[2] The shoer of

[1] Histoire de France, vol. i. p. 556.

[2] ' But Witikind had reappeared, and the Saxons took to their arms again. The Saraves, a Sclavonic people living between the Elbe and Sorba, had invaded the neighbouring frontiers of Saxony and Thuringia.

horses not unfrequently bore this honourable distinction, and when the era of chivalry developed itself from the usages of the feudal system, we find him on a different footing, and uniting with his handicraft those functions which the Comte de l'Étable had relinquished—such as the government of the stables and studs, and assuming the title of 'écuyer,' or officer of the feudal lord to whom he was attached. This shows a return to the Celtic customs, and testifies that the Roman and barbarian usages were rapidly disappearing.

'In so far as it was a military institution,' writes M. Martin,[1] 'chivalry descended in a direct line from the Celtic customs. The fashion of receiving young men among the warriors fell into disuse with the Gallo-Romans, but was preserved among the purely Celtic people. Feudality revived it, and gave it the significant title of " chivalry," which indicated that the possession of a war-horse—of a *destrier*,[2] was the distinctive sign of a

Charles quickly despatched three officers to check them : these were Adalgiste, *Cubiculare* or Chamberlain, Gellar, *Comte de l'étable*, and Worad, *Comte du palais;* for already the servile functions which belonged even to the person of the monarch, were regarded as honourable distinctions and gave a title to commanders of armies.'—*Eginhard. Annales*, p. 205. This Comte de l'étable was the origin of ' Constable,' an honourable designation which has been in use for many centuries.

[1] Hist. de France, vol. iii. p. 335.

[2] *Destrier* was the name given to a war-horse, which was also the Latin *destrarius,* or *dextrarius,* of the middle ages ; derived, we are told, from *dextra,* because the horsemen handled their steeds only with the right hand ; or more likely because the war-horse was led by a groom or squire until required for battle. The Troubadours often mention it :

Chacuns d'eux broche son auferrant Gascon.
La peust on voir maint auferrant d'Espagne.
D'Estriers, auferrant et Gascon.

11*

nobleman. The young noble, before attaining the rank
of chevalier, or complete warrior, had to serve many years'
apprenticeship under the designations of *page, varlet,
damoiseau*, and *écuyer.* . .   . It was in the name of
Saint George or Saint Michael that he was armed as a
chevalier.[1] The young nobles filled in the castles of their
lords all kinds of domestic offices, to which the feudal
system, the conservator of Celtic traditions, did not attach
any idea of servility.'[2] The Gauls and Bretons had
already afforded an example of this servitude. The
popular ballads of Brittany, collected by M. la Ville-
marque, and which are supposed to have been sung by
the bards of the fifth and sixth centuries, contain allusions
to it. One ballad says : 'And all the castles he saw were full
of men-at-arms and horses, and each warrior furbished his
helmet, sharpened his sword, cleaned his armour, *and shod
his horse.*' Another song, entitled 'Le Barde Merlin,'
recounts the success of a young noble in a horse-race, the
prize for which was to be Leonora, the king's daughter,
and says : 'He has equipped his red steed, *he has shod it
with polished steel,* he has put on its bridle.'[3]

In connection with this greatly increasing importance

The bards of the 6th century, however, use the word *eddestr* for a
charger, which was of Celtic derivation.

[1] *Varlet, vaslet, vasselet,* under-servant. *Damoiseau*, from *domicellus*,
diminutive of *dominus*, an inferior lord. *Ecuyer*, scutifer, or shield-
bearer. He carried the buckler of his lord, and attended him in combat,
like the Gaulish ' trimarkisia.'

Saint Michael was the chief of celestial chivalry, and Saint George
of the terrestrial.

[2] Hist. France, p. 108.

[3] *Megnin.* La Maréchalerie Française, p. 72.

of the horse, the office of *maréchal*, or farrier, also assumed a higher rank; but of this notice will be taken hereafter.

In the tenth and eleventh centuries, the horse-shoe formed a part of every horse's armour, and, in fact, constituted his state of belligerency. This is manifest in a curious passage occurring in the oath administered to the nobles of Franche Comté by Archbishop Burhard, in the *trève* or Paix de Dieu (A.D. 1027), where it is said: ' I shall neither assail the clerk nor the unarmed monk, nor those who accompany them without arms; I will not seize upon any ox, cow, goat, ass, nor their burdens; I will also respect birds, cocks and hens, that is, if I do not require them, when I will buy them for two deniers; neither will I carry away the " unshod mare " (*jument non ferrée*), nor the untrained colt.'[1]

Megnin thinks the designation ' auferrand,' sometimes given to war-horses, probably arose from this state of the hoofs. It may be remarked, however, that so far as I have been able to trace it, this name has been always applied to grey, or, as we term them, ' iron-coloured horses.' The *ferrant*, *auferrant*, and *blancferrant*, were only different shades of this hue; which was probably due to the early admixture of African and Barbary blood with the indigenous or Gothic race of horses—a breed soon renowned throughout Navarre to the Garonne; and in consequence of the preponderance of greys in it, it received the above names.

The ' ferrant' at a later date is as frequently met with in history as the ' auferrant;' and in one instance we have

---

[1] *Castan.* Origines de la Commune de Besançon, p. 42. Fragmentum Concilii Verdunensis, apud *Chifflet.*

a curious play upon the word.   In the reign of Philip
Augustus, King of France, Count Ferrand of Flanders
was taken prisoner at the battle of Bovines (1214), and
carried in chains behind four shod horses into Paris. The
populace improvised a song for the occasion, the refrain
of which was founded upon horse-shoes (*fers*), horses
(*ferrants*) the Count's title (Ferrand), and his ignominious condition.

> Et quatre ferrants bien ferrés,
> Trainent Ferrand bien enferré.

CHAPTER IV.

HORSE-SHOES FOUND IN SWITZERLAND: THEIR ANTIQUITY, AND
SHAPE. M. QUIQUEREZ'S RESEARCHES AND OBSERVATIONS. VALU-
ABLE INDICATIONS AFFORDED BY THE SHOES AS TO THE BREEDS
OF HORSES, AND THE DIFFERENT RACES OF PEOPLE. FORGES IN
THE JURA ALPS. VERY ANCIENT SHOE. PREVALENCE OF SHOES
WITH CELTIC REMAINS. ROMAN CAMPS. HORSE-SHOES OF DIF-
FERENT FORMS. THE BURGUNDIANS AND GROOVED SHOES. INCREASE
OF SIZES. SHOES OF THE MIDDLE AGES: THEIR CHARACTERISTICS.
FARRIERS' MARKS. SHOES FOUND IN BELGIUM. GERMANY. HORSE-
LOVING TRIBES. INFERIOR HORSES. ANCIENT HORSE-SHOES OF
LARGE AND SMALL SIZES. GROSZ'S DESCRIPTION. ROMAN CAMP
OF DALHEIM. THE BURGUNDIAN GROOVE. STEINFURT. MONUMENT
WITH RUNIC INSCRIPTION AND FIGURE OF A HORSE-SHOE. THE
BURGUNDII. THE FARRIER AS ARMOURER. THE DWARF REGIN.
SAINT ELOY'S DAY AT THE BURGUNDIAN COURT. THE PATRON
SAINT. GERMAN HISTORY. WIDE PREVALENCE OF THE GROOVED
SHOE. SCANDINAVIA. THE SMITH'S ART. GOLDEN SHOES. PEAT-
MOSSES AND THEIR CONTENTS.

IN Switzerland, as has been noticed, shoes of the form
peculiar to the Celtic, Roman, and subsequent periods,
have been found. Those discovered by M. Troyon[1] in
the supposed sacrificial mound of Chavannes, have been
described as differing only in the absence of calkins from
the majority of those already considered. They were
five in number, and very primitive in shape. Their

[1] *Troyon.* Colline de Sacrifices de Chavannes-sur-le-Veyron, p. 5.

measurement appears to have been—length, 4½ inches ; width, 4⅛ inches. The strongest branch, which may be looked upon as that for the outer border of the hoof, had the holes punched *coarsely* (that is, farther from the external border) ; and the inner or weaker branch, *finer*, or nearer the outer edge. The holes were a little more rectangular than is usually seen in these primitive specimens. M. Troyon was in doubt as to the epoch to which this mound, and the bones, spurs, bits, and other articles, belonged ; but elsewhere he appears to refer the shoes to the second 'iron age,' or the Helveto-Roman period [1] (see fig. 22). In speaking of these articles, this able antiquarian remarks : ' A horse-shoe has been discovered, with arrow-heads and lances, in a tumulus in the neighbourhood of Aussée, which appears to me to resemble that of Chavannes. Another has been found in a tumulus in the Canton Berne, but its form is exactly that of those met with in the Roman ruins. We see horse-shoes like those of Chavannes, but of more advanced workmanship, from the battle-field of Cressy, and preserved in the Artillery Museum of Paris.' [2] Baron Bonstetten gives a drawing of a fragment of a shoe of this description, obtained by workmen who were demolishing a tumulus standing between Sariswyl and Murzelen, Canton Berne. It is merely the toe-piece of the shoe, without holes or any other indication of its antiquity. In three other tumuli explored by this archæologist, arms and several objects in bronze were recovered,

---

[1] Rapport sur les Collect. d'Antiq. du Musée Cantonal à Lausanne, 1858.

[2] Colline de Sacrifices, p. 12.

which were classed as belonging to the Helveto-Roman age.[1]

The Museum of Avenches exhibits many shoes obtained from the Roman ruins of Avencium, the ancient capital of Helvetia. They have all, with one exception, six nail-holes; the largest has eight.[2] In the excavations made at Grange, near Cossonay (Canton Vaud), relics of the same kind have been picked up. The figure of one designed by M. Bieler, gives its size as barely 4 inches in length and 3 inches in breadth (fig. 27). It has low calkins, and a slight groove runs from heel to heel. Altogether, it looks a much more recent shoe than any of those usually ascribed to the Celtic or Gallo-Roman age; though M. Bieler is of opinion that it belongs to the third century. A specimen in the Berne Museum, and which was dug out of a tumulus at Garchwyl, near

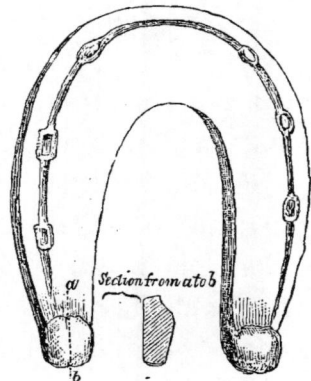

fig 27

Berne, does not differ much in appearance from the last. It was found with a very fine specimen of a vase and other articles, but their age is uncertain. The tumulus was supposed to be very old—anterior, it was surmised, to our era, and at any rate not dating any later than the third or fourth century.[3] In appearance it is more modern, and is chiefly remarkable for having the groove

[1] Recueil d'Antiq. Suisses.
[2] *Bieler.* Journal de Méd. Vét. de Lyon, vol. xiii. p. 246.
[3] Ibid.

passing continuously from toe to heel—in having four
nail-holes on one side and three on the other, and showing also a toe-piece with six marks proceeding from it
(fig. 28).[1]   The Roman camp on Mount Terrible has

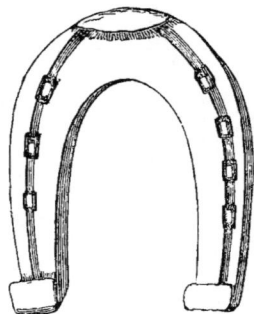

fig 28

also furnished a number, which are
in the private museum of M. Quiquerez.   M. Bieler thus sums up
the general characteristics of the
shoes he has examined : 'The shoes
of the Roman epoch have usually
six holes (*étampures*), and very
rarely the largest have eight. These
rectangular holes are generally distributed along a groove analogous to that of the English shoes, and without interruption at the toe; but the
holes are much larger than the grooves, and cause
bulgings on the external border.   The *ajusture* (fitting
to the shape of the foot's surface) is null, or nearly
so.   Lastly, the heels are rolled over in some shoes, others
have rude calkins, and some have also a *crampon*, or toe-
piece.   With regard to the nails, they differ essentially
from our own, and are more of the Arab form.   The
head is flat, about half a line in thickness; its shape is
nearly semicircular, and it is from one-half to three-
quarters of an inch in diameter; the shank or body
(*lame*) is square and rather strong.   When the head has
been worn to the surface of the shoe, the part buried in
the cavity of the aperture is in outline like a T.'

From the excellent memoir on the horse-shoes found

[1] *Jahn. Antiquarisch Gesellschaft. Zurich, 1850.*

in the Jura Alps, by M. Quiquerez,[1] who has distinguished himself by his researches into the situation and mode of working the Celtic forges, we will make a few extracts, which are perhaps as satisfactory as they are lucid. ' For a long time,' he says, ' there have been remarked various kinds of horse-shoes in the monuments belonging to several ages, without our having been able until the present time to make them serve as a guide to recognize with precision the period in which they were used. They have also been collected from the pastures, forests, and cultivated lands, at such depths that it could not be admitted they belonged to modern times. Some particular forms, and especially the diminutiveness of these shoes, indicated a smaller race of horses, or a breed with small feet, such as are yet noticed in certain kinds of well-bred animals. At any rate, the meagre quantity of metal employed seemed to point to a light race, or perhaps the scarcity of iron, or even these two causes combined. It is very remarkable that these small shoes are not limited to one portion of the Swiss Jura, but are found from the banks of the Rhine to Geneva, throughout the whole extent of the Alps, on both its slopes, as well as in its central valleys. We may then be assured that these are the shoes of the indigenous horses which have pastured over the whole of this country at various periods, during a long space of time. They ought, therefore, to afford a characteristic index of those Gaulish horses so renowned in bygone ages, but which have been

[1] Les Anciens Fers de Chevaux dans le Jura. Mém. de la Soc. d'Emulation du Doubs, 1864, p. 129.

modified by crossing with strange breeds during the Roman and barbarian conquests. A more attentive study of these shoes, and of the localities from whence they were procured, permits their being divided into at least two classes, belonging, if not to different epochs, at least to people shoeing their horses diversely in the same country. These differences of form correspond also to an augmentation in size, thickness, and weight, and in such a way that those we look upon as the most ancient weigh scarcely more than from 90 to 120 grammes;[1] while those of the following ages also increase in weight and dimensions, so that for the time of the Romans they reach from 180 to 245 grammes; then to 365; and lastly, in our own days, they weigh from 490 to 850 grammes, and even more. These modest objects of antiquity thus reveal facts no less interesting to archæology than to agriculture. Under the last head they seem to indicate a progressive augmentation in the height of the horses, and an amelioration in the indigenous species, arising from the progress of agriculture and commerce, as the two began to require horses with more strength than elegance or lightness. In an archæological point of view, they furnish a material proof of the persistence of the usages of a country in its mode of shoeing horses; so that the invasions and foreign occupations could not cause them to be entirely abandoned by our native farriers. This last fact also testifies to the existence of the same people in these regions, and their surviving the

---

[1] The gramme is equal to 15.4 grains troy, or 16.9 grains avoirdupois.

Roman and barbarian domination. Nevertheless, it is not only the permanence of the shape of the horse-shoes which has given rise to this opinion, but also the persistence that the people and the artisans of the country have shown in the reproduction of the forms of ordinary articles, instruments, or arms; and to such a degree is this the case, that the hatchets of stone, for example, and those of bronze and iron, are found, after long intervals, to be so similar in form and dimensions that the difference of material could not be taken into account. This evidently proves the influence of habit in the use of utensils of a certain form. The hatchet of bronze remains as small as that of stone; and it is the same with the weapon made of iron—apparently for the same reason, that the untempered instrument of iron was scarcely better than the one made of bronze. Drawings of Roman antiquities and those of the middle ages represent iron arrow-heads, keys, knives, and designs of vases, which are exactly the same. The same fact is noticed in certain details in architecture; for instance, the church of *Moutiers-Grand-Val,* built in the 7th century, we find the same details that may yet be discerned in the theatre of Mandeura.

'The shoes we look upon as the oldest, show, to commence with, that the Celts were already acquainted with siderurgy; the examination we have made of the ancient forges in the Jura furnishes us with important indications in this respect. (More than 160 siderurgical establishments of various epochs have been already discovered, and some of them have furnished antique objects which serve to determine the age of the iron. The furnaces and crucibles disinterred by us are peculiar in form, and appear to testify that the use of the blast to hasten the combustion of the fuel was then unknown.)'

It may here be remarked that Mr T. Wright shows that the Romans in Britain smelted their iron very imperfectly. 'It is supposed that layers of iron ore, broken up, and charcoal mixed with limestone as a flux, were piled together, and enclosed in a wall and covering of clay, with holes at the bottom for letting in the draught, and allowing the melted metal to run out. For this purpose they were usually placed on sloping ground. Rude bellows were, perhaps, used, worked by different contrivances.' Mr Bruce, in his account of the 'Roman Wall,' has pointed out a very curious contrivance for producing a blast in the furnaces of the extensive Roman iron-works in the neighbourhood of Epiacum (Lanchester). A part of the valley, rendered barren by the heaps of slightly-covered cinders, had never been cultivated till very recent times. 'During the operation of bringing this common into cultivation,' Mr Bruce says, 'the method adopted by the Romans of producing the blast necessary to smelt the metal was made apparent. Two tunnels had been formed in the side of a hill; they were wide at one extremity, but tapered off to a narrow bore at the other, where they met in a point. The mouths of the channels opened towards the west, from which quarter a prevalent wind blows in this valley, and sometimes with great violence. The blast received by them would, when the wind was high, be poured with considerable force and effect upon the smelting furnaces at the extremity of the tunnels.' This primitive mode of smelting is still in use among some peoples unacquainted with the improvements of civilized nations. The ancient Peruvians, for example, built their furnaces in this manner. Mungo Park also noticed a similar practice in Africa, and it has also been described as existing in the Himalaya mountains of Central Asia.

'The shoes of the first period are small, narrow, and scant of metal, constantly pierced with six holes, whose external opening is strongly stamped in a longitudinal form, to lodge the base of the nail-head. The slight thickness, and especially the narrowness of the metal, causes it at each hole to bulge, and to give a festooned appearance to the external border of the shoe. The thickness of the latter is from one-eighth to one-seventh of an inch, and the width from six to seven-tenths of an inch between each hole, thus indicating the dimensions of the bar of metal before stamping. The form of the stamped holes indicates the employment of a steel punch, and consequently a knowledge of the manufacture of steel at the period when these horse-shoes were made.

'One of these shoes (fig. 29) has been found, with a portion of the bones of a horse, in a peat-moss near the old abbey of Bellelay, at a depth of twelve feet, resting on the primitive soil. There was, therefore, every reason to believe that this horse had not been buried in the peat, but that, on the contrary, it had perished in this place before the formation of the heap, inasmuch as its scattered bones testified to the work of carnivorous animals gathered around their prey. Many of these shoes have been found at various depths in the turf-beds of the Helvetic plain, but we have not been able to obtain pre-

cise information with regard to them. This turf-pit has
yielded numbers of coins from the first half of the 15th

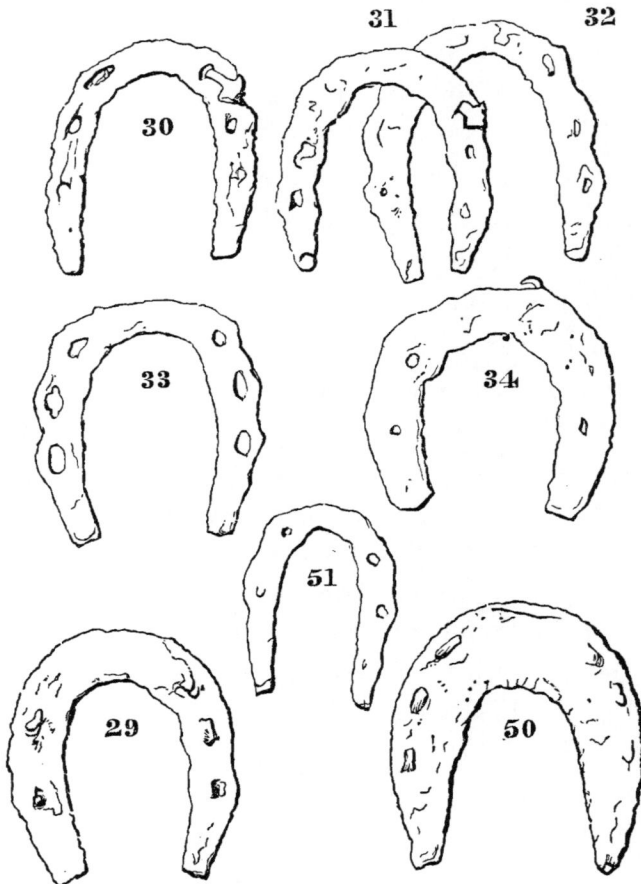

fig. 29

century to the year 1480. These were only covered by
$23\frac{1}{2}$ inches of turf, still spongy, but which had nevertheless taken at least four centuries to form. Taking
this particular case into consideration, and reckoning the
overlying deposit as accumulating at the rate of 6 inches
in a century,—far too low an estimate by reason of the

density the turf assumes as it becomes old and forms the inferior layers,—the shoe discovered at the bottom ought to have lain there at least 2400 years. These same turf-beds enclose, or rather cover, a place where there is charcoal beneath 19 feet 8 inches of peat, and this being on the primitive ground, gives a period of more than 4000 years since it was laid there. In the neighbourhood there are iron scoriæ indicating an ancient forge, and in this country, where iron mines only exist, wood is carbonized for no other purpose than to work that metal, and all the ancient forges used nothing else.

'More than twenty of these shoes have been collected in the soil of a Celtic establishment between Delémont and Soyhiere, on the right bank of the Byrse, territory of Courroux, and near Vorbourg (fig. 51). There were no traces of Roman articles, nor yet those of a posterior age, but only antiquities of the stone, those of the bronze, and, lastly, of the iron periods. The last was characterized only by horse-shoes, and by two discs resembling the iron money of the Spartans. On the other bank of the river similar shoes were also found (figs. 30, 31, 32), and two beautiful lance-heads or Gaulish javelins. Near the first shoes was a pointed spur. Another shoe of the same form has been met with in the track of an antique road, near Saint-Braix, not far from one of those ancient forges where objects belonging to the stone age have been dis covered. A neighbouring hamlet is called Césais or Cæsar, a characteristic name also given to a ridge or mound near which passes a Roman road joining the plateau of the Franches-Montagnes with the enclosure of Doubs, and which shows traces of military works. The

Jurassian Society of Emulation is about to publish what we have written on the new discoveries made in this portion of our mountains (figs. 33, 34).

'Other shoes, always like the former, are frequently met with in pastures, forests, and cultivated lands, but constantly at somewhat considerable depths. They often also mark the ancient narrow road-ways, which have ruts worn into the rock, and where the short axle-tree has scraped away the stone at the sides in its passage, at a height of from 12 to 13 inches (Celtic roads). We have rarely found this description of shoes in the Roman camps; in fact, only on that of Mount Terrible, which was formed on an *oppidum;* we believe, however, that the shoes from this place belonged to the same category as the Celtic objects of the three ages, and which have been found in such large numbers. Nevertheless, it is very remarkable that one of these shoes has been gathered in the ruins of the castle of Asuel, supposed to have been built in the 11th century and destroyed in the 15th (fig. 33). But it might well belong to an earlier period, as we have found a similar specimen in the walls of the château of Sogron, where a horse certainly never planted foot (fig. 35). This building dated from the 8th century, and was burned in 1499; in its vicinity we have found a stone hatchet and two Celtic coins of Togirix.

'We might also mention the discovery of one of these shoes with undulated borders at a great depth near the glass-works of Moutier, on the track of a Celtic road at the entrance to the passes of Court, and also farther away at the level of the river Byrse (fig. 52). We have seen *débris* of shoes on the continuation of this road near the mill of the Roches de Courrendelin, and also near Grellingen, always beside deep ruts, and sometimes beside transverse grooves and cuttings in the rock, in the bed of these passages, intended to prevent the horses slipping. These same shoes are also found at the bottom of the *tourbières* of the Swiss plain, in the Gaulish monuments of Alesia, in the plains of Champagne, on the battle-field where Attila is said to have been defeated in 451.[1] The Cossacks, the descendants of the ancient Scythians, or Huns, yet shoe their horses in the same fashion. We might cite many other discoveries of these same shoes, as well in Switzerland as elsewhere, and particularly in the districts of the Jura. We think that these are assuredly the shoes of the indigenous horses which wandered or pastured on the mountains of our country, long before the arrival of the Romans; and they have remained in use with the Jurassic people during the Roman domination, and still later, concurrently with those we are about to describe. It may have happened that the shoeing of the Gallic horses was derived from the relations of the Gauls with Asia, where nail-shoeing is said to have been of high antiquity; and if we, as well as our neighbours, regard these small shoes as of Hunnic, Saracenic, or even of Swedish origin, it is simply because people confound the epochs of the invasions which have desolated the country. Even now, these articles are attributed to the Cossacks in 1814.

'In the numerous Roman camps whose remains occupy

---

[1] *Camu-Chardon.* Notice sur la Défaite d'Attila, Mém. de la Soc. Acad. de l'Aube, 1854.

the summits of the mountains or hills of the Jura, along
Upper Alsace, as in the chain of Lomont, in the castles of
the same period, perched on culminating points, in the
ruins of Roman villas buried beneath nearly every
village, on the track of roads of the like date, and also
scattered over the country, we have gathered horse-shoes
of a different form to those already noticed, but whose
dimensions yet resemble them, though they are always
more circular. They are also stronger in metal, and
consequently more heavy, varying from 180 to 245
grammes. They are with or without calkins (*crampons*),
and pierced by six holes—three on each side, placed farther
from the external border than in the preceding. The
heads of the nails are still oblong, but not so high or
salient, and indeed are nearly hidden in the holes counter-
sunk for this purpose. There are other shoes which, in
form, in weight, and in dimensions are allied to these, and
are found in the same places; but they offer a characteristic difference. This consists in a groove (*rainure*, Angl.
fullering) extending around the outer border of the shoe
from the heels to the toe, and sometimes deep enough to
completely lodge the heads of the six nails with which
they are furnished. At other times, this groove is scarcely
noticeable, and would appear only to have been used to
indicate the line on which the farrier sought to make the
holes. Shoes with a deep groove are yet in use in England; but with us they seem to have been older than, or
contemporaneous with, the cutlasses with wide blades,
sharpened only on one side, and provided with one or two
of these longitudinal grooves. Knives of the same period
are similarly ornamented, and these certainly belong to

the end of the 4th or the commencement of the 5th century. The weight of these fullered shoes amounts to about 265 grammes each (about 9½ ounces).

'These two varieties of shoes are not only met with in Roman establishments, civil and military, but also in the Burgundian tombs of the 5th century, and in ruins of the 7th and 8th centuries; as also in the dwellings of the middle ages, and in all the districts over which horses of this epoch have passed. According to all appearances, during the Roman period the people of the country had preserved the mode of shoeing practised by their ancestors of Celtic origin, and the breed of horses had scarcely increased in size; while the Romans, or rather the foreign troops attached to the legions, had imported stronger horses, and employed shoes different from those of our nation. Such is at least the opinion that we derive from the facts and the circumstances accompanying the discovery of these articles. We possess some shoes found with a heap of horses' bones, the hoofs of which yet remained shod, and which were lighted upon when repairing the road from Courtemantruy to Saint-Ursanne, not far from the Roman camps of Moron and Mount Terrible (figs. 36, 37). Another shoe, almost identical with them, has been gathered in the last-named camp, on the same level with Roman relics (fig. 38). A fragment was also found in the same place (fig. 39). The ruins of the Roman villas of Debilliers and Fourfaivre contained a considerable number of the type represented in figures 40 and 41. It would be superfluous to offer any more descriptions or drawings, because in nearly all the Roman sites in the country, shoes of the same, or of slightly dif-

ferent form have been collected.   It is at all times necessary to remember, however, that the majority of the Roman

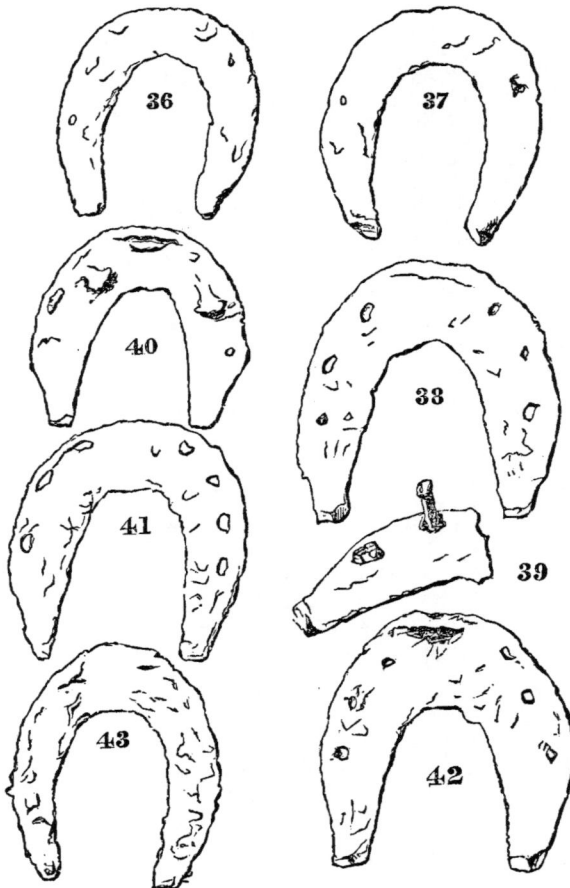

villas destroyed during the first invasion of the barbarians
have been subsequently more or less repaired to serve as
habitations, either by the Gallo-Romans, or by the Burgundians, when these last established themselves in the country.
We have already given numerous proofs of these restorations of the 4th and 5th centuries by the Burgundians,
and recovered many of the relics of these warriors of six

feet in height, still armed with their grooved " scramasacs," the pointed spur at the heels, and wearing great girdle-plates of iron damascened with silver. One of these " six-feet" people of the 5th century was laid in a tomb formed of large masses of tuff roughly chiselled, and near him were found the bones of a horse, which had pro bably been that of the giant, the shoes of which yet exist-ed; they had six oblong holes and were "fullered" (*à rainures*) (fig. 42). Not far from this many other graves, of the same or an earlier epoch, have furnished horse-shoes ; the one we give a drawing of is the smallest, the others are wider in metal, so as to cover the greater part of the sole. This is not an exceptional form, for we have a number of the same kind. In addition, these shoes differ but little from those of the Roman period, and show a continuation of the same manner of shoe-ing, with the slight modifications the farriers adopted according to circumstances. There are always shoes with six nails, sometimes fullered, but not undulated as in the first period. In the foundation of the church of Mou-tiers-Grand-Val, built in the 7th century, a similar shoe has been found (fig. 40). To the shoes of certain origin, we add another form which has also been admitted at divers epochs, though more rarely, and appears to in-dicate a mode of shoeing strange to the country. We give as a type of these shoes (fig. 44) a specimen found on the track of the ancient road from Aventicum to Augusta Rauracorum by Pierre Pertius, and in the valleys of the Byrse, between Laufon and Bâle. They are par-ticularly distinguished by the massive form of the calkins, which appear like a great protuberance a little in front of the extremities, which become sharp. The one repre-

sented is the thickest we have found; it was associated
with more than twenty others mixed up with some Ro

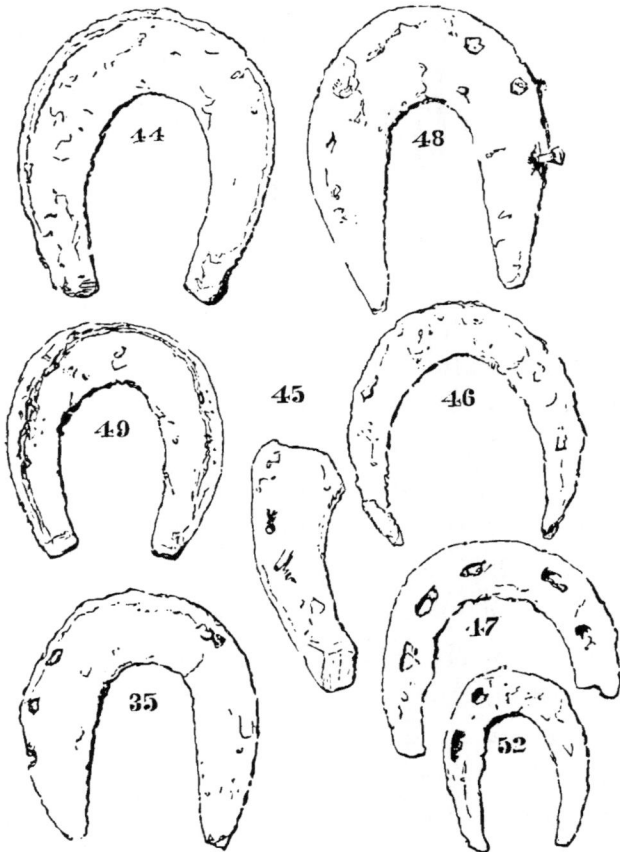

man remains and coins of the 4th century.   This variety
is found in the middle ages, in the ruins of various castles,
as that of Sogron (fig. 45); a circumstance which leads
us to think that they commence in the barbarian epoch,
and continue during the middle ages, not regularly or as
a generally adopted style, but rather as a foreign importation whose origin is unknown.

'Shoes really of the middle ages, and anterior to the

15th century, are characterized in those (figs. 45, 46, 47), from the Château of Sogron (8th to 15th century); and also those of Asuel and Vorbourg (figs. 48, 49). One of them is peculiar in having a very primitive toe-clip (*pinçon*), formed by the toe of the shoe being a little elongated and bent upwards (fig. 49); and another has the calkins inverted, or turning towards the heel of the foot (fig. 46). The specimen from Vorbourg (fig. 49) closely resembles that from Souboz (fig. 50); and yet the latter was found at such a great depth in a quarry, that the workmen believed the rock must have grown since it was deposited. But there can be little doubt that it was lost in the pasture on this part of the mountain traversed by a Roman road, and at a very remote date had slipped through a crevice in the rock.

'It has already been remarked that in the ruins of various castles, as elsewhere, shoes have been gathered like those of early times, but we have emitted doubts as to their employment at a later period. The shoe from the Château of Asuel weighs 425 grammes, and it has six nail-holes like those of the 12th century, mentioned in the *Roman du Renard* (edit. Willems, p. 241), when the cunning fox engaged the wolf Isangrin to read, under the feet of a mare, on what conditions she would surrender the flesh of her foal! This description of shoe, stronger in metal and of similar dimensions, appears to characterize the horses of the middle ages, which had to carry heavy caparisons of iron and riders covered with weighty armour. They sometimes offer an important indication, consisting in the mark of the farrier who forged them. This is very distinctly seen on the shoe from Asuel, and on those of Vorbourg and Sogron. That from Asuel reminds us of

the time when the last owner of that place fought for
Charles le Téméraire against the Swiss and their allies.
The size of the shoes of these various epochs is not the
only thing to consider in the determination of the species,
for the dimensions must necessarily have varied a little.
Nevertheless, it is very remarkable that those of the first
period scarcely vary, and they might be confounded with
the shoes of mules and asses found sometimes with the
more noble steed.   Certain small light shoes, bearing the
characteristics just described for each epoch, may have
belonged to some palfrey or hackney ridden by a young
Gaul or Gallo-Roman, as well as to the steed of the fiery
Châtelaine of the middle ages.

'This notice of the horse-shoes which have been worn
in the Jura in ancient times is far from being complete;
and it has no other merit than furnishing specimens of
ascertained origin, and offering as closely as possible
types rather than exceptions, for we have been careful to
choose those for our drawings which represent the most
characteristic and usual forms.'

In Belgium, shoes of this ancient type have also been
discovered.   In making a road at Jodoigne, in a cutting
at a certain depth from the surface, some Roman pottery
and four of these plates were discovered in a bronze vase.
They were described by M. Schayes, who remarks: 'The
horse-shoes were, like the pottery, in perfect preservation.
I believe them to be of Roman origin.   They are less
regular in form than our modern shoes, and are no
more than from 4 to $4\frac{1}{4}$ inches long, and $3\frac{3}{4}$ and 4
inches wide.   The vessel containing these was supposed to
be no older than the 15th century, and it was surmised

that the articles had been put into it from some tomb and again buried. The previous year bones had been found in the place in which this collection was discovered.'[1] No drawings accompany the description.

In the Royal Museum of Antiquities at Brussels is a shoe, found in 1863, during excavations carried on at Wundrez-lez-Binche, Hainault. With it were several antiquities, and notably a bronze coin of Faustina (A.D. 175). Four inches in length and width, this specimen of farriery (fig. 53) has only four nail-holes, and though broad in the cover, is yet thin and light, and unprovided with calks.[1] The outer border is even, the holes quadrilateral and well placed.

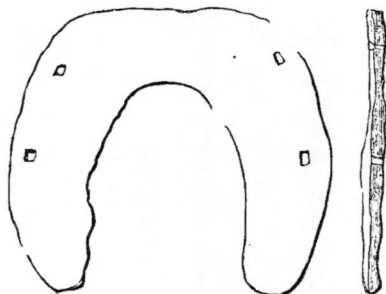

fig 53

A very interesting discovery was made in 1848, during mining operations at Lede, a village near Alost, Eastern Flanders. Three shoes were found along with relics which authorities have stated to be Frankish, and to belong to about the 6th century. One of these relics is an earthenware vase (fig. 54), which certainly bears a striking likeness to one type of that ware pertaining to that age and country. The first

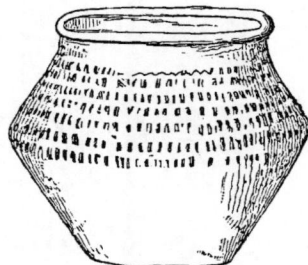

fig. 54

horse-shoe we might designate a Romano-Frankish speci-

---

[1] Bulletin de l'Académie des Sciences de Belgique, vol. xiii. p. 193.

men, from its resemblance to those we have named Gaulish
and Gallo-Roman (fig. 55). It has the usual irregular

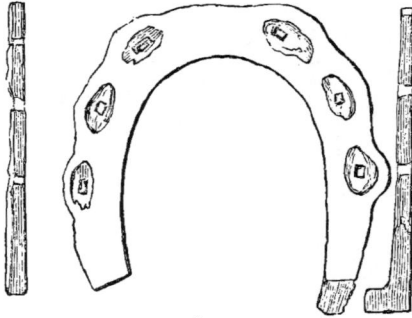

fig 55

outer border, the six
peculiar nail-sockets,
only one calkin, and
is light in form. It
measures four inches
in length and width.

The second exam
ple has a more modern
appearance; has curi-
ously shaped calkins on both heels, an even border,
and six quadrilateral nail-holes. It is a little larger
than the first specimen, and it will be seen from a
side view that it bends up towards the heels of the foot
(fig. 56). The third shoe is of the same width, but an

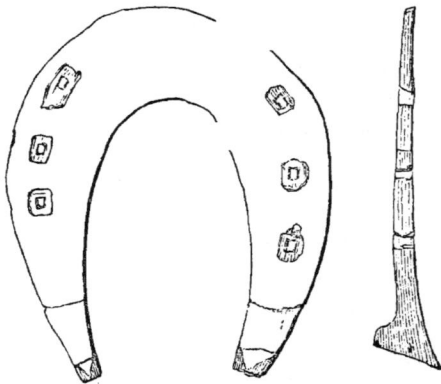

fig. 56

inch longer than the
last, and is particularly
striking from its being
coarsely grooved, hav-
ing calkins which are
strong exaggerations of
those already described,
and being greatly curv-
ed towards the heel and
toe, so that the mid-
dle of the shoe is on the
same level with the ground face of the calk (fig. 57). In
this respect it bears a marked resemblance to the *ajusted*
shoe introduced by Bourgelat in the last century. It is
somewhat remarkable to find these three types of shoes

in the same place, along with Frankish remains, though neither of them differ from those described by M. Quiquerez. All these specimens are now in the Royal Museum of Antiquities, Arms, and Artillery, at Brussels, to the obliging curator

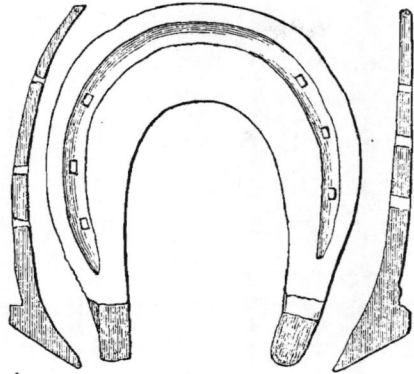

fig. 57

of which I am indebted for information relative to them.

In Germany, we find the same traces of antique shoes as are discovered in France, Switzerland, and Belgium. The Germans, like the Celts, represent one of the most remarkable races of early times ; and though their history does not extend so far back as that of the Celtæ, yet the ancient writers made very little distinction between them, and when they first encountered them found they were also in possession of iron. The Cimbri or Germans, then, wore mail armour, had polished white shields, two-edged javelins, and large iron swords. They were also to some extent a horse-loving people ; and when they fought with Marius they numbered 15,000 cavalry magnificently mounted. Each had a fine lofty helmet, and bore upon it the head of some savage beast, with its mouth gaping wide ; an iron cuirass covered his body, and he carried a long lance or halberd in his hand. The Teucteri, a tribe on the banks of the Rhine, were famous for the discipline of their cavalry. Their ancestors, in the early ages of tradition, established this force, and it was maintained by posterity. Horsemanship was the sport of their children, the emulation of their youth, and the exercise in which they persevered to old age. Horses were bequeathed along with the domestics, the household gods, and the rights of inheritance, and unlike other things, they did not go to the eldest, but to the bravest and most warlike child.[1]

Their horses were neither remarkable for beauty or swiftness, nor were they taught the various evolutions practised by the Romans. The cavalry either bore straight before them, or wheeled once to the right in so compact a body that none were left behind. 'Who are braver than the Germans?' asks Seneca,[2] 'who more impetuous in the charge? who fonder of arms, in the use of which they are born and nourished, which are their only care? who more inured to hardships, insomuch that for the most part they provide no covering for their bodies—no retreat against the perpetual severity of the climate?' Cæsar tells us that they passed their whole lives in hunting and military exercises.[3] The chief's companions or select followers required from him 'the warlike steed and the bloody and conquering spear.' Their presents from neighbouring nations were most valued when they consisted of fine horses, heavy armour, rich housings, and gold chains.

The Suevi had, according to Cæsar, poor and ill-shaped horses. Yet they must have proved very efficient, for the Suevi, 'in cavalry actions, frequently leap from their

[1] *Tacitus,* cap. 32.   [2] On *Anger,* i. 11.
Bell. *Gall.* vi. 21.

horses and fight on foot, and train their horses to stand still in the very spot on which they leave them, to which they retreat with great activity when there is occasion; nor, according to their practice, is anything regarded as more unseemly or more unmanly than to use housings. Accordingly, they have the courage, though they be themselves but few, to advance against any number whatever of horse mounted with housings.' [1]

In the last century, shoes were dug out of graves, which were to all appearance pre-Roman. One of these shoes has been described as having the catches or calkins projecting in a peculiar manner upwards instead of downwards, as if to grasp the hoof; but it is not stated whether there were also nail-holes. [2]

Many years ago, veterinary surgeon Plank [3] mentioned finding shoes in Bavaria, which, from their antique form and the situation they occupied when discovered, he believed to have been worn by Roman cavalry horses. Schaum also speaks of ancient shoes as being found in his district. [4] At Willerode (Mansfelder Gebirgskreise), Rosenkranz [5] speaks of a variety of old iron work being found in grubbing up a forest called Wolfshagen. This consisted of rusty spikes, *unusually large horse-shoes* (ungewöhnlich grosse Hufeisen), a battle-axe, and a kind of sharp knife, made of flint, which he thought might be a sacrificial knife.

[1] Bell. Gal. iv. 2.
[2] *Beckmann.* Beschreibung der Mark Brandenburgh. Berlin, 1751. *Arnkiel.* Heidnische Alterthümer.
[3] Veterinärtopographie von Baiern, p. 18.
[4] Alterith. S. von Brauenfels, S. 39.
[5] Neue Zeitschrift. Halle, 1832. Band 1. Heft 2.

Klemm[1] remarks: 'The horse must have been equally valuable to the war-loving German as the intelligent and trusty hound was to the huntsman. The German horsemen were respected by the Romans. They displayed great affection for their steeds and had them under excellent control, although Tacitus does not praise the horses for either their beauty or speed. The Germans had saddles and horse-shoes; the latter are often found in the soil of the fatherland. They indicate a small race of horses then in existence. The horse-bones dug up by Dr Wagner were also small.'

Arnkiel,[2] speaking of the supposed horse-shoe found in Childeric's grave, notices that the most ancient shoes discovered 'are small and thin, very much oxydized, and have neither toe-pieces (griff) nor toe-clips, but small calkins at the heel, and the nail-holes are near the centre of the shoe.'

Ludwig Lindenschmidt,[3] who has so ably, and almost exhaustively, explored the ancient grave-mounds of Sigmaringen and its vicinity, is puzzled at the presence of single horse-shoes in graves, without the bones of horses, spurs, or equipment. 'They form one of the unsolved mysteries of the graves, and are in no way accounted for

[1] Handbuch der Germanischen Alterthumskunde, p. 133. Dresden, 1836.

[2] Cimb. Heidenrel. p. 164.

I much regret that I have been unable to refer to a paper by S. D. Schmidt on what were called *Swedish* horse-shoes: 'Ueber Sogenannte Schwedenhufeisen, mit Nachtr. v. Prof. Renner,' in Jena Variscia, iii. 61.

[3] Die Vaterländischen Alterthümer der Fürstlich Hohenzoller'schen Sammlungen zu Sigmaringen. Mainz, 1860.

by the supposition that they may be intended as a sign
of the former occupation of the deceased—as, for example, that of a smith. The Royal Museum contains
several such single horse-shoes, discovered in graves, all
of different kinds, and from different places. These objects
buried in the tomb seem rather to bear some relation to
symbols of old heathen superstitions—such as the practice
of nailing a horse-shoe on the threshold of the door, which
yet lingers in some places. Certainly the subject requires
further investigation and explanation.' The very old grave-
mounds of Gauselfingen yielded many primitive curiosities,
such as celts, arm and finger-rings, glass beads, &c., of
the Celtic or early German people. 'The third grave-
mound contained two horse-shoes (figs. 58, 59), an iron

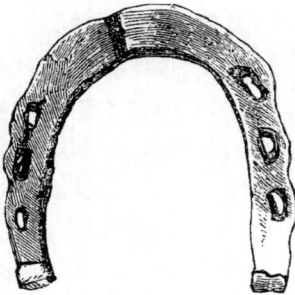 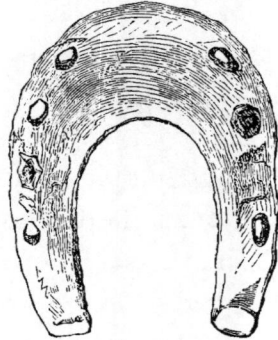

fig 58   fig 59

arrow-head, a fine iron dagger, the handle of which was
much damaged. Beside these lay the remains of a
leathern girdle, ornamented with metal knobs.'

In the Grand-Duchy of Luxemberg, there are remains of what is known to archæologists as the Roman
camp of Dalheim, which for many centuries have consisted in nothing more than substructures, though
everything connected with them demonstrates that they

13

constitute the *débris* of one of the most considerable establishments the Romans founded in this region. Many ancient thoroughfares, still known to the peasantry as *pagan roads*, abut on these ruins. The archæologists, from various proofs, but chiefly those derived from the presence of coins, attribute the final destruction of this important villa to the barbarian hordes under Attila, about A.D. 450. It has proved particularly rich in antiquities, which have been referred to the interval between Augustus and the fall of the Roman empire, and for many years excavations on its site have been carried out with great care.

In 1851, this camp commenced to be intersected by a new public road, and the excavations instituted by the Board of Public Works were placed under the direction and surveillance of the Archæological Society of the Grand-Duchy. Among other objects, evidently Roman, recovered from these remains, were four horse-shoes of a comparatively modern form—that is, more of the Burgundian than the Gaulish or Celtic shape. They were not all of the same dimensions. Figures 60 and 61, de-

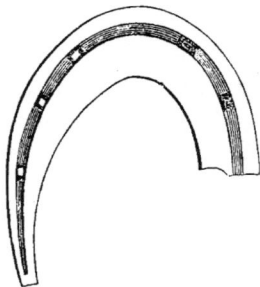

fig 60

lineated by M. Fischer, a veterinary surgeon of Cessingen,[1] represent the smallest and largest of the four. The former is about the usual size of the early period to which they are supposed to belong, but the latter is large. All had been worn, and bent nails yet remained in the holes. They were very much cor-

[1] *Annales de Méd. Vétérinaire,* p. 28. Bruxelles, 1853.

roded, and the two smallest were broken. The 'Burgundian' groove was present in the four specimens, and
was continued from one extremity to the other. This
mode of *fullering* is not now practised in this part of
Europe. The least of these articles appears to have
had six holes and no calkins ; but M. Fischer represents
the largest as furnished with *nine*
apertures, and two square, well-
formed calkins. M. Namur, the
archæologist who described the
antiquities found in the camp,
asserts that they each had *eight*
holes.[1] In 1852-3, the excavations being continued, a small
shoe of the same shape was
found, but it had only *four* nail-

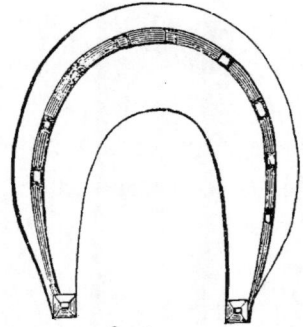

fig. 61

holes ;[2] and in 1854-5, the same antiquarian rescued several
more, but they did not, it appears, differ from the others.
M. Namur gives no drawings or descriptions of them, but
merely states that they were of the ordinary form, and
were found associated with Roman *reliquæ* of various
kinds and dates.

It may be noted that these specimens of antique shoes
bear much resemblance to shoes found in various parts of
Würtemberg, which Grosz figures, and which will be
alluded to presently. He thought they belonged to the
middle ages.

It is also somewhat remarkable, that at Steinfurt, in

[1] Publications de la Soc. pour la Recherche et la Conservation de
Monuments, etc., vol. vii. p. 185. Luxembourg, 1852.
[2] Ibid. vol. ix.

the same Duchy of Luxemberg, Engling [1] found two
iron plates which had been horse-shoes, and he figures
them among Roman urns and vases from this antique
locality, believing them to be Roman.   Each shoe possesses six nail-holes, and has the *rainure* circling from
heel to heel.   In shape they are not very unlike those
from Dalheim (and which are now in the Archæological
Museum of Luxemberg).   They are described as so
remarkably small that they were surmised to have been
worn by mules; but, from their form, they were undoubtedly intended for the small indigenous horse (figs.
62, 63).   This grooved shoe is perfectly distinct from

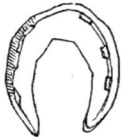 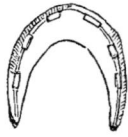

that of the Gauls or Celts, and is
certainly a great advance in workmanship.   The rough, bulging
border gives place to an uniform
one; and the groove, as well as

fig 62   fig 63

the nail-holes and general form of the shoe, evidence skilful
manufacture.   From these discoveries, we are led to believe that the powerful equestrian nation of the Suevi,
as well as the German tribe which in after-times constituted the Burgundi, shod their horses immediately
after, if not before, the Christian era.   How they acquired
the art we know not; but it is well to remember that, in
the 3rd century B.C., the Gauls passed along the line of
the Danube as conquerors, and in their course left colonies
among the Suevi, who, even in the time of Tacitus, still
spoke the Gaulish tongue; [2] and also that it was often

[1] Le Tombeau de Childeric I., p. 158.
[2] *Tacitus,* lib. xliii.

the Suevian cavalry, under Ariovistus, that the Sequani either fought with or against, in the wars between them and the Ædui or Romans.

Colonel Smith, in noticing the universality of horse-shoeing, says for Germany : 'We have seen it sculptured in bas-relief with a Runic inscription certainly as old as the 9th century, accompanying a figure of Ostar, upon a stone found on the Hohenstein, near the Druden altar in Westphalia, a place of Pagan worship that was destroyed by the Franks in the wars of Charlemagne. Had the horse-shoe been invented in that age, it could not already have become an object of mysterious adaptation in the religion of barbarians, which was on the wane at least a century earlier.'[1]

Grosz[2] mentions that, in the years 1730, 1744, 1761, and 1820, a somewhat large number of horse-shoes was found at certain places in Bavaria, during excavations. Some of them were very deeply buried, and thickly covered with rust. Though he does not altogether coincide in the views of several antiquarians as to the antiquity of these objects, yet his remarks are not without interest, particularly as he describes the different varieties which have been noted in Germany. 'The horse-shoes which have come down to us from remote periods, having been found in several parts of the country at various depths, show in general three essential varieties.

---

[1] Op. cit., p. 131. The *horse-shoe arch* occurs frequently as a figure on the sculptured stones left by the Celts, and which are found in England, Scotland, and elsewhere.

[2] Lehr- und Handbuch der Hufbeschlagskunst. Stuttgart, 1861.

'The most numerous is that shown in figure 64.   At

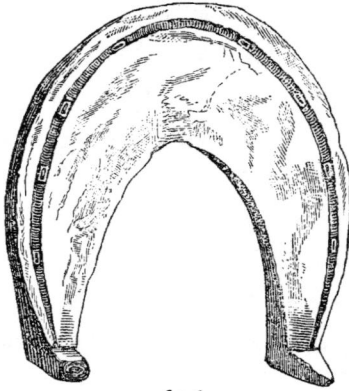

fig. 64

the toe it is more than twice
as broad as at the heel, but
it is thinner throughout than
a German shoe of now-a-
days.   All shoes of this kind
are furnished with calks at
the heels, and sometimes at
the toes, some of which have
been welded on after the
shoe was made, and others
formed from the shoe itself.   The greater number have a
groove, in which there are generally eight nail-holes.   The
seat of the shoe is flat.   The heads of the nails are sometimes narrow and sometimes broad, and project beyond
the shoe.   This variety of shoe is of several sizes, and no
difference can be perceived between those of the fore and
hind feet.   According to tradition, it has been assumed
that these broad shoes dug up in certain places were
brought into the country by foreign armies, particularly
by the Swedes (1632-48); but if one considers that not
quite a hundred years ago there were no high roads in the
country, and that horses were used mostly on badly-con-
structed paths, it is then probable that with us such a
broad shoe was customary and necessary for special protection to the hoof.   Still less should it be assumed that these
shoes, as some would wish us to believe, were introduced
by Roman armies; for the Romans have been expelled
Germany since the 3rd century, and it might well be asked
whether iron would remain so long in the ground (1500
years) without becoming entirely destroyed by rust.

Shoes of the second type, as shown in figure 65, are not
unfrequently found in the
neighbourhood of Stuttgart.
They are of medium size,
broad at the toe, with six or
eight nail-holes, and partly
grooved for the nail-holes.
The sole is in some instances
a little hollowed out towards
the inner circumference ; the
calks are high, square, and

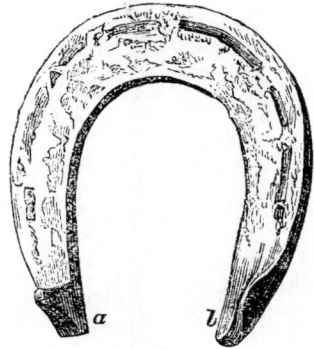

fig. 65

placed towards the ends of the branches, something like
slipper-heels (*Pantoffelstollen*), cut off obliquely, and in
some very much prolonged. Some of these shoes have
only one calk (*a*), which is long and pointed, while the
other heel of the shoe (*b*), has merely an edge bent downward to match it. This shoe has a seat (*richtung*, curve to
fit the foot) quite peculiar, the heel extremity being quite
thin and tapering, and curving up towards the back part of
the foot (fig. 66,*a*). The Oriental and Arab shoes have the
same bend given to them
even in the present day.
Since these articles correspond with the descrip-
tion of Spanish shoes
both in their form and
curve, and since Stuttgart

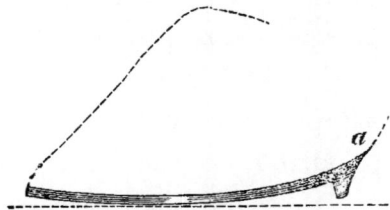

fig 66

was alternately besieged and occupied by the Spaniards
in the years 1546 to 1551, and in 1638, it may
be assumed with reasonable certainty that they are of
Spanish origin.'

'Figure 67 exemplifies a form of shoe of somewhat rarer occurrence. The specimens found are generally small, cer tainly never larger than mid dle size; they are narrow throughout, some being grooved and furnished with six or eight nail-holes; opposite to which the outside edge bulges a little. Instead of having calks, the heel-ends of

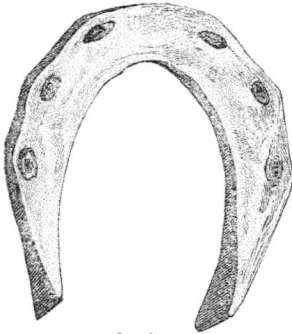

fig 67

the shoes become gradually narrower and thicker towards the extremities. The nail-heads are wedge or chisel-shaped, and project beyond the face of the shoe. Judging from the size and shape of these objects, and from the character of the nail-heads, they appear to have served as winter shoes for riding-horses, and without doubt were introduced by foreign cavalry. (From the end of the 13th to the close of the 18th century, Stuttgart and its vicinity was often visited by foreign troops, such as Im perialists, French, Spaniards, and Swedes.) These shoes are so oxidized and incrusted that they may well be looked upon as several hundred years old.

'Besides the horse-shoes just described, antique shoes of peculiar shapes and different construction have been found here and there in several places in and outside Würtemberg; so that it is evident that at the period to which they belong, the art of shoeing was in a very primi tive condition. Some few examples are provided with a groove, while others have long quadrangular nail-holes, often with oval countersinking; some, again, are furnished

with heel and toe calks of unusual shape, others are plane,
but, at the same time, as a rule, they are of exceedingly
coarse workmanship : a fact which may still be perceived
despite the ravages made by rust.   . Universal as the
practice of shoeing is at the present day, there are yet
places, such as North Germany, Hungary, and others,
where it is not always necessary, and where horses are
seldom shod, except on the fore-feet, or only in winter ;
others, on the contrary, as the horses of the rich, being
shod merely as a kind of luxury on all four feet.'

The 'ajusted' or curved antique shoes are peculiar to
Germany, it would appear. They have not been found in
France, so far as I am aware; neither, as we will see hereafter,
have they been met with in this country. It will be remembered that two specimens were found in Belgium. They
seem to be generally grooved, and have peculiar calkins.
Grosz's last illustration gives us the primitive undulating-
bordered shoe.

We have seen from M. Quiquerez's report, that the
earliest traces of grooved or 'fullered' shoes are found
with remains of the Burgundi, and constitute a new and
characteristic form. This ancient people—one of the
principal branches of the Vandals, originally inhabiting
the country between the Oder and Vistula—have left
numerous traces of their passage through, and sojourn in,
various regions of Switzerland and Gaul in the 4th and
subsequent centuries. They established themselves to
the west of the Jura, about the same time that the Goths
entered Aquitaine,[1] and appear to have been, from the
remotest times, distinguished from the other German

---

[1] *Aug. Thierry.* Lettres sur l'Hist. de France, vi.

tribes by living together in villages or *burgen* (from whence their name); which caused them to be looked down upon by the Teutonic race, and accused of degeneracy, in leading a life more adapted for the business of blacksmith or carpenter than that of a soldier. Sidonius Apollinaris, nevertheless, speaks of them as an army of giants;[1] and it appears certain that they were not only good artisans, but also brave warriors, in the intervals of peace earning a sufficient livelihood by their handicrafts; and that at the period of their residence among the ruined Gallo-Roman villas they shod their horses' feet with iron shoes. The discovery, in the tombs of these warriors, of the 'scramasax'—a large cutlass, sharpened only on one edge, and a characteristic weapon of the ancient Germans, with knives belonging to the same period (between the 4th and 5th centuries), all having long deep grooves on both sides corresponding with that in their horse-shoes—indicates that with the Burgundians, as with the Gauls and Celts, the same individual was at once armourer and farrier. The earliest tradition we have of this people, and which belongs to the period preceding their invasion of Gaul, would lead us to believe that they were skilled horsemen and workers in metals. 'The dwarf Regin fled from the Burgundians to the court of the Frankish king Hialprek (Chilpéric), who reigned on the banks of the Rhine, and there he undertook the duties of 'maréchal' (master of the horse and farrier). At this time he met the young Sigurd, son of King Sigmund, a descendant of Odin, who had miraculously escaped from the murderers of his father. The

[1] Carmen xii. apud Scrip. Franc., i. 811.

dwarf directed the education of this prince, and spoke to him of the wonderful treasure of the Nibelungen, raising in him the desire to carry it off to Tafnir. He forged for him the sword 'Gram,' the blade of which was so sharp, that, when plunged in the Rhine, it cut in two a lock of wool carried against it by the current. He also attended to the incomparable steed 'Grani.'[1] This skill in fabricating arms, and in the management of the horse, appears to have been a particular feature in the history of this people. In the middle ages, so highly were the services of the farrier esteemed, that at the court of the Dukes of Burgundy, on Saint Eloy's day, a piece of silver plate was given to the individual who shod the ducal horses.[2]

St Eloy, Eligius, or Euloge, was Bishop of Noyon in the 7th or 8th century, and by some means or other became the patron saint of farriers, and a gentle name to swear by in the days of Chaucer, who, in his 'Canterbury Pilgrims,' speaks of the 'Nonne'

> 'That of hir smiling was full simple and coy;
> Hir greatest othe n'as but by Seint Eloy.'

The prioress's very tender oath, which custom of swearing was not at all an indelicate one for ladies, even for some centuries after Chaucer's time, has excited much contention among the commentators of the old poet. Warton declares that St Loy (the form in which the word appears in all the manuscripts) means, St Lewis: but in Sir David Lyndesay's writings St Eloy appears as an independent personage, in connection with horses or horsemanship, in

---

[1] *A. Reville.* Etude sur l'Epopée des Nibelungen.
[2] *E. Houel.* Hist. du Cheval chez tous les Peuples.

the way he occurs in the above and other traditions relating to horses or farriery. Lyndesay says:

> ' Saint Eloy, he doth stoutly stand,
> Ane new horseshoe in his hand.'

And again:

> ' Some makis offering to Saint Eloy,
> That he their horse may well convoy.'

Horsemen also appear to have sworn by the good bishop; for Chaucer makes the carter in the 'Friar's Tale,' when he had been assisted out of the mud into which his horses and cart had stuck fast, to thank his assistants by the best animal in his team, and to exclaim:

> ' That was well twight (pulled) my owen Liard boy,
> I pray God save thy body, and Saint Eloy.'

The saint was supposed to work great miracles among diseased animals. We will have more to say about him, however, at a later period.

So far as I am able to ascertain, we have no *written* evidence to show that the Germans shod their horses before A.D. 1185. According to Anton,[1] about that time mention is made of the shoeing of two horses (II. *equorum ferramenta*, Kindliger). In some old German records, given on the authority of Shopflin, there is a notice that the smith was obliged to deliver sixteen horse-shoes and the necessary nails. And in another writing (Sachsen Spiegel), it is ordered that 'the horses of messengers (die Pferde der Boten) shall only be shod on the fore-feet.'

---

[1] *Geschichte der Teutschen Landwirthschaft von den Ältesten Zeiten bis zu Ende des Funfzehnten Jahrhunderts*, p. 37. Gorlitz, 1802.

Grosz[1] says that the shoeing of two horses is noticed in a Westphalian record of 1085.

In the year 1336, we find the Abbot of Waltersdorf, in Bavaria, making the following contract with his smith concerning the work to be accomplished, and its payment. ' He (the smith) is to make for his (the Abbot's) riding-horse three new steeled shoes (*gestaehlte eisen*) for two pence ; and to repair three old ones for one penny. For two or three nails to fasten them, he is to receive nothing . . . . . and the work above stated is to be done with the Abbot's iron,' &c.

In 1400, a tax was fixed at Stuttgard for smith's work, and among other items, ' 6 heller (halfpennies or farthings) was to be paid for forging a new shoe.'[2]

Horses appear to have been early employed by the Germans to draw carriages or carry litters, for it is recorded that in the campaign of Arnulph or Arnold, Emperor of Germany, in Upper Italy, in 896, when returning across the Alps, a disease broke out among his horses which was so fatal, that, ' contrary to custom, oxen were employed to draw the litters instead.'[3] The use of horses in draught or carriage would have been very limited for Alpine travelling had they not been shod.

In Germany, as elsewhere at this early period, the blacksmith held a good position, if we may judge by the price of his *wehr-geld*, or ' blood-money.' The law of Gondebaud or Gombette, the most ancient of the barbarian codes, makes it manifest that the life of a smith

---

[1] Op. cit., p. 8.   [2] Ibid., p. 9.
[3] *Annales Fuldens.* Pertz M., i. p. 411.

was valued at five times the amount of a labourer or shepherd, and equal to that for the murder of a Roman slave belonging to the king.[1] The German and Salic laws also show that the duty of the 'maréchal' or 'mariscalcus' was to attend to twelve horses.   'Si mariscalcus, qui super xii. caballos est, occiditur,' &c.[2]

From the Rhenish provinces as far as Russia, what is termed the German shoe is in use.   This is the model figured by Quiquerez, and which is flat on both sides, and with the fuller or groove for the nail-heads so far from the edge of the shoe, as to make the nail-holes very *coarse*.   Immense calkins, and even toe-pieces of various shapes, are as much in vogue with the Germans as they are with the waggoners of Manchester, Liverpool, and other large cities in England and Scotland.

The Dutch and Russian shoes are coarse imitations of the German ones.

For Scandinavia, I am not aware of any discoveries which would show that this handicraft was practised at a very early period.   If we are to give credence to the historians, archæologists, and anthropologists of that country, the Celtæ inhabited this region of the north ; and if they did so, they doubtless preserved the same arts and usages as their nation in other parts of Europe.   The 'Duergars were their traditional workers in metals ; and these fabricated steel and iron implements in secret caves.   I can find but little mention of shoes, however, though doubtless these cunning workmen armed the hoofs as well as the bodies of the warriors, who were essentially an equestrian race.

[1] *Martin.*   Op. cit., i. p. 437.   [2] Lex Alemannor.   Lex Salica.

The high antiquity of the iron-worker's art is made apparent in the Voluspa, a poem containing the oldest traditions of the Northmen yet discovered, and which is an outline of the earliest Northern mythology. We are told how—

> The *Asæ* met on the fields of Ida,
> And framed their images and temples.
> They placed their furnaces. They created money.
> They made tongs and iron tools.

At a later period, to be a proficient in metallurgical operations was the ambition of princes. Harold, for example, in the poem entitled his 'Complaint,' when describing his address as a warrior, relates: 'I am master of nine accomplishments. I play at chess; I know how to engrave Runic letters; I am apt at my book, *and I know to handle the tools of a smith ;* I traverse the snow on skates of wood; I excel in shooting with the bow, and in managing the oar; I sing to the harp, and compose verses.'[1]

From the Sagas and the history of this region, it is evident that in Sweden, Norway, and Denmark horses were shod at an early period. At first only the rich and noble, perhaps, resorted to the use of shoes for their steeds, and some of these only for display, others when they had to travel on hard roads or during frosty weather. When used for agriculture, the horses may have been deprived of these defences.

Col. Smith states that horse-shoes were in use in Sweden before the Norman conquest of England, since the figure of one is struck on a Swedish coin without

---

[1] *Mallet.* Introduction à l'Histoire de Danemarc. London, 1770.

inscription, and therefore older than the use of Runic letters on medals.

In the eleventh century, shoes appear to have been in general use, for it is recorded that Oluf Kyrre, the first Norwegian king, caused those who sought his court to shoe their horses with golden shoes.

Recent discoveries in the peat-mosses of Thorsbjerg and Nydam in Sleswig have exposed remains of men and horses, supposed to have found their way there in the ' early iron period of the third and fourth centuries ;' but no shoes were found, though there were bridles, spurs, and nose-pieces to protect the horse's nose. Skulls and bones of horses, sometimes almost complete skeletons, were noted, and the state in which they were found is curious. ' Near a tolerably complete skeleton of a horse, were found, besides shield-boards, shafts of lances, and other wooden objects, several beads, two iron bits, several metal mountings for shields, an iron spear-head, a whetstone, several arrow-heads, an awl of iron, and a Roman silver denarius. Not far from it were two skulls and other remains of horses, and near them some iron-bits. The skulls of horses, which, just as those last mentioned, appeared to have been deposited without the other parts of the animals, had still their bits in their mouths, one of the bits being incomplete and evidently deposited in that state. And if there could still be any doubt as to the skeletons being contemporaneous with the antiquities, it must yield to the fact that several of the skulls have been exposed to a similarly violent and inexplicable ill-treatment as the vast majority of the other objects deposited.' The bones were examined by Professor Steenstrap, the Director of the Museum of Natural History of Copenhagen, who pronounced them to have been the remains of three stallions of middle size. But the strangest thing is, that the skulls show the marks of heavy sword-cuts, which we are told could not have been inflicted while the ánimal was alive. Other portions showed that the horses had been pierced with arrows and javelins, while some of the bones had been gnawed by wolves or large dogs. There is here clearly something more than the mere death of the horse in battle. The enemy in such a case would never have taken the trouble to hew away at the skull, ' lying,' we are told, ' on the ground before him,' and that, Professor Steenstrap is inclined to think, when the lower jaw had been separated from the upper, and when the bones were no longer covered with flesh. All this leads us irresistibly to think of some sacrificial ceremony, and of the famous proscription of horse-flesh by the Christian missionaries. Horse-flesh must have been held to be an unchristian diet only because it was in some way connected with the idolatrous worship of the Northmen; the Mosaic prohibition could not have been urged by men who doubtless ate hogs, hares, and eels, without scruple. But then Professor Steenstrap tells us, that no ' such marks have been discovered on the horse-bones from Nydam as could indicate a severance of the limbs, or that the flesh had been eaten." [1] These appear to have been war-horses, and possibly at this time shoes may not have been worn at all frequently. We have seen that in France and Germany, long after shoeing was known, it was not universally practised.

[1] Denmark in the Early Iron Age, by Conrad Engelheart.—*Saturday Review*, Oct. 13, 1866.

CHAPTER V.

AT what period Eastern nations first began to apply an iron defence to their horses' feet, and attach it by nails, it is impossible to fix with certainty. An anonymous writer in the United Service Magazine for 1849, quotes the form of the most ancient Asiatic horse-shoe as being exemplified in the brand-mark of a renowned breed of Circassian or Abassian horses, known by the name of

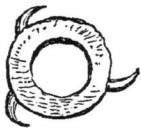

fig. 68

Shalokh. 'The shape is perfectly circular, and instead of being fastened on by means of nails driven through the corneous portion of the hoof, it is secured by three clamps (fig. 68), that appear to have been closed on the outside, or on the ascending surface. Of the antiquity of this form of shoe there is no possibility of judging, because the exact counterpart of it existed already at the period when the Ionian Greeks had established fixed symbols as types of their cities and communities. It occurs on the coins of Lycia, and is known to numismatists by the name of Triquetra (fig. 69). If there

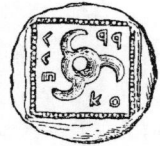

fig. 69

be any difference, it is in a row of points on the Lycian type, as if the shoe had been perforated with holes for small nails (fig. 70); and what makes the selection of this object for a symbol of the region in question the more remarkable is, that, in remote antiquity, it was there Celtic breeders are reported to have first commenced their trade in mules. The horseshoes of early historians, since they do not

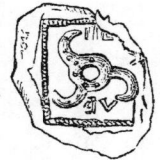

fig. 70

mention farriers, appear to have been of this Lycian form, or were not fastened with nails driven through the horny hoof. It is difficult to escape an admission that horse-shoes of this kind are as old as the Ionian establishments in Asia Minor, unless by denying that neither the Circassian brand-mark nor the Triquetra of Lycia represent them; a conclusion which at least is totally at variance with the denomination of the mark by which the Kabardian breed is known, time out of mind. . . . The round shoe of the old Arabian method is evidentiy a modification of the Circassian or Lycian, the outside clamps being omitted, and nail-holes substituted.

That the Arabs of the Hegira (A.D. 622), or within a generation later, shod their horses, is plain, if we believe the received opinion that the iron-work on the summit of

14 *

the standard of Hosein, at Ardbeil, was made from a horse-shoe belonging to Abbas, uncle of Mohammed, by order of his daughter Fatima. " It was brought," says the legend, " from Arabia by Scheik Sed Reddeen, son of the holy Scheik Sofi, who was son of another holy villager, after the manner of the Moslem!" If the intention had been to advance a mere falsehood, it is to be wondered that Fatima, or the Prophet himself, should not have furnished a sacred shoe of one of the celebrated mares, from which sprung so many of the first breeds of Arabia, according to the assertions of devout Moslems. A horse-shoe most likely it was,' adds this writer, ' but how an uncle of Mohammed should possess horses when the Bein Koreish, as a tribe, were without, and the Prophet himself in the beginning of his career had only three, is quite another question.'

It appears very unlikely that such an article as that shown in the Circassian brand-mark could ever have been employed as a shoe, or fixed to the hoof by the three clamps indicated above ; but to show that the Lycian triquetra could not be intended to represent a horse-shoe, I have copied in figures 68, 69, 70, and 71, this and similar impressions of coins. Figure 69 is the plain triquetra, from the original in the British Museum, and resembling Col. Smith's (who is, I believe, the author of the article just quoted from) Circassian shoe, in having no dots or points ; 70 is the triquetra that the writer refers to ; the original is in the Bibliothèque at Paris, but a drawing of it is given in Sir Charles Fellows' work on the Coins of Lycia.[1]   It will be seen that the points could not

[1] Coins of Ancient Lycia before the Reign of Alexander.   London,

correspond to holes for small nails, wherewith to attach
a shoe to a hoof, as they extend along the clamp which
Col. Smith says was employed to grasp the front of the
hoof. Fellows also gives a copy (No. 30) of a four-
limbed figure belonging to this class (fig. 71), the original

being in the British Museum, and which
could never be meant to represent a shoe.
Sir Charles Fellows does not attempt to
explain the origin or import of the triquetra, and it would certainly require a lively
imagination to associate it in any way with horse-shoes.

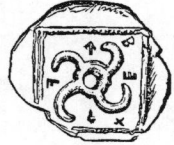

fig. 71

On the contrary, a very frequent device on the ancient coins
of Pamphylia is three human legs, arranged like the hooks
on the triquetra, and the same as borne by the currency
of the Isle of Man. Figure 72 is a copy of an ancient

coin in the British Museum, which has
neither prongs nor men's legs, but cocks'
heads! Surely there is nothing here to
offer the remotest conjecture as to the
origin of Eastern shoeing!

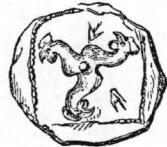

fig. 72

Col. Smith asserts that 'there are indeed ancient
Tartar horse-shoes of a circular form, apparently with
only three nails or fasteners to the outside of the hoof;'[1]
but we may be pardoned for doubting the correctness of
this statement.

That shoeing was known among the Arabs as early as
the days of Mohammed, appears certain. In the chapter

1855. Fig. 25. I am greatly indebted to Mr *A.* T. Murray of the
British Museum, for tracings and impressions of these interesting and
rare coins.

[1] The Natural History of Horses, p. 130.

of the Koran entitled 'Iron,' it is written: 'We formerly sent our apostles with evident miracles and arguments; and we sent down with them the scriptures, and the balance, that men might observe justice; and we sent them down iron, wherein is mighty strength for war, and various advantages unto mankind, that God may know who assisted him and his apostles in secret.'

Sale explains the sentence, 'And we sent them down iron,' as follows: 'that is, he taught them how to dig the same from mines. Al Zamakhshari adds, that Adam is said to have brought down with him from paradise five things made of iron, viz. an anvil, a pair of tongs, two hammers (a greater and a lesser), and a needle.[1]

In the chapter on 'Horses' we are also led to infer that shoeing was known. 'By the war-horses which run swiftly to the battle, with a panting noise; *and by those which strike fire, by dashing their hoofs against the stones;* and by those which make a sudden incursion on the enemy early in the morning,' etc.[2] Unshod hoofs, one would be inclined to think, could not strike fire against the stones.

Heusinger[3] quotes the names of several authorities who were of opinion that the art of shoeing was carried to Constantinople by the Germans. Certain it is, as has been already noticed, that the 'Tactita' of the emperor Leo VI., written at Constantinople in the ninth century, is the first writing in which modern shoes and nails are mentioned. The Byzantine emperors had a guard of honour composed of Saxons from a very early period of the empire.

---

[1] *Sale.* Koran, vol. ii. p. 365.   [2] Ibid. p. 440.
[3] Op. cit., vol. i. p. 9.

Under the Emperor Michael of Constantinople (1038) the horses of the Greek cavalry were shod. The Sicilian horses also at that period had their hoofs protected in this manner.

The Arabs themselves say their first farriers came to them from towns on the sea-board: such as Fez, Tunis, Masarca, Tlemcen, and Constantine, since when their knowledge and their calling have been perpetuated in certain families from generation to generation.

The practice of shoeing among these people is curious, and would almost indicate an independent origin, as well as a high antiquity. Contrary to the accepted opinion, says General Daumas,[1] the Arabs of the Sahara are in the custom of shoeing their horses, whether on the two fore-feet, or on all four, according to the nature of the ground they occupy. Those who shoe them on all four feet are the inhabitants of the stony districts, and these constitute the majority. It is the universal practice to take the shoes off in the spring, when the animals are turned out to grass; the Arabs asserting that care must be taken not to check the renewal of the blood which takes place at that season of the year.

The horse-shoes are kept ready made, and always command a sure sale, the Arabs being in the habit of laying in their supply for the whole year, consisting of four sets for the fore-feet, and four for the hind-feet. The nails are likewise made by the farriers. When a horseman goes to a farrier, taking his shoes with him, the latter is paid by his privileges, and when the horse is shod, its master gets on its back, merely saying: ' Allah, have mercy on

[1] Les Chevaux du Sahara. Paris, 1862.

thy fathers!' He then goes his way, and the farrier returns to his work. But if the horseman does not bring his
shoes with him, he gives two *boudjous* to the farrier for
the complete set, and his thanks are couched in the simplest
formula of Arab courtesy. 'Allah give thee strength!'
he says, as he takes his departure.

In the Sahara, in Syria, and throughout Arabia, the
shoes are fitted in a cold state. In the foot of the horse,
say the horsemen of these regions, there are hollow interstices, such as the frog, the heel, etc., which it is always
dangerous to heat, if only by the approach of the hot
iron. This aversion, founded on the destructive action of
an extreme degree of heat on the delicate parts of the
foot, is so strong among them, that in bivouacs, when the
Arabs of the Sahara saw the French shoeing their horses,
and fitting the red-hot shoes to the hoofs, they exclaimed,
'Look at those Christians pouring oil upon fire!' In a
word, they cannot understand why—especially in long
marches, when exercise makes the feet more vascular, any
one should wish to increase this natural heat by the action
of hot iron.

The shoes are very light, but made of well-hammered
iron. In the fore-shoes, only three nails are driven in each
side, through round holes which are close together. The
toes remain free, as the Arabs say nails in that part of the
foot would interfere with its elasticity, and would cause in
the horse, when he sets the hoof on the ground, precisely
the same sensation a man experiences from wearing a tight
shoe. Many accidents, they assert, thence ensue. The
hoofs are neither pared nor shortened, adds Daumas, and
the horn is allowed to grow freely, the very stony ground

and incessant work sufficing to wear it off naturally as it tries to get beyond the iron. The necessity for paring the feet is only perceived when horses have been for a long time fastened in front of the tent without doing any work, or have remained long in the Tell. In such a case, the Arabs simply make use of the sharp-pointed knives which they are never without. This method has the further advantage, that if a horse casts a shoe he can still proceed on his journey, as the sole remains firm and hard. 'With you,' they say, 'and with your practice of paring the foot, if the horse casts a shoe you must pull up, or see him bleeding, halting, and suffering.'

In Syria, however, the hoofs are shortened, and the wall pared level with the sole. The shoes are somewhat circular, or pear-shaped, and riveted, welded, lapped over, or left open at the heels. The annexed figures represent a Syrian shoe and nail (fig. 73); shoes and nails worn in the provinces of Constantine, Oran (fig. 74),

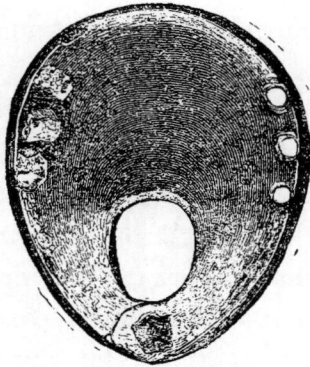 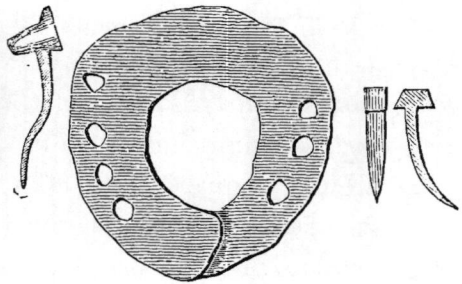

fig. 73   fig. 74

and Algeria (fig. 75); also a shoe from Morocco, found in a Moorish farrier's tent after the battle of Isly (fig.

76). The African shoes, it will be observed, are somewhat

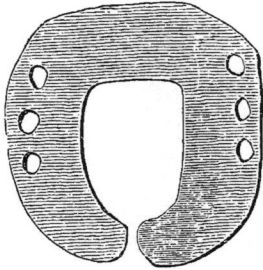
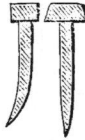
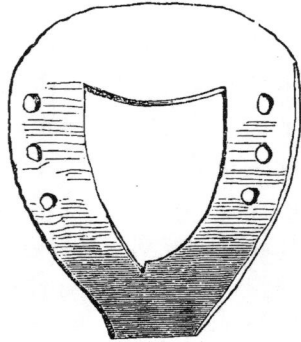

fig. 75   fig 76

square at the toe and approaching the little V in shape.
The central opening is somewhat triangular, and in the
Moorish shoe the heels are welded and bent up towards
the frog.   As the horse can only suffer in the part that is
most sensitive, they think, and not in the part that is hard,
it is, of course, the frog that should be shielded from
accident.   The shoes should therefore cover the frogs.
But this practice, and the undue curvature they give to
the heels of the metal plate, is productive of great injury
to the parts they were intended to protect; pebbles and
gravel insinuate themselves between the shoe and the
frog, and seriously damage the latter; while the point of
the shoe, pressing unduly on the heels, produces such pain
that the poor horse is often compelled to walk on his toes.
The sole pressure exercised by the shoe is decidedly beneficial, and explains in a great measure the almost total
absence of contracted hoofs and various lamenesses which
are the bane of our horses.   They give to the nail-heads
the form of a grasshopper's head, the only shape, they
allege, that allows the nails to be worn down to the last

without breaking. They approve of our method of driving the nails into the hoofs and clenching them on the outside, which prevents a horse cutting himself; but their scarcity of iron obliges them to content themselves with hammering the nail-points close to the face of the hoof, sometimes in a curled fashion, like the Celtic nails, so as to preserve them in a state fit for use a second time, by making a new head. If a horse over-reaches himself, they cut away his heels and place light shoes on his fore-feet, but heavier ones on his hind-feet. They are careful not to leave one foot shod and the other unshod. During a journey, if a horse chances to cast one of his fore-shoes, and his rider has not a fresh supply with him, he takes off both the hind-shoes and puts one of them on the fore-foot; and if the animal is shod only on his fore-feet, the rider will take the shoe off the other foot, rather than leave him in such a condition. Should a horse, after a long journey such as the horsemen of the desert not unfrequently make, require to be shod, it is no uncommon thing to place a morsel of felt between the shoe and the foot.

The necessity, caused partly by the nature of the ground, and partly by the length of their excursions, of shoeing the horses of the Sahara, has shown the expediency of accustoming the colt to let himself be shod without resistance. They therefore give him kouskoussou, cakes, dates, &c., while he allows them to lift his foot and knock upon it. They then caress his neck and cheeks, and speak to him in a low tone; and thus, after a while, he lifts his feet whenever they are touched. The little difficulty experienced at a later period, thanks to this

early training, has probably given rise to the Arab hyper-
bole : 'So wonderful is the instinct of the thoroughbred
horse that, if he casts a shoe, he draws attention to it
himself by showing his foot.'   This exaggeration at least
proves how docile these horses are to be shod, and further
explains how every horseman in the desert ought to have
the knowledge and the means of shoeing his own horse
while on a journey.   With them it is a point of the
highest importance.   It is not enough to be very skilful
in horsemanship, or to train a horse in the most perfect
manner, to acquire the reputation of a thorough horseman ; in addition to all this, he must likewise be able to
put on a shoe if necessary.   Thus, on setting out for a
distant expedition, every horseman carries with him in his
djebira shoes, nails, a hammer, pincers, some strips of
leather to repair his harness, and a needle.   Should his
horse cast a shoe, he alights, unfastens his camel-rope,
passes one end round the kerbouss of the saddle, and the
other round the pastern, and ties the two ends together
at such a length as will make the horse present his foot.
The animal stirs not an inch, and his rider shoes him
without assistance.   If it be a hind-shoe that has been
thrown, he rests the foot upon his knee, and dispenses
with aid from his neighbours.   To avoid making a mistake, he passes his awl into the nail-holes, in order to
assure himself beforehand of the exact direction the nails
should take.   If, by chance, the horse is restive, he obtains for the hind-feet the help of a comrade, who pinches
the nose or ears of the animal.   For the fore-feet, he
merely turns his hind-quarters towards a thick prickly
shrub, or extemporizes another mode of punishment with
a nose-bag filled with earth.   Such cases, however, are rare.

The Saharenes declare that the French shoes are much too heavy, and in long and rapid excursions must be dreadfully fatiguing to the articulations, and cause much mischief to the fetlock joints. 'Look at our horses,' say they, 'how they throw up the earth and sand behind them! How nimble they are! How lightly they lift their feet! How they extend or contract their muscles! They would be as awkward and as clumsy as yours did we not give them shoes light enough not to burden their feet, and the materials of which, as they grow thinner, commingle with the hoof, and with it form one solid body.' When to these remarks General Daumas has answered, that he did not discover any of the inconveniences pointed out in the European mode of shoeing, the Arabs have replied: 'How should you do so? Cover, as we do, in a single day, the distance you take five or six days to accomplish, and then you will see. Grand marches you make, you Christians, with your horses! As far as from my nose to my ear!'

Petrus Bellonius Cenomanus,[1] more than two hundred years ago, says that the shoes used by the Turks for their horses were in his day scarcely one-half the weight of the European shoes—one of the latter having material enough to make two of the former. The Turks were accustomed to buy the large and small shoes ready made, as at present, but the holes were not made in them. They were fitted to the feet, and the holes formed when required for use. The smith sat like a tailor with his legs doubled under him; and bending over the anvil, with a well-tempered punch and hammer the shoe was perforated, and another sharp square punch was twisted round in them to widen

[1] *Aldrovandus.* De Quadrupedibus, p. 50.

them to the proper size. The shoes had no calkins, as the horses did not require them either when at rest or when going at full speed, because of the nails with which they were fastened on, and which had large oblong heads, in shape like the *heart of a pigeon.* He also mentions that when horses were lightly worked, ' it was thought a good custom to shoe them only for half the year; so that, during war, the hoofs may stand wear a long time without shoeing.'

Though all the Arabs are cognizant of shoeing, and the advantages to be derived from it, yet, as we have seen, among the most valuable properties of a horse, they certainly attach very much importance to hard, strong, and sound hoofs. Abd-El-Kader explicitly mentions, that the best Arab horses for traversing stony ground without being shod, are those of the Hassasna tribe in the Yakoubia. Horses are not shod in Muscat,[1] and nevertheless perform long journeys.

It may well be considered very strange that none of the celebrated Arab hippiatrists of the early or middle ages, and whose treatises are yet extant, speak of the farrier's art. My researches have been fruitless in this respect. Abou-Bekr, the author of Naceri, a popular Arab work on the horse, and which is supposed to have been written in the 14th century, never mentions it save as an orthopodic resource. Hizâm, an ancient veterinary writer, recommends castration for horses whose hoofs are naturally thin and undeveloped, on the supposition that the horn is always thicker and stronger in emasculated animals.

It is curious to observe, that the circular shoe is yet

[1] *Stocqueler.* Fifteen Months' Pilgrimage, vol. i. p. 7.

worn in some of the countries which were invaded by the Moors or Turks in the middle ages. The Portuguese, according to Goodwin [1] and Rey,[2] still employ it. It is the same flat plate of iron, with a sharp ridge round the outer edge, like the Syrian, Persian, Barbary, and Turkish shoes, but in substance it is thicker. It is flat on both sides; the nail-holes are of an oblong square shape, very large, and extend far into the shoe, which is nearly round, covering the bottom of the foot, except a small hole in the centre. The heel, however, unlike the others, is turned down to the ground, for greater security in travelling. The principle of nailing is the same as in the French shoeing, and being flat on both sides, is superior to both, in the opinion of Mr Goodwin (fig. 77).

Spain preserves the upturned heels, the plane surfaces, and the circular, sharp, projecting rim of the Oriental shoe. This may be accepted as a proof that the Moors shod their horses while occupying Spain; but as another proof that shoeing was practised in the 11th century, in the time of the Cid, we have the story of King

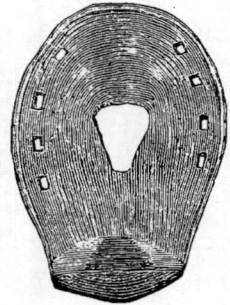

fig. 77

Alphonso escaping from the captivity imposed upon him by Ali Maymon, the Moorish King of Toledo, and a certain Count Pedro Anserez, or Peransures, advising him to have his horse's shoes nailed on in reverse—heels to toe, and so mislead his pursuers. Alphonso effected his escape, though it is not mentioned whether this cunning

[1] New System of Shoeing Horses, p. 167.
[2] Traité de Maréchalerie Vétérinaire, p. 469. Lyons, 1852.

device, which in after-ages was resorted to, had any influence in promoting it.[1] Since the invasion of the Turks, their mode of shoeing has prevailed more or less in Transylvania, though the shoe somewhat resembles that of the Moors, but with more cover. The heels are brought together like the letter V, and welded so as to form a wide patch projecting behind. The holes, three on each side, are circular. 'Wherever the Mussulman has exercised his authority for any length of time,' says Defays,[2] 'some traces of his shoeing remain.'

The Iberian peninsula has been successively invaded by the Romans, who introduced among the Lusitanians a branch of the wide-spread Celts; by the Germanic tribes — Alans, Suevi, Goths, and Vandals; and finally, by the Saracens, who were expelled after the decisive victory of Ourique. As a consequence of these invasions, it appears that at the present day we have traces of the characteristic shoeing existing which was practised by each of the foreign races.

The circular shoe, more or less modified in shape, prevails over a large extent of the continents of Africa and Asia, but we are left in grave doubts as to the origin of this particular form of hoof-armature. It displays a certain amount of originality, yet not sufficient, one would be inclined to think, to warrant the opinion that it was an independent invention. The form is but of secondary importance : garnishing the foot with a metallic plate, and attaching it by means of nails driven through

[1] Chronica de Famoso Cavallero Cid Ruy Diaz Campeador, cap. 42. Burgos, 1593.

[2] *Annales de Méd. Vét.*, p. 260. Bruxelles, 1867.

the horny envelope, is the chief consideration. The paucity of written evidence in regard to the introduction or origin of this art among Eastern peoples, leaves us no room to hope for a satisfactory investigation of the subject. Many nations in Asia, though aware of its existence, yet never require its aid; while others resort to various contrivances instead. Yet among those who shoe their steeds, the practice appears to have been adopted at a comparatively recent period.

In the vicinity of Tomsk, on the upper Obi, far towards the high land of Central Asia, there are scattered a great number of tumuli, which for centuries had occasionally furnished rich spoils to the Calmuck Tartars, the present tenants of the soil. I find that the veracious old Scotchman, John Bell of Antermony, who travelled over-land from St Petersburg to Peking, in 1719, with a Russian embassy, mentions these mounds in the cradle land of our race 'About eight or ten days' journey from Tomsky, in this plain, are found many tombs and burying-places of ancient heroes, who in all probability fell in battle. These tombs are easily distinguished by the mounds of earth and stones raised upon them. When, or by whom, these battles were fought, so far to the northward, is uncertain. I was informed by the Tartars in the Baraba, that Tamerlane, or Timyr-Ack-Sack, as they call him, had many engagements in that country with the Kalmucks; whom he in vain endeavoured to conquer. Many persons go from Tomsky, and other parts, every summer, to these graves; which they dig up, and find, among the ashes of the dead, considerable quantities of gold, silver, brass, and

15

some precious stones; but particularly hilts of swords and armour. They also find ornaments of saddles and bridles, and other trappings for horses; and even the bones of horses, and sometimes those of elephants. Whence it appears, that when any general or person of distinction was interred, all his arms, his favourite horse, and servant, were buried with him in the same grave; this custom prevails to this day among the Kalmucks and other Tartars, and seems to be of great antiquity. It appears from the number of graves, that many thousands must have fallen on these plains; for the people have continued to dig for such treasure many years, and still find it un-exhausted. I have seen several pieces of armour, and other curiosities, that were dug out of these tombs; particularly an armed man on horseback, cast in brass, of no mean design or workmanship; also figures of deer, cast in pure gold, which were split through the middle, and had some small holes in them, as intended for ornaments to a quiver, or the furniture of a horse. While we were at Tomsky, one of these grave-diggers told me, that once they lighted on an arched vault; where they found the remains of a man, with his bow, arrows, lance, and other arms, lying together on a silver table. On touching the body it fell to dust. The value of the table and arms was very considerable.'[']

The Russian government at length sent officers to ex-amine those tombs that had not yet been rifled; and, among others, they discovered one of three stone vaults, contain-ing the skeleton of a man with costly arms by his side, resting on a plate of pure gold several pounds in weight;

['] Travels from St Petersburg in Russia to Diverse Parts of Asia, vol. i. p. 181. London, 1764.

and another of a woman similarly laid on a gold plate, having bracelets and jewels of great value on the arms; while the third held the remains of a war-horse richly caparisoned, with horse-shoes on the feet, and metal stirrups for the rider. This tumulus, no doubt, contained the remains of some mighty Khan, though not of great antiquity, since the stirrups attached to the horse's saddle prove a comparatively late date. The shoes, by the form they displayed, may have been of European workmanship, and the whole deposit of the time of the great Tartar invasion of Russia and Poland, between 1237 and 1241.[1] When the Tartars were visited by mediæval travellers, they were already in what has been called the iron stage of civilization. Marco Polo, who was one of these visitors, when travelling in Badakshan, in the 13th century, remarks that the country was an extremely cold one, but that it produced a good breed of horses, which ran with great speed over the wild tracts without being shod with iron.[2] This notice would almost lead to the belief, that the people among whom he had been previously travelling had resorted to this defence, and it is also an evidence that he was acquainted with the practice in Europe.

Beauplan, travelling among the Tartars of the Ukraine and the Crimea in the 17th century, says that 'when the ground is hardened by frost or snow, the Tartars fasten (*cousent*) under the feet of their horses bits of old horn, with the intention of preventing their slipping and preserving their hoofs from wear.'[3]

---

[1] United Service Magazine, 1849.
[2] Narrative of the Travels of Marco Polo, p. 234.   London, 1849.
[3] Voyage au Midi de la Russie, 1680.   'Lorsque la terre est durcie

Pallas writes of the Cossacks of Jaïk (Orembourg), that their horses are not shod, because the dry soil induces them to have very fine and very hard hoofs.[1]

Wood, who travelled in Turkestan six centuries later, informs us that the Uzbeks shod their horses on the fore-feet, ' and the shoes are in shape a perfect circle.'[2]

In one of the oldest Astrakan Tartar songs, composed towards the end of the 14th century, entitled 'Adiga,' and written in the Nogay-Tartar dialect, the extravagant fashion of shoeing is alluded to. A Mongol Khan was jealous of Adiga, a Tartar chief, who was in consequence compelled to fly to the desert. He was brought back, however, and offered a numerous stud of mares, that he might drink kumiss, and have the meadows of Karaday for the pasture of his hunting-horses, where they would be made fat as ' lions' thighs.' The Mongol, full of wrath because he would not accept this splendid offer, ordered many horses to be killed and a great quantity of mead to be brewed, in order to feast all the tribes whom he wished to assemble in conference before going to war with Adiga's people. None of his nobles could advise him; but they referred him to a sage named Sobra, who lived some distance off, and who could give advice. ' If so,' said the Mongol, ' then bid the horse be put to my golden chariot (*kûs*). Let the horses be shod with *golden shoes and silver*

par la gelée ou par la neige, les Tartares cousent sous les pieds de leurs chevaux des morceaux de vieille corne, afin de les empêcher de glisser et d'empêcher l'nsure des pieds.'

[1] Voyages, vol. ii. p. 107. ' On ne les ferre pas, parce que le sol sec leur procure un sabot tres-beau et tres-dur.'

[2] Journey to the Source of the Oxus.

nails; and, having covered them with golden trappings, let them go and fetch Sobra.'[1]

That horses were shod in this part of the world with plates like those now in use in Europe, in the 16th century, we find testified in another Tartar song on the capture of Kazan by the Russians in 1552. Alluding to the famous war-horse of a prince, it relates that 'under the feet of Argamack the *horse-shoes look like new moons.* Its tail and mane are painted with hennah; on its back hang silk trappings; on its neck, in a talisman, round like a ring, is a prayer.'[2]

It is a remarkable circumstance, that in the neighbourhood of Peking, and from thence throughout Eastern Tartary, as far as I have travelled, shoes resembling in shape those of this country are in general wear. I could learn nothing of the antiquity of the custom in this remote part of the world; but the shoes are extremely primitive, and very like those we have been describing as Celtic. In journeying toward the eastern termination of the Great Wall, 'you cannot help bestowing a passing glance at the operations of the *Ting-chang-ta,* as the shoer of hoofs is denominated, for you may require his assistance frequently during your travel to secure your pony's clanking shoes, or to adjust a new pair; and you are certain to find him busy in the most crowded thoroughfare, or in the most stirring corner of the market-place. He is not, generally, a very bold man in his calling, nor has he much patience with skittish or unmanageable solipeds; for he too often makes it his practice to secure the unruly or vicious brute in the old-fashioned " trevises,"

[1] *Chodzko.* The Popular Poetry of Persia. [2] Ibidem.

or stocks—exact counterparts of those employed by
country farriers in Britain and the Continent half a century ago—where it is firmly bound and wedged in by
ropes and bars, and a twitch—an instrument of punishment still tolerated in other lands—twisted to agony round
the under-lip of the subdued beast, until its extremities
have been iron-clad. The more docile and submissive
animal is less harshly dealt with, for it is allowed to stand
untied, with one of its feet flexed on a low three-legged
stool, while the workman shaves off great slices of superfluous horn from the thick soles, with an instrument which

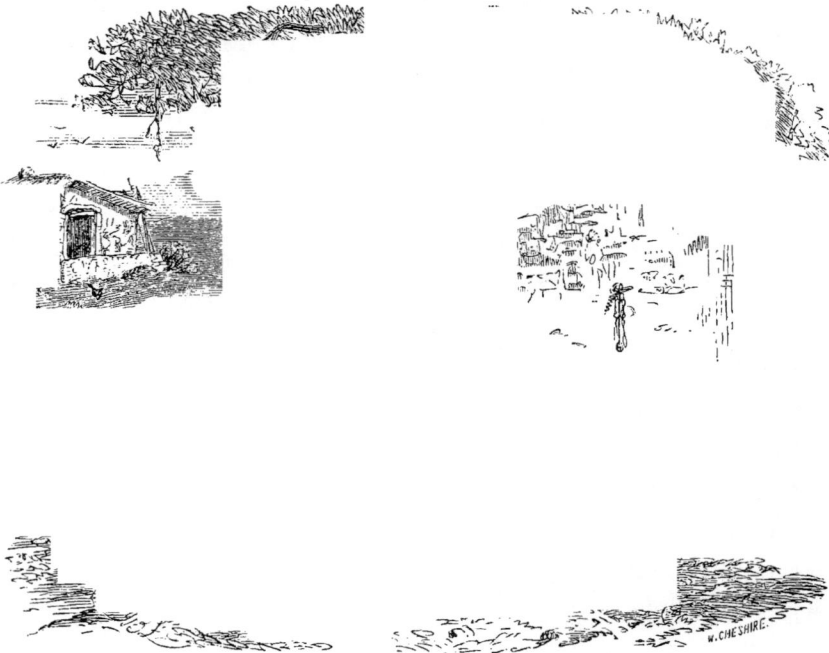

fig 78

differs in no particular that we can see from the now
obsolete "buttress" of England, or the present *boutoir* of
France (fig. 78). Perhaps a fidgety draught animal does

not quite relish the idea of parting from its worn-out shoes;
and the squeamish shoer, to avoid sundry uncomfortable
contusions on his shins, stands some distance off, and
hammers at the end of a long thin-pointed poker, inserted
between the useless plate of iron and the hoof, to twist
it off. Whether aware of it or not, like the French, the
Chinese seem to prefer the foot in process of shoeing
being held up by an assistant, instead of courageously
grasping it as our farriers do. The Tartar ponies being
light-paced and small, and the roads not very stony,
the shoe is light, thin, narrow, and quite ductile. It is,
in fact, nothing more than a slight rim of tough iron,
pierced by four nail-holes, with a separate groove for the
reception of each nail-head; and the heels are drawn so
thin, that when the shoe is nailed on the foot they are bent
inwards to catch each angle of the inflection of the hoof,
and in this way support the nails (fig. 79). Altogether, it is
far more like one of our own horse-
shoes than those of the Afghans, the
Arabian or Barbary, or the Persian
and Turkish curiosities, and certainly
very far superior to the straw sandal
everywhere used in Japan to protect

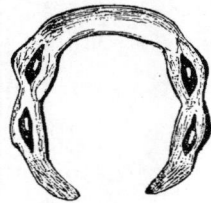

fig 79

the horses' feet. There is little care and a great deal of
dexterity exhibited in nailing on one of these iron plates.
The excellent strong feet of the ponies afford every facil_
ity for a rough-and-ready job. The overgrown horn is
shaved away to a level surface; a single blow makes the
shoe narrower or wider without heating: it is applied to the
solid crust, and one by one the unbending nails are sent
through the whole thickness of the insensitive part of the

hoof with a few sharp taps, the tips of the nails being only simply twisted and hammered close to the face of the hoof; and the Wayland smith has earned his groat. At odd interva's one comes upon a group of these tinkers arming the hot, painful, road-worn toes of prostrate struggling bullocks with a nearly semicircular plate of metal on the outer margin of the hoof; and so smartly, that the bellowing creatures have hardly been thrown on the ground and secured than they are up again, proof against the hard, sun-baked roads.' [1]

Perhaps we are not making a very wide ethnological jump, if we pass from this part of the Old World to the Rocky Mountains of the New Continent, and note the customs among the equestrian, though not horse-loving, tribes of Indians in that wild region. The horse has had but little influence in civilizing the many clans who have become horsemen since that animal was introduced by the early Spaniards, and they have done as little in attempting to prevent its degeneracy in their hands. Iron shoes are never worn on the hoofs, but when travelling over rock ground, and the unfortunate animals become footsore, a substitute for the metal is found in what is termed 'parflêche.' This is the untanned, sundried hide of the buffalo or elk, in which the pounded flesh or 'pemmican' made from these beasts is wrapped up and preserved, and on which these people largely subsist. The thick, hairy skin, I am informed, makes an excellent temporary covering for the foot, forming, when tied round the pastern, a convenient hoof-buskin, like that made from camel's hide in the Soudan.

[1] See my 'Travels on Horseback in Mantchu Tartary,' p. 399.

233

CHAPTER VI.

BRITAIN, ITS EARLY POPULATION. THEIR MANNERS AND CUSTOMS.
EQUESTRIANS. CÆSAR'S INVASION. GREAT NUMBERS OF HORSES.
WORKING IN IRON. CHARIOTS. RARITY OF ANCIENT HORSE-SHOES.
BRITISH BARROWS. SILBURY HILL AND ITS ANTIQUITIES. THE
GREAT KING. OLD HORSE-SHOES. CLARK'S SPECIMENS. BECK-
HAMPTON RELICS. SPRINGHEAD AND ITS REMAINS. YORK SPECI-
MENS. COLNEY, LONDON, AND GLOUCESTER. EXCELLENT ILLUS-
TRATIONS. COTSWOLD HILLS. ROMAN VILLA AT CHEDWORTH.
CIRENCESTER. PEVENSEY CASTLE. HOD HILL AND ITS STORY.
SPURS. HOOP-PICK. URICONIUM AND CONDERUM. LIVERPOOL
EXAMPLES. REPULSE OF THE BRITONS. LAWS OF HOWEL THE
GOOD. DIVISION OF WALES. TRINAL SYSTEM. WELSH KING'S
COURT. THE JUDGE OF THE COURT AND GROOM OF THE REIN.
DUTIES, PRIVILEGES, AND PROTECTION OF THE SMITH. THE
THREE ARTS. VALUE OF THE HORSE'S FOOT. LIST AND VALUA-
TION OF SMITHS' TOOLS. TRIADS. SONS OF THE BOND. THE
SMITH'S SEAT AT COURT. SIR WALTER SCOTT AND THE 'NORMAN
HORSE-SHOE.' KING ARTHUR'S STONE. TRADITIONS OF HOOF-
PRINTS. RENAUD AND THE BLACK ROCKS OF ARDENNES. THE
CHEVALIER MASON. SCYTHE-STONE PITS OF DEVONSHIRE.
STRANGE IMPRINT. THE SEAT OF A ZOOPHYTE. THE ANGLO-
SAXONS. THEIR HORSE-SHOES. EQUESTRIAN HABITS. MONKS
AND MARES. SPORTING PRIESTS. ANGLO-SAXON LAWS. VALUE
OF HORSES. SAXON CAVALRY. HAROLD AND THE DANES AND
NORMANS. SAXON WEAPONS. GRAVES. FAIRFORD, CAENBY,
BRIGHTON DOWNS, GILLINGHAM, BERKSHIRE. BATTLE FLATS.
ANGLO-SAXON ILLUMINATIONS. MATTHEW OF PARIS. SHOEING
FRONT FEET. FROST. SHOEING IN SCOTLAND. NORMAN INVA-
SION. A NOBLE SAXON FARRIER. BAYEUX TAPESTRY. SHOEING

WITH THE NORMANS.   ARMORIAL BEARINGS.   SIMON ST LIZ.
EARL FERRERS AND OKEHAM.   CURIOUS CUSTOM.   DEATH OF
WILLIAM THE CONQUEROR.

BRITAIN probably received its earliest population from
Gallia Celtica some centuries before the Christian era, and
these Belgiæ or Cimbri were what we now term the ancient Britons.   The island, however, was in all probability
populated before the arrival of these wanderers, though we
know little of its history until the advent of the Romans.
At Cæsar's invasion it was well populated, and the interior
was inhabited by people who believed themselves to be
autochthones.   The southern and eastern coasts were more
particularly occupied by the emigrants from Belgic Gaul,
who had crossed the channel and the northern sea, attracted by the prospect of plunder.   After having obtained a
footing they became agriculturists.   They possessed the
same manners as the Gauls, though their social condition was less advanced ; the Celts in Gaul having
attained a comparatively high degree of civilization.   They
were also more fierce than their kindred on the other side
of the channel, and were altogether, perhaps, in a more
degraded condition than those tribes we have been considering.   Their religion was the same as that of the
Gauls, and Tacitus tells us that they had the same worship and the same superstitions.[1]   Druidism found a congenial home in Britain when banished from the continent, though it had existed in this country, in all
likelihood, from the landing of the nomads ; and with its
mysterious and dismal rites, it no doubt claimed the same

[1] *A*gricola, ii.

amount of metallurgic skill that it secretly practised at Alesia and elsewhere.

Fierce and undaunted in battle, the ancient Britons were also a horse-loving people, and largely employed horses in peace, as well as in war. They appear to have been passionately fond of horses, as the fragments of their poetry that have reached us abundantly testify: and it would almost appear that all their fighting men were mounted on spirited steeds.[1] Whether ridden by their fearless masters, or harnessed to the multitudes of chariots so conspicuous in their armies, the little hardy British steeds appear to have been well trained. Cæsar's first impression of them was anything but favourable to the expected success of the Roman arms. When attempting to land upon our coast, he thus describes them: 'The barbarians (as was then the fashion to designate our valiant woad-stained forefathers), upon perceiving the design of the Romans, sent forward their cavalry and charioteers (*essedarii*), a class of warriors of whom it is their prac tice to make great use in their battles; and following with the rest of their forces, endeavoured to prevent our men landing. In this was the greatest difficulty, for the following reasons, namely, because our ships, on account of their great size, could be stationed only in deep water; and our soldiers, in places unknown to them, with their hands embarrassed, oppressed with a large and heavy weight of armour, had at the same time to leap from

[1] For proof of this, see that most interesting collection of traditional poetry translated from the Welsh by Mr Skene, entitled 'The Four Ancient Books of Wales.' Edinburgh, 1868. The poem designated the 'Triads of the Horses' is very remarkable.

the ships, stand amid the waves, and encounter the enemy; whereas they, either on dry ground, or advancing a little way into the water, free in all their limbs, in places thoroughly known to them, could confidently throw their weapons, and spur on their horses, which were accustomed to this kind of service.   Dismayed by these circumstances, and altogether untrained in this mode of battle, our men did not all exert the same vigour and eagerness which they had been wont to exert in engagements on dry ground   But the enemy, who were acquainted with all the shallows, when from the shore they saw any coming from a ship one by one, spurred on their horses. and attacked them while embarrassed; many surrounded a few, others threw their weapons upon our collected forces on their exposed flank '"[1]

Their cavalry and chariots often awed the valorous Romans, and frequently defeated them.   They used the 'Essedum,' or war-chariot, much as the Greeks did in the heroic ages; but this chariot was more ponderous than that of the Greeks, and opened before instead of behind. The wheels were armed with scythes, and the pole was wide and strong, so that the warrior was able, whenever he liked, to run along its top, and even to raise himself upon the yoke, then retreat with the greatest speed into the body of the car, which was driven with extraordinary swiftness and skill.   Contrary to the custom with the Greeks, the drivers ranked above their fighting companions.   These chariots were much esteemed by the Britons, and were made purposely as noisy as possible, so that by creaking and clanging of wheels they might strike dismay.

[1] Bell. *Gall.*, lib. iv. cap. 24—26.

'Their mode of fighting with their chariots is this: firstly, they drive about in all directions, and throw their weapons, and generally break the ranks of the enemy with the very dread of their horses and the noise of their wheels; and when they have worked themselves in between the troops of horse, leap from their chariots and engage on foot. The charioteers in the mean time withdraw some little distance from the battle, and so place themselves with the chariots that, if their masters are overpowered by the number of the enemy, they may have a ready retreat to their own troops. Thus they display in battle the speed of horse, together with the firmness of infantry; and by daily practice and exercise attain to such expertness that they are accustomed, even on a declining and steep place, to check their horses at full speed, and manage and turn them in an instant and run along the pole, and stand on the yoke, and thence betake themselves with the greatest celerity to their chariots again.'[1]   Thus they filled the middle of the field of battle with their tumult and wheeling and careering. The Britons appear to have been the only people in Europe who fought from chariots, a circumstance which affords the early British historian, Geoffrey of Monmouth, an argument to prove that they were of Trojan origin.

The immense number of horses they possessed may be judged from the fact, that Cassivelaunus, the British chief who was invested with the supreme command of the forces of the island, in order to oppose Cæsar, after dismissing all his other troops, yet retained no fewer than 4000 war chariots about him. And their cavalry was

[1] *Cæsar.*   Op. cit., lib. iv. cap. 33.

not to be despised. 'The mode of fighting on horse-back threatened equal danger to those who gave way, or those who pursued. They never engaged in close order, but in small parties, and with great intervals, and had detachments placed in different parts, and then the one relieved the other, and the vigorous and fresh succeeded the wearisome.' 'The horses and charioteers of the enemy contended vigorously in a skirmish with our cavalry on the march; yet so that our men were conquerors in all parts, and drove them to their woods and hills.'[1] Nothing but the superior organization of the Romans, and the ability of their generals, prevented their being defeated by this equestrian people.

That the Celts in Britain were well acquainted with iron, and placed a high value on it, we learn from Herodian. He says: 'They know not the use of clothing, but encircle their loins and necks with iron; deeming this an ornament and an evidence of opulence, in like manner as other barbarians esteem gold. But they puncture their skins with pictured forms of every sort of animals; on which account they wear no clothing, lest they should hide the figures on their bodies. They are a most warlike and sanguinary race, carrying only a small shield and a spear, and a sword girded to their naked bodies. Of a breast-plate or helmet they know not the use, esteeming them an impediment to their progress through the marshes.'

A very old Welsh poem, 'Gorchan Cynfelin,' says, in regard to Druid sacrifices: 'When I was devoted to

---

[1] *Cæsar.* Op. cit. lib. v. cap. 15, 16.

the sacrificial flames, they ransomed me with gold, *iron,* and *steel.*'

The Britons made swords and other weapons of iron; their chariot-wheels were shod with iron, and these wheels are, perhaps, the most characteristic memorials of this ancient race. Their remains have been discovered not only in France, but in many English barrows, with iron snaffles for horses' bridles. York Museum contains a good specimen of both. The impressions upon the coins of Cunobelin and others testify that they were proficients in the construction of carriages and wheels.

Archæological researches, so far as they refer to the subject of horse-shoes, have been much less successful in this country than in France. From what we have just noticed of the dexterity of these Celtic horsemen and charioteers, and of the manner in which they used the horse, it is scarcely possible to believe that the hoofs of that animal could have been unshod. The daily practice of their warlike manœuvres, particularly in our climate, must have entailed an amount of strain and wear upon the feet which they could not have withstood, unless protected in some substantial manner; and as the art of shoeing with iron plates and nails was, as there appears to be abundance of archæological evidence to prove, practised by the same race in Gaul at this period, it can hardly be doubted that such was also the case in Britain. The discoveries of iron shoes, however, have here been comparatively few and far between, though for what reason it would be difficult to say; but perhaps the little attention given to such an apparently trifling matter may be the cause.

Sufficient evidence has been collected, however, to prove that shoes were in use at a very early age, and if not before the Roman invasion, at least during the Roman occupation of Britain ; and that now about to be offered will, it is anticipated, effectually dispose of the assertion made by Dr Pegge, Sir F. Meyrick, Bracy Clark, Youatt, and many other writers, that the art of shoeing was first introduced into England by the Normans. It may also tend to correct the equally erroneous opinion enunciated by some of these and other authorities, to the effect that the Goths and Vandals who overthrew the Roman empire were the first to make this practice of arming the hoofs known to the western world. The Goths and Vandals at any rate did not reach Britain, and although the proofs that shoeing was known before their arrival in Italy and Gaul are strong enough, the testimony is still more decisive as to the employment of iron hoof-plates in this country at an earlier period than that invasion. Neither have any Tartar hordes ever crossed the sea to deposit the shoes of their steeds in our soil, as on the continent of Europe.

Some good specimens of the pattern we have referred to as being Celtic and Gallo-Celtic, have been found in situations and under circumstances which lead us to the conclusion that they also belong to that epoch, and were manufactured by kindred hands.

Sir Richard C. Hoare found the halves of two horse-shoes in a British barrow,[1] but as they are not described

[1] History of *A*ncient Wiltshire, London, 1812—21. Fosbroke is the authority for this statement. I have carefully looked through Hoare's splendid work, but can find no mention of these articles ;

or figured, so far as I am aware, nothing can be said as to their characteristics. This authority was of opinion, however, that few, if any, interments in barrows took place after the Roman invasion in Britain; so that these articles must have been in use before or soon after that event. He also discovered an urn in a barrow, with an ornament on the rim in relief like the shape of a horse-shoe.[1]

The able veterinary surgeon, Bracy Clark, in 1832, described what he termed 'two ancient horse-shoes,' found near Silbury Hill, Wiltshire. This hill, which is situated on the road from London to Bath, is nothing more than a mound of large size, and is believed to be of great antiquity; by some it has even been supposed to be the appendage of a Druidical temple, it being placed exactly due south, and possessing other characters of a similar kind. It is to be much regretted that no me-thodical and careful examination has yet been made of this tumulus, for at various times objects of great age and antiquarian value have been obtained from it. An opening was made in it in 1723, when a human skeleton, the antlers of a deer, a knife with a horn handle, and a horse's iron bit were found. Stukely thought the hill was the grave of a great king, and that these were his remains. 'In the month of March, 1723, Mr Holford ordered some trees to be planted on this hill, in the middle of the area at the top, which is 60 cubits (103 feet 9 inches) in diameter. The workmen dug up the body

neither is any notice of them to be found in his Guide to the Wiltshire Barrows.

[1] Ibid., p. 121.

of the great king there buried in the centre, very little below the surface; the bones were extremely rotten, so that they crumbled them in pieces with their fingers. The soil was altogether chalk, dug from the side of the hill below, of which the whole barrow is made. Six weeks after, I came to rescue a curiosity which they took up there, an iron chain, as they called it, which I bought of John Fowler, one of the workmen: it was the bridle buried with the monarch, being only a solid body of rust. I immersed it in a limner's drying cloth, and dried it carefully, keeping it ever since very dry. It is now as fair and entire as when the workmen took it up. There were deer's horns, an iron knife with a bone handle, too, all excessively rotten, taken up along with it.'[1] Bracy Clark described the bit in his 'Treatise on Bits.'

Hoare asserts that the majority of the Wiltshire barrows, of which this Silbury Hill was undoubtedly one, were the sepulchral memorials of the Celtic and first colonists of Britain; and some may be ascribed to the subsequent colony of Belgæ who invaded the island. Roberts[2] plainly indicates that this immense cairn must have been erected before the arrival of the Romans; for the Roman road which traverses this county, and which passes in a tolerably direct line, when it reaches the mound turns out of its course to avoid it, and in doing so cuts through a large barrow in its vicinity, part of which is yet standing between the avenue and the hill. It was in the vicinity of this mound that these shoes were met with.

[1] *Gough.* Camden's Britannia.
[2] Pop. *A*ntiquities of Wales.

The person who presented them to Mr Clark, says of the first shoe (fig. 80) that it was found upon the down on the opposite side of the road, at the distance of nearly half-a-mile from the place where the other shoe was found, under a heap of flints. These flints, it is probable, were taken at some former period from the above spot, and were deposited upon the down, probably for mending

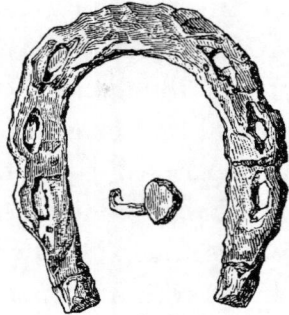

fig 80

the roads; for, from the perfect accordance and similarity of both these shoes, in their peculiar make and fashion, says Bracy Clark, and from other circumstances, there can be no reasonable doubt of their having been constructed at the same period, and in all probability belonged to the same animal, the one being a hind, and the other a fore shoe, and of nearly the same size. They had also perfectly similar nails. Being looked upon by the labourers who removed the flints as mere old iron, they were passed unnoticed by them, as they sometimes found in these localities Roman and other coins of some value.

Of the second shoe (fig. 81), he says it was found 'by the levelling of a bank, in Silbury Hill mead, for the purpose of watering it. The soil removed on this occasion was principally chalk, to the depth of a foot or

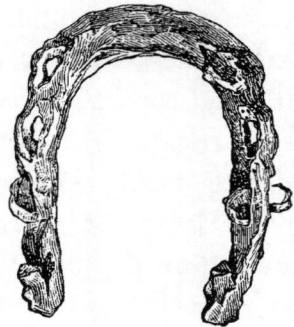

fig 81

16 *

two.' No mention is made of bones of horses, or other articles, being found with it, but the skeleton of a man was found at some little distance.

Mr Clark, who was somewhat of an enthusiast in the matter of shoes and shoeing, and appears to have lost no opportunity of examining old specimens, though he previously believed that this art was only introduced into Britain by the Normans, confesses these Silbury shoes to have been the oldest he ever saw or heard of, and appears to have been rather puzzled by them. In all likelihood, as he remarks, the animal to which they belonged had been buried with them, since the nails were present in them, as in many of the Gallic specimens, with the clenches quite perfect and in their flexed state, which would not have been possible had the shoe been torn off while the horse was alive. This veterinarian acknowledges the shoes as truly exhibiting an early period in the history of the art. 'Their mould or general form is neither broad nor heavy, as in the oldest French shoes we have ever seen, but they are rather what would be called a light shoe. In their upper surface (foot surface), flat, a little concaved, however, inwards, and at the inflections perfectly flat. The under surface of the shoe is rounded a little and convex, or rising in the middle, having in each of the quarters three immense deep oval or oblong stamp-holes or countersinks, as mechanics would call them, not very near to the outer rim of the shoe, and perforated through in the middle of these cavities, with three large, almost square, perforations; the size of these, which time and oxydation may perhaps have a little enlarged, gave abundant opportunity for the early artisan to direct his nail as much obliquely outwards as he wished, which a more confined aperture, or greater thickness of metal, would not have allowed him so readily to do. Now these stamp-pits must have been done with a very rough, clumsy tool, for the rim or outer margin of the shoe has been terribly disturbed by it, and thrown out into bulges of a surprising size, disfiguring the shoe very much, and also endangering the horse's legs. The heels of the shoes are provided with very prominent calkins, made by doubling or turning over the iron, and lapping and welding it; finding, no doubt, the great advantages which attended this plan. The wearing line of the shoe at the toe in No. 1 (fig. 80) was considerably worn away, but in No. 2 (fig. 81) hardly so much. These shoes, generally speaking, are thickest forwards, and go declining in thickness till reaching the calkins. Their insides are thicker than the outside. The nail-heads are very remarkable for their size, and projecting high from the shoes; and that part of the head next the aperture in the shoe is formed with a very abrupt broad shoulder, and nearly straight, but a little inclining, however, towards the shank. The sides of the head of the nail are nearly straight and perpendicular, forming an obtuse angle to the former line; upwards it passes by another converging line towards the summit, or top of the nail, which is made flat, and is of the length of about a quarter of an inch, for receiving the blows of the hammer; the head itself stands beyond the shoe, and if embraced by the finger is flat, and shows a thickness of only about, or perhaps less than, the eighth of an inch. The shank of the nail is short, compared with modern nails, and is square, tapering all the way to the point, but is made rather flatter and broader on one side, viz., that side which corresponds to the flatness of the head.'

The nails were not *pointed*, as now-a-days; and appear to have been driven only a short distance in the hoof, and the end that had passed through was bent round and lay close to the side of the foot for safety. The sharp point was not wrung off, as is now the custom, but passing along the face of the hoof, was turned round like a carpenter's nail, and probably buried slightly in the crust, to give it a hold. 'The excellent preservation in which these shoes are found can only be accounted for by their having been for a long time defended, perhaps, by the hoofs to which they were attached, and secondarily, from their being deposited among flints and chalk, the most indestructible and undecomposable materials of all the earthy substances.'

These relics are certainly extremely crude attempts in workmanship, and betray a very primitive period—the very infancy of the art,—more so, indeed, than any specimens that have yet been met with. Some time after they were discovered, the late Dean of Hereford obtained a horse-shoe similar in form, which had been found with others, and a skeleton, a short distance north-west of Silbury Hill. This was figured in the Transactions of the Salisbury Institute.

Two specimens of similar construction, and which were found at Beckhampton, are now in the Museum at Cirencester, Gloucestershire. One of them (fig. 82) is much more primitive-looking than the other, and is of smaller size, agreeing very closely in this respect with those described and figured by Bracy Clark. The rolled-over calkins are particularly conspicuous. The other (fig. 83) is of larger size and more circular in shape, and shows

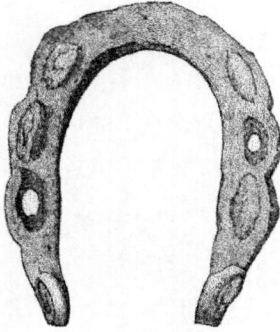

fig. 82

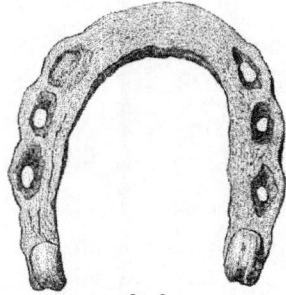

fig 83

a nail-head worn down to the surface of the shoe. Beck-hampton, we must remember, is near the Druidical circle or temple of Abury, the western avenue of that structure extending towards this village; and that the stupendous mound of Silbury is within the plan of Abury, and may have been a component part of the temple. It is some-what remarkable that this portion of Wiltshire, so famous for its ancient British monuments, should furnish such a number of these primitive horse-shoes.

Three-fourths of a shoe, in excellent preservation, and evidently of the same period, was found at Springhead, near Gravesend, Kent, some years ago, and is now in the possession of Mr Sylvester of that place. It was found imbedded in compact chalk, and, from its appearance, has been scarcely worn; it had broken through at one of the nail-holes soon after being fastened on the hoof. From the situation of this relic, and the accompanying remains, there can scarcely be a doubt as to its belonging to the Roman, or even pre-Roman, period. Its length is $4\frac{1}{8}$ inches; width, $3\frac{3}{4}$ inches; breadth at toe, $\frac{5}{8}$ths of an inch; and at heel, $\frac{1}{2}$ inch. The plate is thin; at the toe, where it is strongest, it is scarcely $\frac{1}{4}$th inch. The iron is of excellent quality; and the calkin, which is formed by doubling over the end of the branch, projects about $\frac{1}{4}$th inch above the ground surface of the shoe (fig. 84). The nail-holes, three of which are yet intact, have been three on each side, and of the usual form. A small lump of rust indicates the remains of a nail-head filling up the middle hole of one branch. The border of the shoe, particularly the external one, is markedly undulating, owing to the large

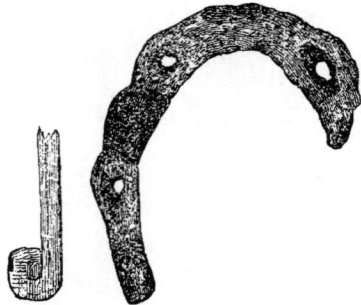

fig 84

size of the cavity made to contain a portion of the nail-head. This cavity is $\frac{2}{4}$ths of an inch long, and $\frac{3}{8}$ths wide; and the hole for the reception of the nail-shank is nearly circular, and has a diameter of $\frac{1}{4}$th inch: certainly the nails must have been very thick for the small hoofs shoes of this kind would fit. The weight of this excellent specimen is 3 ounces 7 drachms; so that the entire shoe may be calculated to have weighed about 5 ounces. There are no retaining clips, and the ground and hoof surfaces are flat and rough, as if carelessly and scantily hammered. Springhead, where this antique scrap was found, stands near the Roman Watling Street; and from the soil in its vicinity, which is chalky, great numbers of coins—many fibulæ, some fictilia, etc.—belonging to various periods in the early history of our

country, but particularly the Roman, have been picked
up during a number of years. The coins are chiefly
brasses, some of them very old. Only one gold coin has
been discovered—that of the Roman Emperor Valentine.

The three specimens next exhibited (figs. 85, 86, 87)

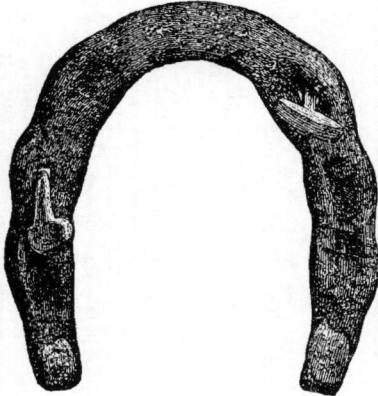

fig. 85

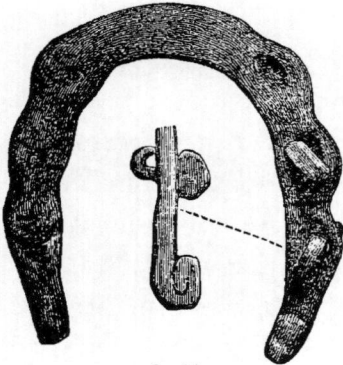

fig. 86

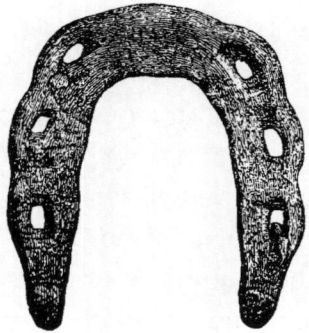

fig. 87

are from the York Museum, and were found a few years
ago under a cobble-road, near the bridge which crosses
the foss of that city, at a depth of eight feet below the
surface. A number of these shoes were discovered in
this situation; and it has been conjectured by some one

that very long ago there may have been a ford at this place, and that these articles were then lost in the clay by horses in crossing. They are evidently Celtic, or Romano-Celtic, if we compare them with those from the graves in Gaul. Of the three represented, figure 86 is apparently the oldest; next, figure 85; and lastly, figure 87. All have been worn; all have the irregularly undulating border, the peculiar groove, nail-holes, and calkins, and the characteristic nail-heads. Figure 85 is a comparatively large shoe, and figure 87 a small one. They are very thin, and do not exceed ¼th of an inch in thickness. The nails in 85 and 86 have the points turned in a similar manner to those of Silbury Hill; and figure 87 alone appears to have been wrenched off while the horse that wore it was alive. The stalks or bodies of the nails are shorter and more square than we now use them, and the heads are of the semicircular T pattern. The calkins stand about ¼th of an inch higher than the shoe.[1]

It may be observed, that in the same museum are the remains of a chariot, and the bones of a man, horse, and pig, which were collected in a barrow not far from York; but I cannot ascertain that any shoes were found. With specimens of Romano-Celtic shoes—that is, of shoes of this pattern found associated with Roman remains—we are more liberally furnished; for it must be confessed that those which we might at a hazard term 'pre-Roman' are extremely scarce.

At Colney, in Norfolk, were discovered Roman urns,

---

[1] I am indebted to A. J. Owles, Esq., Enniskilling Dragoons, for photographs of these fine specimens.

iron spear-heads, and 'a horse-shoe of unusual shape'—
round and broad in front, narrowing very much backwards, and having its extreme ends brought almost close
behind, and rather pointed inwards, with the nail-holes
still perfect.'[1] No drawing accompanies this description.

In making a deep excavation at Lothbury, London, in
1847, at a depth of 16 feet below the surface, the workmen
came upon a number of Roman *reliquiæ*, consisting of
iron keys, Samien and other pottery, and various other
articles, amongst which was an iron horse-shoe (fig. 88).

It is of the usual fashion of
that epoch, is only three inches
six-eighths long, three inches
five-eighths wide, and about
three-quarters of an inch at
the broadest part of the toe.
It narrows very much towards
the heels, and there are but
faint traces of calkins. The
one branch is a little longer

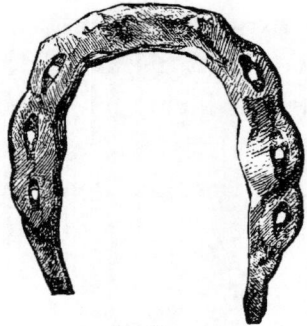

fig. 88

than the other, and altogether the specimen is thin and
light. The peculiar shape of this horse-shoe, the depth
at which it was discovered, and its being mingled with
undoubted Roman remains, proves that it must be of
high antiquity, pointing to the Roman-British period as
the age of its fabrication.[2]

Another shoe of the same character was found in
Moorfields, in the line of the old London Wall, some

[1] Archæologie, vol. xiv. p. 4.
[2] Journal of the *A*rchæological *A*ssociation, vol. vi.

years ago. It is about 4¼ inches long, has the six oval cavities, and calkins rolled-over and welded (fig. 89).

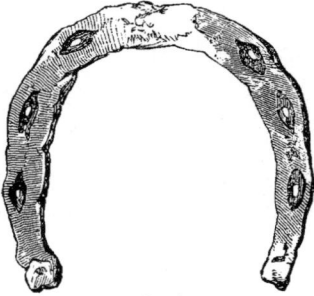

fig. 89

In the British Museum there is also a specimen, procured while making a sewer in 1833, in Fenchurch Street, London. Fragments of Roman pottery, *boars' teeth*, and other articles, were found with it. It is thin and light, has the nail-holes of the characteristic number and shape; narrows a little towards the heels, where there are calkins, and shows marks of wear. It measures four and three-eighths inches long, and four inches wide. It is narrower across the toe than several of the others examined, and resembles somewhat the third York specimen (fig. 90).

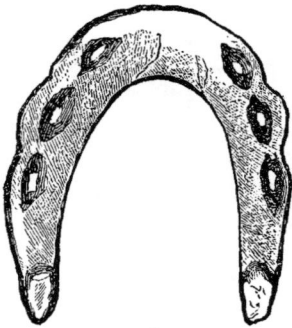

fig. 90

In August, 1854, there was discovered at Gloucester, at the depth of some nine or ten feet from the surface, and mingled with numerous fragments of Roman *fictilia*, the outer half of a strong iron horse-shoe, with one of the large flat-headed nails already described remaining in one of the three holes. It is exactly similar in size and make, to the last-mentioned shoe.

Another shoe precisely like it, but of rather larger dimensions, was met with beneath a Roman road at Inneravon, Linlithgowshire, Scotland, when the old pavement was being removed to prepare the ground for macadam izing. This shoe is in the possession of the Society of Antiquaries of Scotland.[1]

Gloucestershire, indeed, has long been famous for the Roman and other ancient remains discovered in it from time to time. The town of Gloucester boasts of a high antiquity, it being the Caer Glowe or Glev of the Celts, the termination *-um* being afterwards added, *euphoniæ gratia,* to form the Glevum, the name by which the Romans designated this large colonial city; subsequently it was the Gleow-ceaster of the Saxons. Its importance to the ancient Britons and Romans may have been owing not only to its situation on the banks of the Severn, but also to its proximity to the great iron district of the Forest of Dean. It is not to be wondered at, then, that some of the finest specimens of farriery I have been able to inspect should be discovered in this county. Some years ago, when laying down sewers in the town of Gloucester, many relics of antiquity were disinterred in the excavations. In Northgate Street, at a depth of eight or ten feet below the present level, which is also the usual depth at which all other Roman remains, such as tesselated pavements and the like, are found, and some seven or eight inches below the pitched Roman road (*via strata*), were found a number of horse-shoes and other articles of the Roman period. Two of the shoes I have had the opportunity of inspecting, and they correspond in every particular with those already described as belonging to

[1] Journal of the *Arch*æological *A*ssociation. vol. xiv.

this period. One of them (fig. 91) is the most perfect specimen I ever saw, and is so little affected by its long sojourn underground, that but for the fact of its having been found with fibulæ, a lamp (*lucerna*), and other characteristic memorials of the Roman æra, together with its peculiar form, one would be perfectly justified in asserting it had quite recently come from the anvil

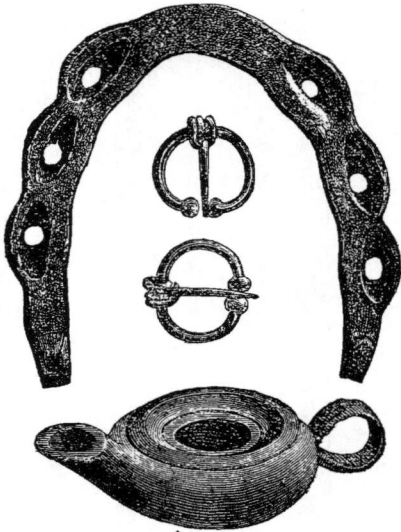

fig 91

of the blacksmith. It has never been worn, a circumstance to which its high preservation is partly due; the edges are perfectly clean and sharp, and every stage in its manufacture can be readily traced, as there is not the smallest speck of rust upon it. The iron of which it is composed is of the very purest description, and so white and ductile, that it was at first conjectured to be silver. This, however, has been ascertained to be owing to the presence of a somewhat large proportion of nickel,[1] which has most largely contributed to the exemption from oxidation. I am informed that iron of this character, with much nickel in it, is found on the surface of the ground in Wilts. The outside of the shoe

[1] An analytical chemist who examined it, informed me that it was the rarer metal titanium.

is black, as all iron work is when just from the hammer.
The specimen weighs only $4\frac{1}{4}$ ounces, and is $4\frac{1}{4}$ inches
long, and $3\frac{7}{8}$ inches wide. The calkins are rolled-over in
the usual way; the immense oval depressions for the nail-
heads are stamped nearly through the substance of the shoe,
and have been made by a blunt tool when the iron was
very hot. There is nothing to indicate that the shoe had
ever been placed on the bick or beak-horn of an anvil to
give it its shape. The *round holes* pierced for the passage
of the nails appear to have been punched through when
the iron was in a cold state, as the round holes in the
horse-shoes are made at the present day in Syria, Turkey,
and the East generally. These apertures are only six in
number, and there is no indication of attempts at raising
a toe-clip. Both surfaces of the shoe are plane, and the
workmanship is not of a very high order, but appears to
have been executed in a hurried manner.

The other shoe I examined had been found a short
distance from it. It is very perfect, though slightly worn
(it had been on the left fore foot), is precisely similar in
figure, size, and other particulars, and is made of excellent
iron. Accompanying these two shoes was a most interesting specimen [1] found on the surface of the ground,
on a high hill, one of the Cotswolds, which has been
recently ploughed up by permission of the owner, who
on that occasion discovered this shoe. The hill is in the
parish of Haresfield, and is known as Broadborough
Green, or Ringhill; and the spot where it was found is

---

[1] I am deeply indebted to *J*. D. T. Niblett, Esq., M.A., F.S.A., of
Tuffley, near *G*loucester, for an inspection, and the particulars connected
with the discovery of these three specimens.

by the side of the ancient trackway, leading through the British to the Roman camp, the remains of which are still discernible. Being so near the surface of the soil, which is there very thin, and overlying the rock, the iron is very much corroded, but the form of the shoe, which is identical with the other two, is perfect. It is narrower, longer, and heavier than the two specimens just described, and the three nail-heads of one side are yet in the shoe. They project nearly as high as the calkins, and are of the shape always observed with these shoes. Its small size, and staple-like form, caused it to be designated a 'mule shoe.'

· A very interesting discovery of a Roman villa has been recently made at Chedworth, a place on the great Foss Road, sixteen miles from Gloucester. With a very fine tesselated pavement, have been found a great number of articles, such as a silver spoon; two silver coins, on the obverse of which are the words 'Imperator Cæsar Antoninus Augustus;' a coin of Heliogabalus, and another of Valens; bronze fibulæ; rings; implements; bone hair-pins; bronze coins of Constantia, Constantinus, Urbs Roma, &c.; nails, armlets, twisted chains with swivels · styles, and steelyards with lead weights; iron implements, knives, chisels, spear-heads, crooks to suspend a kettle and three pigs of iron. The presence of the latter articles would tend to show that they had been manufactured on the spot. There were also various kinds of pottery; bones of the horse, ox, sheep, and pig, and antlers of a large herd of deer, as well as two fragments of human skulls. There are proofs that the villa has been destroyed by fire, and 275 coins, mostly Roman, fix the date; no

Saxon coins have been discovered, and Mr Roach Smith informs me that the relics are entirely Roman. It would appear, from various evidences, that the villa had been built or repaired after the time of Constantine the Great, and an inscription 'Prasatia' leads to the surmise that it belonged to the husband of Boadicea.

But the most important feature in this discovery is connected with our present subject: the recovery of one whole shoe and several fragments, which are said to have been with the other remains. But not one of these shows the outline we have hitherto been studying, and which has, with a few exceptions, so far as I have been able to learn, been characteristic of the shoes found with Roman or supposed pre-Roman objects. On the contrary, all exhibit what we would consider evidences of more recent manufacture. We no longer have the undulating border, the long and wide oval depressions, the narrow cover, the rolled calkins, and the large semicircular nail-heads. The nails and nail-holes are very like those now in use; the latter are stamped close to the margin of the shoe, the nails have been driven through the hoof, and the points twisted off and clinched in the usual way. The workmanship is entirely different to that we have been considering, and is much more advanced. One perfect specimen (fig. 92) measures $3\frac{5}{8}$ inches long and 4 inches wide, an imperfect one (fig. 93) $4\frac{1}{4}$ inches long and the same in width, while another half-shoe (fig. 94) is $4\frac{5}{8}$ inches long, and must have been equally wide. The breadth of it is extraordinary, measuring no less than $1\frac{3}{4}$ inch, and the shoe when complete must have nearly covered the whole of the horse's sole; it shows four nail-holes, two of which are occupied by the remains of nails.

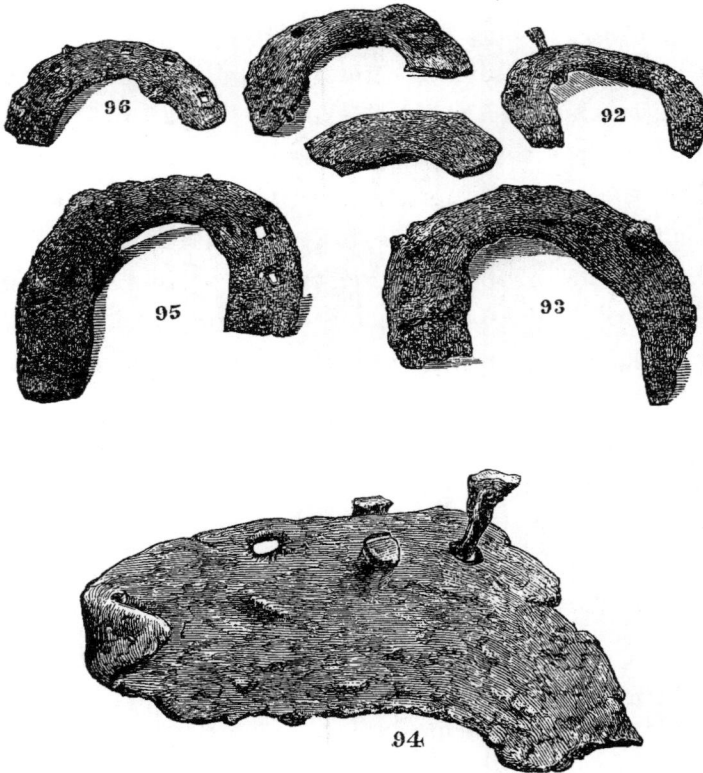

The only peculiarity I can discern between this and the shoes of a much later age, is the curious attempt at a calkin, which is here formed by the iron having been drawn to a point and bent forward on the ground face of the shoe.   This specimen is extremely clumsy and heavy, and quite unlike the light, and we might almost say elegant, shoe hitherto found.

Figures 95 and 96 are similar to 92.

It is impossible to account for the presence of these unusual specimens with Roman remains.   Mr Roach

Smith informs me that the discovery of the villa was, of course, accidental, and the excavations were not carefully conducted by any one likely to note the position of the articles found. If such be the fact, there is a probability that these shoes may have belonged to a much later date than the other relics discovered, and which they in all likelihood overlaid.

It is necessary to mention, however, that at Cirencester (the Roman Corinium, the Corimon of Ptolemy, and the Duro-Cornovium of the Antonine itinerary) various important Roman remains have been found, such as altars, querns, coins of all dates, from Claudius (A.D. 42) to Valentinian (A.D. 424), Samian and common pottery, bronze fibulæ, articles of bone, ivory, and glass, and great numbers of iron nails. Many of the latter have the peculiar head of the Roman horse-shoe nail, and others have the modern head fitted for the stamped and fullered shoe.

In the museum of this town are several shoes, two or three of which closely resemble those found at Chedworth, but none of the undulating-border type. These are said to have been found with the Roman remains, but there appears to hang some doubts as to the truth of this.[1]

The ruins of Pevensey Castle, in Sussex, furnishes us with another example of the early type. This castle, one of the most remarkable in the country, has been garrisoned and fortified by the Romans, Saxons, and Normans—the

---

[1] In the Catalogue of the Museum, it is stated that 'some of the iron objects are not Roman, but mediæval, and to one or two a still more recent date must be assigned.'

ruins of each occupier telling such a tale of 'mutability' as one spot has seldom told; but, as is nearly always the case, the Roman has left his mark indelibly fixed on those walls and towers that at one time stood proudly above the low shore, when the sea almost washed their base. The Roman Castrum has an area of seven acres, but the irregular form of the walls would indicate that here was a British stronghold before the arrival of the Romans. The shoe found within these ruins, and which is now in the museum of Lewes Castle, Sussex, is larger than the specimens we have yet examined, being $4\frac{1}{2}$ inches long and $4\frac{1}{4}$ wide. It does not appear to have been much worn, and yet its thickness does not exceed $\frac{1}{3}$ of an inch; it has no calkins, and both surfaces are flat. The border is undulating, and the nail-cavities and holes are like those of the Gloucester shoes. The workmanship is good, and the nail-holes, six in number, well placed (fig. 97).

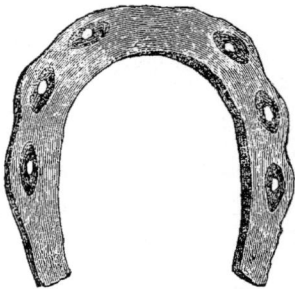

fig 97

A horse-shoe has been discovered within the interesting Roman encampment on Hod Hill, Dorsetshire. This camp appears to have been a Celtic fastness made subservient to the Roman system of castrametation, and was made a great military post by the Romans. In it weapons, implements, and personal ornaments have been found in considerable numbers, all manifesting an extraordinary predominance of iron over bronze. One of the iron manufactories or smelting-places was discovered near this camp, and from evidences attending the discovery, it was established probably as early as the reign of Claudius. From the coins found in this camp, and which range from ancient British, through Augustus, Agrippa, Tiberius, Germanicus, Nero and Drusus, Caligula and Claudius, up to Trajan, as well as from other testimony, Mr R. Smith is led to assert, that not the 'slightest evidence has been afforded of the tenure of the camp at any period after the Roman occupation of Britain.'[1] In iron, there have been discovered numerous varieties of spear-heads, arrow-heads, swords, the cheek-piece of a helmet, knives, agricultural implements in great variety, bridle-bits, chains, and keys.

To the courtesy of Mr Durden, of Blandford, who possesses this, and very many of the other Roman antiquities found in the castra, I am indebted for an inspection of the interesting shoe (fig. 98). That gentleman writes to me as follows : 'It was found within the Roman castra on Hod Hill, about three miles from Blandford, associated with many domestic articles of Roman manufacture. The coins hitherto found there belong to the first century, and it is presumed the shoe belongs to the same period.' Less primitive-looking than some of our other specimens, especially those from Springhead and Silbury Hill, it yet belongs to the same type. Its width is $3\frac{3}{4}$ inches, length $4\frac{1}{8}$-inches, and its breadth is a

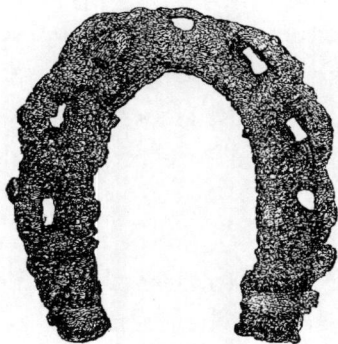

fig. 98

[1] Collectanea *Antiqua,* vol. VI. p. 10.

little more than that of the Springhead example. Though much oxidized, it yet retains the undulated border, and it is perforated by seven nail-holes of very large size, with the oblong socket to lodge the nail-head. Three of the holes are on each side, and one in the centre of the toe has doubtless been intended to act like the modern toe-clip, and prevent the shoe from being driven back. This feature in these antique shoes is very rare, indeed this is the only instance in which I have been able to trace it. The aperture for the shank of the nail, instead of being nearly circular, as in the Springhead shoe, is quadrilateral, and of immense size, in proportion to the shoe ($\frac{3}{8}$ths long, by $\frac{3}{16}$ths wide). One of the nails yet remains in the shoe, but the head is much worn; though sufficient is left to prove that it was of the flattened, high, and wide T pattern. The shank is almost square like a carpenter's nail, and fills the hole; and at a distance of only $\frac{1}{4}$ inch from the foot surface of the shoe it bends suddenly forward as if to form a clench on the outside of the hoof. The excessive thickness of the nail, and the very short hold it had of the hoof, are easily accounted for. The shoe has evidently been for the near (left) fore foot, and the inner branch towards the heel is narrower than the outer one; it shows faint traces of a calkin, but the outer heel has a well-defined calkin formed by doubling over the extremity, as in the other specimens of this period, though this has been more clumsily done than in some of those we have noticed. The foot-surface is slightly concave from the outer to the inner rim.

In the large collection of undoubted Roman remains brought to light in this castra, are three spurs of antique shape, two of iron (figs. 99, 100), and one of bronze (fig. 101). 'Had they been found unaccompanied by objects

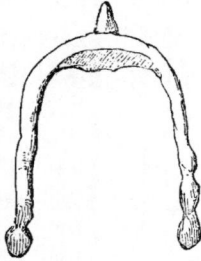 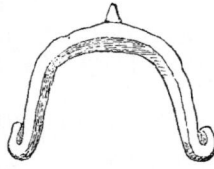 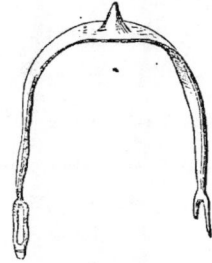

fig 99   fig 100   fig 101

so exclusively Roman,' remarks Mr Roach Smith, 'they would, and with reason, have been called Norman or late Saxon.' These spurs are remarkable for their short neck or 'prick,' which is even less than the Anglo-Saxon specimens, and much more so than those of a later date. C. Caylus [1] figures an ancient bronze spur with apertures at the ends of the branches to fasten it on, like those represented in this bronze relic from Hod Hill.

At Shefford, in Bedfordshire, what was called a hoof-pick was encountered with Roman relics : ' Of Roman relics no place in Bedfordshire has furnished the quantity or quality equal to Shefford. About four dozen Samian cups, dishes, and *pateræ* of various shapes and patterns have been there discovered, and at Stanford Bury, in its immediate vicinity. A vast variety of other reliquiæ were found with these ; some splendid articles in glass, a beautiful radiated amber-coloured vase, quite perfect; a splendid blue jug, or simpulum, of elegant form, and the sacred knife that accompanies the simpulum on the reverses of coins of Antoninus and other emperors, as emblems of the impe-

[1] Recueil, vol. iii. plate 9.

rial and pontifical dignity. A few yards from hence was dug up the bones of a horse, and the ashes of his rider, together with an iron implement, evidently formed to pick the horse's hoofs, and fasten his shoes. With these were found a small silver musical instrument, a denarius of Septimus Geta, representing him at the age of nine or ten years ; another also of Geta was found near, apparently two or three years older ; these coins were of fine workmanship and in beautiful condition."

We may be allowed to entertain doubts as to the article named being a hoof-pick; such an instrument would scarcely be necessary, if at all, with such narrow shoes, which had no concavity between them and the sole, as at a later period.

At Uriconium or Viroconium, now Wroxeter, in Shropshire, and which was one of the largest and most important Roman towns before its destruction in the middle of the fifth eentury, a fragment of a small horse-shoe has been gathered, but it is so oxidized and imperfect that none of its details can be made out. It is now in the Shrewsbury Museum.

A horse-shoe, supposed to be Roman, has been found at the ancient Conderum, Northumberlandshire. There is a drawing given of it in the Archæologia Æliana (vol. vi. p. 3), but no particulars as to its discovery or its dimensions. It resembles somewhat, if one can judge from the figure, those in the Cirencester Museum and at Chedworth, the cover of the shoe being wide, the borders even, and the foot-surface concave.

In the Rolfe collection of the Liverpool Museum is a

---

[1] *Gentleman's Magazine,* p. 518, 1848.

shoe four inches long and the same in width, which evidently belongs to the era of undulating borders, small calkins, and nail-holes with deep sockets (fig. 102). Unfortunately there is no history attached to it.

This is all the evidence, so far as I can discover, which we may bring forward in favour of shoeing being in vogue in Celtic, or pre-Roman, and Roman times in this country. The wide extent over which the

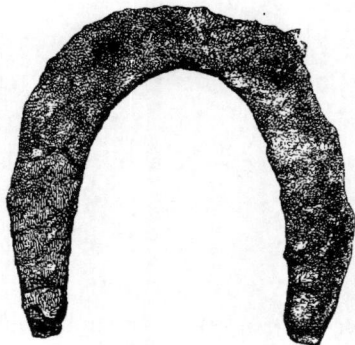

fig 102

remains of hoof-armature has been traced, the relics, in the majority of cases, accompanying them, and the singular uniformity in size and character of most of the specimens, can scarcely leave a doubt as to the fact of shoeing being known at that early stage in our national history.

The ancient Britons were, to a large extent, driven out of England by the Anglo-Saxons, and either fled to the continent of Europe, where they gave their name to Brittany, or retired to Wales (A.D. 447)—the *Britannia Secunda* of the Romans—where, amid their inaccessible mountains, they defied their treacherous invaders, and for many centuries retained their peculiar customs and laws. The fact of the former may be inferred from the traces of the Cromlech, the sacrificing-stone, and the Druid-circle; while from the latter, part of which may have existed long ages before, but were revised by Howel Dha, or the Good, on the banks of the Tav, in A.D. 911, we have written evidence to prove that this handicraft was not only known and practised, but that they who followed it were privileged individuals, holding somewhat high rank at Court, and treated as if their art was one of great value.

That remarkable method of division or enumeration of the ancient Celtic nations, the trinal system, had divided Wales, between the years 843 and 876, into three dynasties,—North, South, and Powysland; and it is in the code of laws applicable to each of these, that we discover the link in the chain of evidence required to bring our history into harmony with the relics just described. These laws altogether show a very advanced agrarian condition, and much beyond that of any other nation at this period. In the 'Dull O Gwynedd,' or Venedotian Code of North Wales, it is ordained that the judge of the court 'is to have from the chief groom his horse, *complete from the first nail to the last,* and saddled, and brought to him when he rides.' Amongst the other privileges and duties of the groom of the rein, 'he is to have his land free, his horse in attendance, and his clothing like the rest; his woollen clothing from the king, and his linen clothing from the queen.' He is 'to have the king's rain-caps in which he shall ride; his old bridles, his old hose, his spurs, his brass-mounted saddles, and all his horse equipage. He is to officiate in the absence of the chief groom. He is to hold the king's stirrup when he mounts and when he alights, and lead his horse to the stable, and bring it to him on the following day. He is always to walk near the king, that he may serve him when necessary. *He is to shoe the king's horse.* . . . .
His protection is, from the time the smith of the Court

shall begin to make *four horse-shoes, with their comple-ment of nails, until he places them under the feet of the king's horse,* to convey away an offender.' The duties of the smith were:—'He is to make all the necessaries of the palace gratuitously, except three things: these are, the suspending irons of the rim of a caldron, the blade of a coulter, the socket of a fuel-axe, and head of a spear; for each of these three things he is to be paid the value of his labour. He is to do what is wanted by the officers of the palace gratuitously; they are to present him with clothes for each piece of work. He is entitled to the "ceinion."[1] His seat in the palace is on the end of the bench, near the priest of the household. His protection is, from the time he shall begin his work in the morning until he shall finish at night.'

There were three arts which the son of a *taeog* (or villain) was not allowed to learn 'without the permission of his lord; and if he should learn them, he must not exercise them, except a scholar, after he has taken holy orders: these are scholarship, *smithcraft,* and bardism.'

To show the value put upon the extremity of a horse's limb, it is enacted that 'the worth of a horse's foot is his full worth.'[2]

'Four horse-shoes (*Pedeyr pedhol*), with their com-plement of nails, are two pence in value;' a small sum, if the Welsh money bore a like value to that then current among the Anglo-Saxons, five of their pence making one shilling.

[1] The *ceinion* was the first liquor that came into the hall.

[2] Book iii. chap. 4. We are reminded by this of the saying of Jeremiah Bridges, 'No Foot no Horse;' or, as our French friends have it, 'Pas de Pied, pas de Cheval.'

Then follows a list and valuation of the appliances of a Celtic smith :—

'The tools of a smith, six-score pence :

The large anvil, three-score pence :

The brick-orne anvil, twelve pence :

The bellows, eight pence :

The smith's pincers, four pence :

The smith's sledge, four pence :

A paring-knife (for the hoofs ?—Cammec-pedeyr Keynnyanc), four pence :

A bore (or punch—Kethraul), four pence :

A groover (Knysyll), four pence :

A vice, four pence :

A hoof-rasp (Carnllyf), four pence.'

This enumeration is curious, as we observe in the list several of the articles found in the Druidical mound at Alesia, in Gaul.

The Dimetian, or 'South Wales Code,' is in some respects similar to that of the Venedotian. 'The protection of the groom of the rein is, *whilst the smith of the Court makes four shoes with their complement of nails, and whilst he shall shoe the king's steed.*'[1] The protection of the groom of the rein to the queen was the same.

The smith of the Court was to have the heads of the oxen and cows slaughtered in the palace, and food for himself and servant from the palace; as well as the feet of all the cattle,[2] and other privileges. The worth of his tools was also six-score pence.

---

[1] Book i. chap. 7.

[2] The ancient Welsh used the legs of cow-hides for shoes. In the Venedotian Code, it is specified that the king's apparitor is to have ' the

'Three arts which a taeog is not to teach to his son without the permission of his lord: scholarship, smithcraft, and bardism: for if the lord be passive until the tonsure be performed on the scholar; or until the smith enter his smithy; or until a bard be graduated in song,—he cannot afterwards enslave them,' proving that the smith was a freeman.

The trinal, or tripartite, system was sometimes curiously applied:—'There are three fires, kindled by a person on his own land, which are not cognizable in law: the fire of heath-burning, from the middle of March to the middle of April; the fire of a hamlet kiln; and the fire of a hamlet smithy, that shall be nine paces from the hamlet, and having either a covering of broom or of sod thereon.' [1]

In these laws we find the smith and his craft, horse-shoes, and horses, remarkably mixed up in those triads that seem to be so strangely related to the symbolism of the ancient world:—the mystic number 3, the pyramid, triangle, the basis of the mysterious ogive; the number that was considered holy at the first dawn of civilization, that is found wherever variety is developed, and that meets us everywhere. The Welsh laws afford us a striking instance of the influence of this wonderful numeral. 'Three things for which, if found on a road, no one is bound to answer (or be responsible for taking possession of): a *horse-shoe* (*pedol*), a needle, and a penny.' 'There are three *one-footed* animals: a horse, a hawk, and a

legs of the oxen and kine obtained by his information, to make boots to the height of his ankles.'
[1] Book ii. chap. 8.

greyhound: whosoever shall break the leg of any one of them, let him pay his whole worth.'

In the Gwentian Code, applicable to the district inhabited by the Silures, it is written: 'The protection of the groom of the rein is, to conduct the person *while the smith of the Court makes four shoes, with their sets of nails, and shall shoe the king's steed'* 'The groom of the rein has the king's daily saddle, his panel, his bridle, his spurs, his hose, and his rain-cap when discarded; also his *old horse-shoes* (*hen pedolen*), and his *shoeing-irons* (*heyrn pedoli*).' [1] In the triads of the 'Cyrethian' we find: 'Three free sons of the bond: a clerk, a bard, and a smith. Three bond sons of the free: the sons of the above.' Of the king's hall it is ordered: 'The servants are apportioned in three parts, one third to the queen. . . . . The smith (*gof*) of the Court is to sit in a chair before the judge (near a column), which column the silentiary is to strike, on the side furthest from the king, when commanding silence.' In the 'Leges Wallice,' of about the same date, there is also another paragraph relating to our subject: 'Refugium gwastrant awyn (equisonis) est, conducere hominem tanto tempore quanto faber curie faciet IIII[or] *ferra cum clauis,* et cum eo *ferret* dextrarium regis.' [2]

Oxen alone were used for the plough: 'Neither horses, mares, or cows, are to be put to the plough; and if they should be put, and abortion should ensue to either mares or cattle, or the horses be injured, it is not to be compensated.' [3]

---

[1] Book i. chap. 6.   [2] Book i. chap. vii.
[3] Venedotian Code.   Book iii. chap. 24.

These extracts from the ancient laws of Wales which may have been—and we have every reason to believe were—in existence centuries before the reign of Howel the Good, show in the most unmistakable manner that farriery was practised and held in high estimation by the primitive people of Britain, that the Court farrier was a sacred sort of personage, on whose shoulders the mystic mantle of the Druid iron-workers had fallen, and whose handicraft was not to be practised by every one.

It is very strange that, in relation to this subject, these laws of Wales have never before been examined.

Sir Walter Scott appears to have sanctioned the popular opinion, afterwards maintained by Sir F. Meyrick, Bracy Clark, and other notabilities, that these ancient Britons, the Welsh, did not shoe their horses. In one of his miscellaneous poems, the ' Norman Horse-Shoe,' composed in 1806, he relates an engagement on the banks of the Rymny, between the Norman Lords-Marchers of Monmouthshire, Clare, Earl of Striguil and Pembroke, and Neville, Baron of Chepstow, and the Welshmen of Glamorgan. The piece is prefaced by the announcement, that the Welsh, inhabiting a mountainous country, and possessing only an inferior breed of horses, were usually unable to resist the shock of the Anglo-Norman cavalry. On this occasion they were successful, notwithstanding that the horses of the latter were shod:—

> ' Red glows the forge in Striguil's bounds,
> And hammers din, and anvil sounds,
> And armourers, with iron toil,
> Barb many a steed for battle's broil.
> Foul fall the hand which bends the steel
> Around the courser's thundering heel,

That e'er shall dint a sable wound
On fair *Glamorgan*'s velvet ground!

.   .   .   .

Old Chepstow's brides may curse the toil,
That arm'd stout Clare for Cambrian broil;
Their orphans long the art may rue,
For Neville's war-horse forged the shoe.
No more the stamp of arméd steed
Shall dint *Glamorgan*'s velvet mead;
Nor trace be there, in early spring,
Save of the Fairies' emerald ring.'

After the evidence we have adduced, there is no reason to suppose that Glamorgan's velvet mead was not as likely to be dinted by the shoe-print of the Welsh horses after, as doubtless it had been long centuries before, this sanguinary skirmish; or that Neville's horse's hoofs were any better prepared for marching and fighting than that of the British chief who defeated him.

Besides all this, there are certain traditions afloat belonging to an early period, concerning hoof-prints and marks of horse-shoes on stones, which, if incorrect, so far as an examination of these impressions proves them to be, yet point to the prevalence of shoeing at a very remote age. For instance, there is an old tradition that, in the west of England, not far from the Devil's Coit, St Colomb, and standing on the edge of the Gossmoor, there is a large stone, upon which are deeply-impressed marks, which a little fancy may convert into the imprints of four horse-shoes. This is 'King Arthur's Stone,' and these marks were made, so says tradition, by the horse upon which the ancient British king rode when he resided at Castle Denis, and hunted on these moors.[1]

[1] Romances of the West of England.   First Series, p. 204.

Sir Walter Scott, in the 'Bridal of Triermain,'[1] describes an adventure of the same King, where he is tempted to drink from a goblet by Guendolen; but when he—

> 'Lifted the cup, in act to drink,
> A drop escaped the goblet's brink—
> Intense as liquid fire from hell,
> Upon the charger's neck it fell.
> Screaming with agony and fright
> He bolted twenty feet upright—
> The peasant still can show the dint
> Where his hoofs lighted on the flint.'

It is remarkable to find this tradition of hoof-prints in existence beyond England, and to note that it refers to nearly as early a date. On the black rocks of the Dame de Meuse, in the Ardennes, Belgium, is still shown the ineffaceable imprint left there by the horse on which Renaud was mounted. This valiant knight was the supposed contemporary of Charlemagne; his astounding deeds of prowess almost rival those of our own Arthur, and towards the termination of his career he became a chevalier mason, carrying on his back all the enormous blocks of stone required to build the 'Sainte Eglise' at Cologne.

My curiosity was considerably excited, when, in the course of recent researches, I found that a correspondent to 'Notes and Queries,' had sent the following letter to that valuable periodical, in January, 1864: 'Can any of your readers inform me when horses were first shod with iron? I have just had brought to me a stone about five inches over, on which is plainly impressed the mark of a pony's or mule's shoe. It was found near the scythe-

---

[1] Canto ii. 10.

stone pits, on the Blackdown Hills, between Honiton and Cullompton.'

With some difficulty, I at length discovered the gentleman into whose hands this geological specimen had fallen, Mr Matthews, of Bradninch, near Cullompton, Devonshire, and on my applying to him for an inspection of it, he most kindly and promptly sent it to me.

The resemblance of the impression to the form of a horse-shoe was undoubtedly most striking (fig. 103), and in

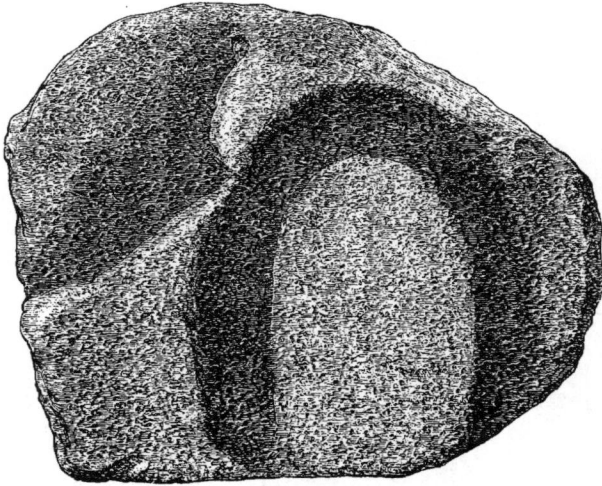

fig 103

size it exactly corresponded to one of the Roman Gloucester shoes then in my possession. There were no bulgings, however, on the outer margin ; and yet it was so remarkably like the shoe, and like the impression it would make on sand or clay, that any one at the first glance, and who was not a geologist, would have had no hesitation in affirming it to be due to that cause. But an examination of the stone effectually demolished such an opinion. It belonged to a kind called in technical language ' chert,' a sand-stone that underlies the chalk formation, and occurs in the lower green sand; and the imprint had been formed long ages before horses or Druid blacksmiths had worn or made hoof-plates on the more recent and superficial strata of our present earth.

Sir C. Lyell has given an opinion with regard to this curiosity. He says, 'Most of the horse-shoe impressions, of which I have seen a great many in the older stratified rocks of Scotland, have been thought to imply the former presence of medusæ, but this is a mere conjecture, derived from finding similar impressions made on the sands on which such gelatinous bodies rest. They have nothing to do with the footprints of horses.'

Professor Tennant, of the Strand, London, most obligingly undertook to explain the nature of the horse-shoe imprint, and the mode of its formation. It was only necessary for him to fit into it a petrified zoophyte, whose base, like the bottom of a champagne bottle, had perhaps made scores of these 'Man Friday' tracks, to settle the question. One of these creatures had settled itself upon the soft sand, when there was nobody present to note the circumstance; the almost circular indent made by its cup-like basis had escaped obliteration, the sand became rock, —fine, close, and hard enough to sharpen a scythe-blade, and to render the Devonshire scythe-stone pits famous; and long after subsequent races of creatures had passed away—even the Druids and aboriginal horses, the whilom resting-place of this half-animal, half-vegetable, had been revealed, and a chip knocked off one of its sides. So much for the traditions of hoof-prints.

After the departure of the Romans from Britain, and the invasion of the Saxons, Angles, and Jutes, we find history for a long period nothing but a tissue of traditions. We may believe that the Saxons occasionally, if not constantly, shod their horses; but whether in the same fashioned shoe that the ancient Britons and Gauls used, is a matter for doubt. Mr Syer Cuming[1] says he has seen a shoe very like in form that which Chifflet describes as found in Childeric's tomb, and which was said to have been discovered with Saxon weapons in Kent. It was of small size, very thin, and much oxidized. Elsewhere, at a later period, he remarks: 'The question regarding the employment of horse-shoes by the Teutonic tribes of Britain has received some slight elucidation. I feel confident that the Anglo-Saxons shod their steeds, and that they called the metal shoe *calc-rond, i. e.* rim-shoe; though Bosworth says the name signifies a round hoof; and my confidence is supported by the fact of the discovery of some horse-shoes in a Saxon burial-place in Berkshire. Mr T. Wills permits me to lay before you a horse-shoe, which there seems good reason to regard as of Saxon origin; it is about three inches and seven-eighths long, exceedingly thin, agreeing in this respect with the previously-mentioned horse-shoe found with Saxon remains in Kent, and the iron of which it is composed is of that peculiar ropy kind, so characteristic of the Anglo-Saxon era. It is sharp at the extremities, has no calkins, and the *six large, square nail-holes* are cut clean through the substance, and not counter-sunk to receive the nail-heads. This curious specimen was recovered from the northern side of the

[1] Journal of the Archæological *A*ssociation, vol. vi.

Thames, about midway between Dowgate and Blackfriars Bridge.'[1]

We may be allowed to entertain some doubts as to the meaning of the Anglo-Saxon term ' calc-rond,' especially as applied to a ' rim-shoe' for horses. The Saxon for shoe is ' sceo' or ' þcoh ;' and the verb to shoe ' þceczan ;' while the smith is written as in German, þmiᵹ.

It would appear certain that, as with the invasion of Gaul by the Franks, another form of shoe gradually came into use in England on the arrival of the Saxons. We have but little to lead us to believe that this German race cared much for the horse, or employed it to any extent at first. In this respect they resembled the Franks. In process of time, however, they became expert horsemen, and placed much value upon the noble beast; in this they again followed the example of the Franks—a change that might be attributed, in both instances, to their having come into contact with another race—the Celtic,—to whom the horse had for ages been an all-important adjunct of existence. This is rendered apparent from the fact, that those of the Britons who cared to remain among the invaders, were intrusted with the studs of the Anglo-Saxon kings. In the laws of Ina, written towards the termination of the seventh or commencement of the eighth century, the ' hors-wealh' stands in high estimation. This functionary was a Welshman, or rather an ancient Briton, who had the charge of the king's stud, his knowledge of horses apparently justifying his being selected to attend to them, as the British inhabitants excelled in the care and management of these creatures,

[1] Op. cit. vol. xiv.

and were therefore preferred as keepers of the royal stables. The ' hors-weard,' or watchers of the lord's horses, are also specially mentioned in the laws of Æthelbirht and Ina (sixth and seventh centuries). The Anglo-Saxon laws, it must be remembered, are far behind those of the Britons, and leave us fewer details concerning the domestic life of the people. We will see hereafter that the smith and his craft occupied a somewhat important position with this people, though perhaps less than with the Britons.

So late as the time of Bede (seventh century) we find it stated that the English only began to use saddle-horses (631), when prelates and others rode on horseback, who till that time were wont to go on foot. But if, he adds, upon any urgent occasion they were obliged to ride, they used mares only. Fosbrooke thinks this notice refers to the heathen Anglo-Saxon priests, who were disgraced by being compelled to ride on mares. It is true that in several parts of the world it is reckoned an indignity to use a mare for this purpose—in South America, for example. And in Java it appears to be looked upon as a punishment, for Crawfurd [1] mentions that, in the 16th century, a rebel chief was subdued by the Prince of Mataram, and the conqueror, without offering him any further injury, directed a *lame mare* to be brought, on which, barebacked, and with a miserable bridle, he mounted his discomfited rival, and in this plight dismissed him to his chief, to tell the story of his disgrace. ' It is necessary to explain,' adds Mr Crawfurd, ' that in Java it is considered a disgrace to ride a mare ; none but the meanest of the people using mares for the saddle.'

[1] Indian *Archipelago*, vol. ii. p. 324.

The indignity of being compelled to ride mares did not continue very long with the English monks, who soon became owners of the best-conditioned horses in the land, and were as devoted slaves to hunting, and other amusements of a similar character, as any beyond the monastery doors. When the archdeacon of Richmond arrived at Bridlington, Yorkshire (in 1216), to be inducted to the priory, he was accompanied by ninety-seven horses, twenty-one dogs, and three hacks. In 1256, Walter de Suffield, bishop of Norwich, bequeathed by will his pack of hounds to the king; whilst the abbot of Tavistock, who had also a pack, was commanded by his bishop, in 1348, to break it up. William de Clowne, abbot of Leicester, who died in 1377, had so good a stud, and was so skilful in hare-hunting, that the king, his son Edward, and several noblemen, paid him an annual pension that they might hunt with him. Wycliffe, who lived at this time, in his 'Trialogue,' inveighs against the priests for their 'fair horses, and jolly gay saddles and bridles ringing by the way.' And Chaucer does as much in his admirable delineation of the monk of his day :—

> 'A monk there was, a fair for the mastery;
> An out-rider that lovéd venerie (hunting);
> A manly man to be an abbot able.
> Full many a dainty horse had he in stable.
> .   .   .   .
> Therefore he was a prickasour (hard rider) a right :
> Greyhounds he had as swift as foul (birds) of flight :
> Of pricking (hard riding), and of hunting for the hare
> Was all his lust; for no cost would he care.'

On the Continent, in 1180, the third council of Lateran prohibited this amusement while bishops were journeying from one abbey to another, and restricted them to a train of forty or fifty horses![1]

But the Anglo-Saxons, even so early as the time of Bede,[2] in their youth or 'childhood,' appear to have excelled in horse-racing. Hunting on horseback was a favourite pastime, and we are told how long the chases were, and how rugged the paths.[3] An ealdorman's[4] heriot or claim to that title was the fact of his possessing four horses saddled and four not saddled, with arms and money; while the king's thegn or baron must own a moiety of that number, and the middling thegn or knight, one-fourth.[5]

Horses must have been numerous and looked upon as an important acquisition, even by the Danish invaders; for in the reign of Ethelred (866) these people made one of their incursions into England in numbers never before equalled, and were allowed by that monarch to locate themselves for the winter in East Anglia. So bold were they in their strength, that they levied demands upon the king; and among the many items he was compelled to furnish was a supply of horses, which mounted the greatest part of their army[6]

Horses also appear to have been very acceptable gifts. For, 926, we read that Hugues, the son of King

[1] *Velly.* Hist. de France, vol. iii. p. 236.

[2] Hist. Eccles., lib. v. cap. 6.

[3] Life of St Dunstan. Cotton MSS. Cleop. B. 13.

[4] The 'ealdorman,' or 'aldormanus,' was, among the Anglo-Saxons, originally a dignitary of the highest rank, hereditarily and officially, and nearly synonymous with that of King.

[5] Leges Anglo-Saxonicæ.

[6] *Asser.* De Rebus Gestis Ælfredi, p. 15. Edit. Oxford, 1772.

Robert of France, presented Athelstan of England with three hundred fine coursers and their trappings, besides other valuables.[1] Athelstan enacted that 'no man shall send any horses over sea, but such as be presents.'[2]

In the reign of this monarch it is probable that horses were used for ploughing; for in one of his laws (16) it is ordained that 'every man have to the plough two well-horsed men.' From these laws we also learn, that a horse was valued at half a pound, 'if it be so good; and if it be inferior, let it be paid for by the worth of its appearance, and not by that which the man values it at who owns it, unless he have evidence that it be as good as he says.'

About this period, too, tournaments began to be popular among the Anglo-Saxons. In 934, Henry the First of Germany published his institutions concerning them, and certain classes and persons were forbidden to engage in them under penalty of losing their horses.[3] Even previous to this period, Nithard mentions that some French gentlemen fought in play on horseback.[4]

It has often been asserted that the Anglo-Saxons had no cavalry in the days of Harold, and that their defeat at the battle of Hastings was chiefly due to the absence of that arm from their force. This would appear, however, to be incorrect. At the decisive battle between that unfortunate monarch and the Danish invader, Hardrada, at Stamford Bridge, in the East Riding of Yorkshire, only a

[1] MSS. Cleop. B. 5.
[2] ' Nemo equum aliquem ultra mare mittat nisi eum donare velit.' —Legis Æthelst.
[3] *Goldastus.* Constitutiones Imperialis, vol. ii. p. 41.
[4] *Turner.* Hist. Anglo-Saxons, vol. iii. p. 130.

few days before the appearance of the Normans and the battle of Hastings, the Anglo-Saxons were so strong in cavalry that the Danes, who were chiefly infantry, had to dispose themselves in a particular order of battle in order to repel the fierce attacks of these horsemen.[1]

After the defeat of the Danes, Harold hurried back to London to meet the Normans, but through disgust at his behaviour, and perhaps owing to the long distance and the fatigue they had already undergone, his northern army appears to have been almost, if not entirely, dispersed. But even at the battle of Hastings, though the footmen formed the chief part of his army, there was a force of cavalry; this, however, was purposely dismounted and incorporated with the other portion, owing to the position of the Anglo-Saxons on hilly ground.

The weapons of our Anglo-Saxon ancestors were purely Teutonic, and so far as the examples furnished by their graves afford evidence, it would appear they borrowed nothing from the Romans. In battle they fought as Saxons; and it was only when they came into contact, socially, with the people who had preceded them, that they felt the superiority of the Romans in the arts of peace.[2] They carried their manners and customs with them into England, as well as their peculiar arms and equipment, and with these also, perhaps, their own form of horseshoe. Certain it is, that from the time of their achieving their supremacy in England, the characteristic bulging-bordered shoe of the earlier ages appears rapidly to have gone out of fashion. A specimen of the new kind of

[1] See Snorre's Sagas.
[2] *Wright.* The Celt, the Roman, and the Saxon, p. 415.

shoe, which was found in Fleet Ditch, in 1847, will make this change manifest (fig. 104). This may have been of a later date than some of the other Saxon shoes, but it was in all probability in use before the Norman conquest. It was very small, thin, and without calkins. Mr Syer Cuming, alluding to this shoe and the alteration in its shape, lays some stress on the form as-

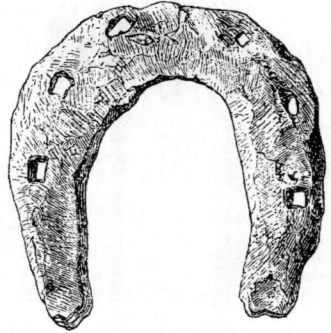

fig 104

sumed by the inner margin, which in the Celtic pattern, he says, is the figure of a Norman arch, and this Saxon shoe that of an arch of the 15th century. The very ancient specimen in the British Museum, however, which was found with Roman remains, is narrow across the toe, and the third York Museum example is the same.

In one of the Fairford graves opened by Mr Wylie,[1] and which apparently belonged to the Saxon period, a small, thin plate of iron 'like a miniature horse-shoe was found.' In the drawing given, however, there are no traces of nail-holes.

At Caenby, near Lincoln, Mr Jarvis[2] reports, that in a tumulus opened by some workmen, there was found a skeleton, a sword-blade, horse-furniture, and a horse-shoe. This was supposed to have been a Saxon grave. No drawing or description is given of this shoe.

Some years ago, a Saxon tomb was opened on Brighton Downs, and with some characteristic remains

[1] Fairford Graves. Oxford, 1852.
[2] *Akerman.* Remains of Pagan Saxondom.

was found a horse-shoe, which fell into the hands of the late Mr Faussett. After that gentleman's death, his collection of antiquities passed to Mr Mayer, of Liverpool, who presented them to the Free Public Museum of that town. Unfortunately, of the dozen specimens of horse-shoes in that building there appears to be but little, if any, history to be obtained; nearly all the specimens belong to the Rolfe collection, and but one to that named the Faussett, and this, I presume, is that from the grave at Brighton. Mr Mayer appears, from the statement given to me by the sub-curator of the museum, to think it might be Roman, but the shoe is not of the usual Roman type. It has apparently eight nail-holes, is $5\frac{1}{4}$ inches long and $4\frac{1}{2}$ wide, and the breadth of the branch is about $1\frac{1}{2}$ inch (fig. 105). It may be added, that in the

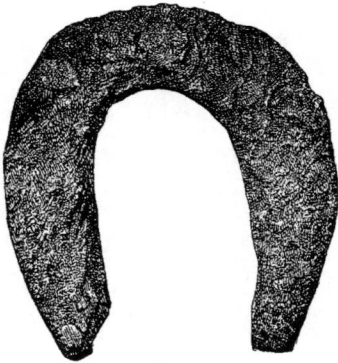

fig. 105

Rolfe collection there are two or three specimens of apparently the same age, and several of a later period. But these lose their value through having lost the history of their discovery.

Two remarkably curious specimens of a similar kind to that from Fleet Ditch were discovered in 1854, at Horred Hill, parish of Gillingham, Kent, deeply imbedded in brick clay. In appearance they look even more primitive than that example, and one (fig. 106) would appear to have been made during the transition from the Roman to the Saxon shape. It is of the same size as the Hod Hill shoe, but has more breadth of iron. The border is not undulated, and the nail-holes, though large, are square; there is no socket for the nail-head. One side, which has no calkin, has four nail-holes; and the other side, which has a calkin formed exactly like

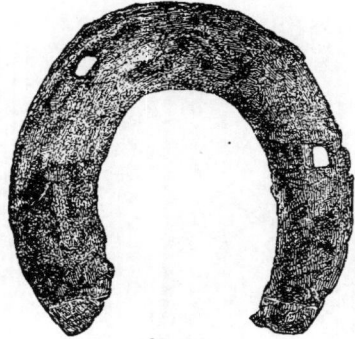

'fig. 106

the Roman and Gaulish specimens by doubling over the extremity of the branch, has only three. The iron appears to be remarkably good and fibrous, and much resembles that of the Saxon weapons made of that metal. The other shoe (fig. 107) is almost identically the same so far as regards size, but it is apparently of more recent date than the other, though still very primitive. It has two calkins raised at the extremities of the branches, and these, though very low and thin, are formed as in modern times. Wide at the toe and sides, it is very nar-

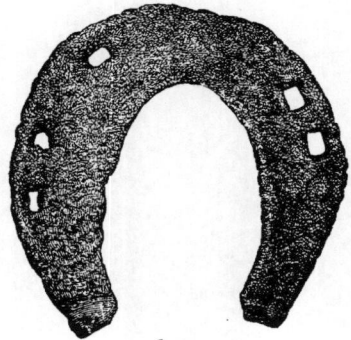

fig. 107

row and light towards the heels, has four square nail-holes on one side, and three on the other. Both specimens are very light, slightly concave to the foot, and convex to the ground surface, and would fit a horse about thirteen or

fourteen hands high. From circumstances connected
with their discovery, they were surmised to be at least a
thousand years old.

Some years ago there were found in a graveyard in
Berkshire (already alluded to by Mr Cuming) three
horse-shoes accompanied by purely Saxon remains.

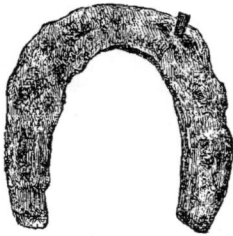

fig 108

Drawings of these and their accompanying relics are now in the
possession of Mr C. Roach Smith,
and to him I am indebted for permission to copy the former. It will
be seen that one of the shoes (fig.
108), the smallest (4 inches in
length and width), is of the primitive type, and still retains
a nail; while the other two (figs. 109, 110) are com-

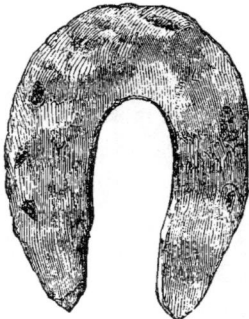

fig. 109

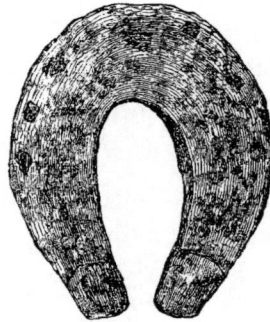

fig. 110

paratively large and heavy, one with calkins, the other
without; both have the even border, and but little to
distinguish them from mediæval horse-shoes. The occurrence of these two varieties in the same place, along with
unmistakable Saxon relics, testifies that they were both in
use at this period, and reminds us of the Frankish speci-

mens found in Belgium. Mr Roach Smith informs me that no particular account of the find reached him.

We have evidence that, in the time of Harold, horses must have been generally shod for service in the field. Dart,[1] in his History of York, says that at Battle Flats, six miles east of that city, the scene of the conflict between Harold and the Danes under Tostig (A.D. 1066), 'the farmers in ploughing frequently turn up a very small sort of horse-shoes, which would only fit an ass or the least breed of northern horses;' and Camden,[2] in speaking of the ancient village of Aldby, remarks : ' Aldby may have been a Roman before it was a Saxon villa. Stanford bridge has the name of Battle Bridge in writings after the Conquest, such as the instrument containing Oswis' translation, but it now keeps its antient name, and has no memorial of the battle except a piece of ground on the left hand of the bridge called Battle Flats, in plowing which of late years they find pieces of swords, and a sort of small horse-shoes that could only fit an ass or the smallest breed of northern horses, but are proofs of the antiquity of shoeing in England.'

It is much to be regretted that no description can be found of these articles.

In the Anglo-Saxon manuscripts of an early date, we have additional proof that horses wore shoes. In the accompanying illustration (fig. 111, next page) of a riding Saint, copied from an illuminated manuscript (Tiberius C. 6. fol. 11.) in the Harleian collection of the British Museum, and belonging, it is surmised, to the 11th century,

[1] Eboracum, p. 84.   [2] Britannia, vol. iii. p. 69.

the horse is shod in the most unequivocal manner, each hoof exhibiting three nails.

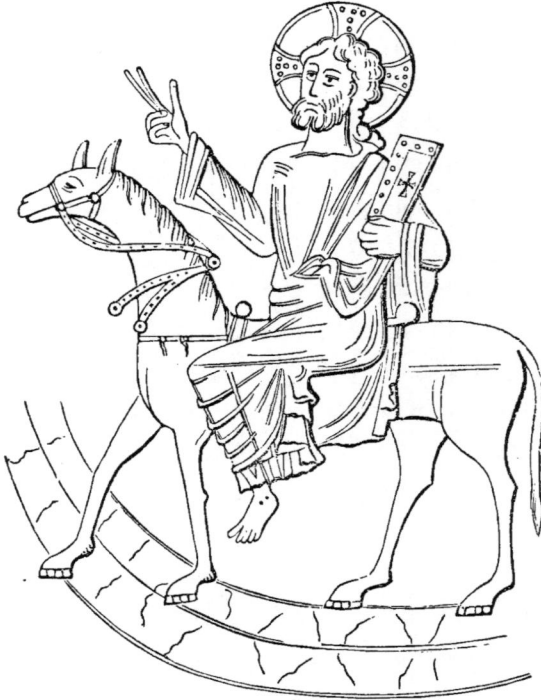

fig. 111

In another (Plut. 2278), representing a group of Anglo-Saxon equestrians, all the horses are represented as shod, the shoes having calkins, and retained on the hoofs apparently by four nails on each side.

In the Cottonian collection is another manuscript (Nero C. 4), with a series of illustrations of the life of our Saviour, in which is a royal cavalcade, whose horses' feet are all protected with shoes ; and also a picture of the flight into Egypt (fol. 7), where the mule or ass has its hoofs yet more distinctly armed.   In the same volume is an

Anglo-Saxon calendar, and for the month of May there is shown a nobleman hawking on horse-back, the feet of the steed being carefully shod, like those of a hawking equestrian of the 14th century, whose portrait will be referred to shortly.

Matthew of Paris speaks of horses both shod and unshod, and is angry with an archbishop who demanded shoes for unshod horses.[1]

In the ' Chronicon Monasterii de Abingdon,' a document probably of the 10th or 11th century, under the head of rents due to the hostillar is the following entry : ' Hi sunt redditus quos habet hostilarius, *ad ferramenta equorum*, ad usum monachorum, pauperum, peregrinorum, emenda.'[2]

In the ' Speculum Saxonica ' (lib. ii. art. 12), it is mentioned that shoes were only applied to the fore-feet. ' Four handsfull of corn shall be given to each horse during the day and night, and the horses shall be shod on the fore-feet (*in anterioribus pedibus equi sufferrentur*).' In the ' Jus Feudale Saxon.' (cap. 34, pt. 15) it is ordained, ' Their horses ought only to be shod on the fore-feet, and not on the hind-feet.'[3]

It would seem that the Anglo-Saxons experienced the same inconvenience from frost that we now do, for we read that in 832, the year began with excessive rains, and a frost succeeded, which was so sudden and intense, that the iced roads were nearly impassable by horses.[4]

Horses were shod in Scotland, in all probability, at as early a period as in England, though perhaps not regularly.

[1] *Fosbroke.* Op. cit.   [2] De Consuetudinibus Abbendoniæ.
[3] *Du Cange.* Glossarium.   [4] Annales Ruberi, p. 56.

The first written evidence I can find that bears upon this point, is in the laws of Malcolm II. (A.D. 1003—1033), which were framed and in force for forty or fifty years before the Norman invasion of England.   In one of these laws it is ordained, that when a man was condemned to death, the Crown took possession of his ' *broken, unshod horses,* and not more than 20 sheep, goats, and pigs,' [1] etc.

More than four centuries later, this statute appears to have been extant ; for in the new law of James III. (1487, Parliament 13, cap. 113), it was limited only to those horses intended for servile work (*operas serviles destinantur*) ; for if they were unbroken (*indomitos*) or intractable ; or broken and shod, or, in fine, capable of carrying saddles, and being ridden upon, they were not to belong to the Crown. [2]

The Norman invasion and conquest of England (1066) appears to have given rise to the supposition in many quarters, that the art of shoeing was introduced into this country by William the Conqueror.   This is quite a mistake, as we have sufficiently shown.   Horses had been shod for many centuries in Britain before the arrival of the Normans ; and though this practice may not have been, for various reasons, a general one, yet its benefits were sufficiently manifest to make it appreciated, and resorted to in particular circumstances.   Another proof, if any more were needed, that the Saxons employed this defence for their horses' feet, would be found in the fact, that Wel

---

[1] Leges Malcomi Secundi, cap. 3.   De Feodo Institiarii, Clericorum, etc. 4. ' *Item,* de homine condemnato ad mortem, Coram Justitiaro, coronator habebit *equos domitos non ferratos ;* oves infra viginti, capras, et porcos, infra decem,' etc.

[2] *Skeene.* Regiam Majestatem Scotiæ.   Edinburgh, 1609.

beck, in Nottinghamshire, was, at the invasion, in the pos
session of a Saxon chief named Gamelhere, who was
allowed to retain two carucates of land in Cuckeney, on
condition that he shod the king's palfreys upon all the
feet, with the king's shoes and nails, whenever he visited
the manor of Mansfield ; and if he put in all the nails,
the king was to give him a palfrey worth four marks ; or
if the horse was lamed in shoeing, the chief had to supply
one of like value to the king.[1] A Saxon nobleman unacquainted with the art of shoeing before the conquest of
England by William, would not have been deemed a very
safe agent in superintending that important operation immediately after that event. If any reliance is to be placed
on the Bayeux tapestry, said to have been wrought by
Matilda, the wife of the Conqueror, or the Empress
Matilda, wife of Henry I. of England, the Normans and
the Saxons are in one part represented with their horses
shod with heavy shoes, while in another part King Harold's
horses have unarmed feet.

The Normans brought many horses with them to
England, and it was their cavalry that enabled them to
defeat the army of Harold II. From a period far ante-
cedent to that conflict, the Normans were acquainted with
the mode of extending the usefulness of the horse by
protecting its hoofs with a metallic rim attached by nails ;
and on their gaining the supremacy in England, the art
of shoeing appears to have received marked attention.
William gave to Simon St Liz, a Norman nobleman who
had accompanied him across the channel, the town of
Northampton, and the whole hundred of Falkley, then

[1] *Thornton's* Nottinghamshire, p. 447.

valued at £40 per annum, to provide shoes for his horses.[1] Another follower, Henry de Farrariis, or Ferrers, is said to have taken his name from the circumstance that he was intrusted with the shoeing of the king's horses, or rather, the control of the shoers; for which his sovereign bestowed upon him the honour of Tutbury, in the county of Stafford.[2] After the Crusades, when it became the custom for families to take coat armour hereditarily, a charge of six horse-shoes was assumed by this great house.[3] These armorial bearings are, without doubt, much older than the regular establishment of heraldry, and were, with the family name, signs of office   'This bearing of horse-shoes in armoury,' says Guillim, 'is very ancient, as the arms of Robert Ferrers, Earl Ferrers, testifieth, who lived in the time of King Stephen, and who bore for his arms, argent; six horse-shoes, sable.'[4] The origin of the family name and office is perpetuated by a curious custom. The town of Oakham, the comparatively insignificant capital of the smallest county in England, also lays claim to horse-shoes in its arms, and Guillim relates that it is the chief town in Rutlandshire, seated in a rich valley, and an indifferent good and well-inhabited town. Here is an ancient privilege or custom which the inhabitants claim, that is, ' if any nobleman enter precinct or lordship, as an homage, he is to forfeit one of his horse's shoes, unless he redeem

[1] *Dugdale.* Baron., vol. i. p. 58.   Blount's Tenures, p. 50.

[2] *Brooke.*   Discovery of Errors in the Catalogue of the Nobility, p. 198.   [3] Ibid. p. 65.

[4] The present Earl Ferrers has, as one of the supporters in his coat of arms, a reindeer *charged* on the shoulder with a horse-shoe.—*Vide* Burke's Peerage List.

it with money; and the truth of this is apparent by the many horse-shoes nailed upon the shire-hall door; and their badge is a horse-shoe.' This shire-hall is one of the oldest mansions in the kingdom, and was built by Wakelin de Ferrers, son of an earl of that name.

Evelyn, travelling in 1654, writes in his Diary: 'I took a journey into the northern parts. Riding through Oakham, a pretty town in Rutlandshire, famous for the tenure of the barons, who held it by the taking off a shoe from every nobleman's horse that passed with his lord through the street, unless redeemed with a certain piece of money. In token of this are several gilded shoes nailed on the castle gate.' And Gough, in his Camden, asserts that the bailiff of the town had power to take a shoe off the horse of any man of noble birth who declined to pay the tribute money; the amount to be paid being left to the equestrian's generosity, while his liberality regulated the size of the horse-shoe inscribed with his name and title, which was set up to commemorate the event.

The origin of this singular impost or tenure is not known. A recent visitor, an army veterinary surgeon, says: 'I was much amused about four years ago, when marching through Oakham, a town in Rutlandshire, to find a very arbitrary law in existence there. On looking over the court-house, I found the walls literally covered with horse-shoes, and some of them of the most exaggerated and fantastic shape, gilt and emblazoned with the heraldic devices peculiar to their donors, and others the simple shoe. When I questioned the worthy old guide relative to the eccentricity of the act, he informed me that it originated with Elizabeth. Her Majesty, when passing through that town, found one of her horses lame from the loss of a shoe, and there was no one who could replace it. She forthwith issued a mandate compelling all peers of the realm to forfeit a horse's shoe when passing through the locality, or the payment of a fine. The proceeds accruing therefrom were devoted to the maintenance of a blacksmith.'[1] This tradition is not a very probable one, as it conflicts with nearly all the others; the custom is, in all likelihood, of an earlier date than the days of Queen Elizabeth.

Blount, in his 'Jocular Tenures,' informs us that a Duke of York once paid a silver horse-shoe to Lord Ferrers, and that a silver horse-shoe is due from every scion of royalty who rides across one of his manors. Of the shoes seen by Evelyn, three at least are said to remain—those bearing the names of Earl Gainsborough, Henry Montagu, and Lord Gray. Among the more notable ones of later date are those presented by the Earl of Cardigan in 1667, Lord Ipswich in 1687, Lord Guildford in 1690, and Lady Percy in 1771. More than thirty years ago, Queen Victoria acknowledged the right of Oakham, as her uncles, the Prince Regent and the Duke of York, had done before her; and the late Duke of Wellington soon followed her example. The law itself has sanctioned this unique species of taxation, Lords Denham, Campbell, and Wensleydale having followed the precedent of the famous Lord Mansfield. The day upon which Lord Campbell's horse-shoe was added to the collection of trophies, was a red-letter one in the chronicles of Oakham Hall, for on that day it recovered its long-lost 'golden shoe.' This

[1] *F. F. Collins, Royal Dragoons.* The Veterinarian, p. 663, 1867.

was not really a gold shoe, however, but a gilt one, that had done duty on the hoof of Lord Willoughby d'Eresby's favourite horse 'Clinker.' Deceived by its appearance, or misled by its popular designation, some rogue stole Clinker's shoe. This happened in 1846, and for twelve years the pride of Oakham Hall was conspicuous by its absence; but in 1858, the bailiff of the town was astonished by receiving the long-missing golden shoe *per rail,* accompanied by some humorous verses; but the thief was never discovered.[1]

The most recent instance of the horse-shoe impost having been levied, is reported in the daily papers for January, 1869 :—

'SHOEING A PEER.—A short time since, Lady Louisa Finch, Lord Redesdale, Mr Campbell (who were on a visit to George Finch, Esq., Burley-on-the-Hill), and G. H. Finch, Esq., M.P. for Rutland, paid a visit to Oakham Castle to inspect the Old Norman Hall (the oldest in England except Westminster Hall) and its horse-shoes. This getting to the ears of the bailiff, he was quickly down upon his Lordship for the honour of a shoe. Lord Redesdale selected one similar to those which of late have been fixed on the walls, and the new shoe will shortly be added to the large number now in the castle. The old manorial custom, from which this arises, took place at the first erection of the castle, on the grant to Walchelme de Ferrars, whose ancestors bore arms *seme* of horse-shoes, as designative of his office of Master of the Horse to the Duke of Normandy. In the early Norman period of our history, grants of customs seem

[1] Chambers's Journal.

to have been on this principle, that the Lords de Ferrars were entitled to demand from every baron, on his first passing through this lordship, a shoe from one of the horses, to be nailed upon the castle gate, the bailiff of the manor being empowered to stop the horses (and carriages also of late years) until service was performed. The custom is still preserved in Lord Redesdale giving a shoe on the 24th September, 1868.'

Soon after the Norman Conquest, we also find that 'Henry de Averyng held the manor of Morton, in the county of Essex, *in capite* of our Lord the King, by the serjeantry of finding a man with a horse, value ten shillings, and four horse-shoes (*quatuor ferris equorum*), one sack of barley, and one iron buckle, as often as it may happen that our Lord the King should go with his army into Wales, at his own proper expense for forty days.' [1] These acts will testify to the high value put upon shoeing by the early Norman kings.

It is rather amusing to read Bracy Clark's history of the introduction of shoeing into Britain by the Normans, and how the evil they had carried with them—for Bracy Clark's sole idea seemed to be that shoeing was an unmitigated evil — recoiled upon themselves, and caused the death of King William. He points the moral by stating, that the conqueror lost his life through his horse falling with him in jumping a ditch where the ground was slippery, for if the animal had not been shod he would not have fallen. 'Thus,' he says, 'the monarch who was the first to introduce the art of shoeing into England, was one of the first and most celebrated victims.' And M. Nicard

[1] Blount's Tenures, p. 16.

believes this statement, and explains how the accident occurred. The death of the king may have been caused by his horse falling with him, though that is a rather doubtful matter, as one account has it that he died from the effects of a wound sustained in France; at any rate, it is certain that he was not the first, by perhaps at least ten centuries, to introduce the art of shoeing into Britain.

CHAPTER VII.

In connection with the archæological discoveries which have enabled us to fix, approximately, the period when shoeing was first introduced into, or practised in, Europe, I have deferred alluding, until now, to another matter which has excited much interest among antiquarians; this is the discovery of what are generally termed 'hipposandals'—objects in iron, of somewhat different shapes, but all apparently designed for the same purpose. In various museums in France, Germany, Switzerland, and Britain, these curious-looking instruments are exhibited under the designation of '*hipposandals*,' or '*soleæ ferreæ*,' owing to its being supposed,—because the Romans did not employ nailed-shoes, and these articles usually presenting themselves with Roman remains,—they were used as sandals for their horses' feet. A large number of archæologists,—at the head of whom are the Abbé Cochet,[1] M. Namur,[2] and Mr Roach Smith;[3] and several Continental veterinary surgeons, with others, Professors Reynal of Alfort,[4] and Defays of Brussels,[5] MM. Fischer of Cessingen,[6] and Bieler of Rolle[7] (Switzerland)—are of this opinion; while others again, as Professor Quicherat of Chartes, MM. Castan and Delacroix of Besançon,[8] Captain Bial[9] of the French Artillery, and M. Quiquerez of Switzerland, are opposed to them, and think that these articles could never have been intended for, or worn as, shoes or sandals. Mr Roach Smith, the eminent archæologist, appears at one time to have held a middle opinion on the subject: 'It has been supposed they were used as temporary shoes for horses with tender feet, and they have been called stirrups; but both these notions are unsatisfactory.'[10] Some of these so-called sandals have been found in Gallo-Roman and Frankish graves; many with Roman remains of various kinds, and others without any accompanying relics.

Though their forms are varied, yet it will be found

[1] Le Tombeau de Childéric I.

[2] Public. de la Soc. Archéol. du Luxemburg, vols. vii. p. 185; xi. p. 92.

[3] Collect. Antiq., vol. iii. p. 129.

[4] Journal Vét. de Belgique, 1853.

[5] *Annales de Méd. Vétérinaire,* 1867.

[6] Journal Vét. de Belgique, 1853.

[7] *Journal de Méd. Vétérinaire de Lyon,* 1857.

[8] *Journal de Méd. Vét. Militaire,* 1866.

[9] *Megnin.* Origine de la Ferrure.

[10] Catalogue of the Museum of London Antiquities, p. 77.

that they chiefly belong to three models which, in all probability, have had the same uses, though they differ in shape. The first model may be described as a somewhat oblong or oval plate, or sole of metal, having a pyriform or circular opening in the middle (supposed to be for the purpose of allowing the moisture to escape from the horse's foot, as well as to give it air !). Transverse or crucial grooves are nearly always noticed on the under-surface of this plate, as if to make it *bite* the ground better. Two clips, sometimes four, rise from its sides, which are terminated at times in rings or hooks bending outwards, and the posterior part of the plate usually ends in a hook that projects more or less upwards.

The second form, found concurrently with the first, is much narrower in the sole, has a longer heel or spur than it, and is besides furnished with one in front which rises like the prow of a galley ; clips also flank the sides, but these are irregular in number, sometimes one on each side, sometimes two, and in one instance I have seen (in the British Museum) only one on one side ; these clips are often rather high, and nearly always terminate in eyes or hooks bending outwards. Sometimes there is an oval opening in the sole, but the grooves are seldom absent.

The third description is more curious. There is no hook in front, but the posterior one yet remains ; and the two lateral appendages are prolonged, gradually tapering and bending towards each other as they incline to the front of the plate, until they meet and are welded together, when they are drawn out to form a strong hook, as if to compensate for the absence of the anterior crotchet of the second model.

So early as 1758, one of the first class was found at Culm, near Avenches, Switzerland;[1] but in this century they have been largely dug up over a comparatively wide expanse of territory. They have been discovered in the departments of the Sarthe and Moselle; in 1853 at Arques, in the Roman establishment of Archelles; at Caudebec-les-Elbeuf (the ancient Uggate); at Riviere-Thibonville (Eure); at Vieux, near Caen (the ancient Argægenus); at Vieil-Evreux (the ancient Mediolanum); at Chatelet, Dijon, Autun, Troyes, Montbeliard, Mandeure, and Seine-Inferieure. They have likewise been found in the Frankish cemeteries of Lorraine and Champagne; and in 1862, at the demolition of the ancient bridge of Reignac (Indre) a number of them were recovered, with a sword-blade, and coins of Adrian and Antoninus. In 1854, two more were extracted from the Roman road between Langres and Rheims; these are now in the Chalôns Museum. Another was picked up at Chateau de Beauregard (Hautes-Pyrénées) in 1856, and was presented to the Cluny Museum by M. Fould; and M. Widranges procured some from excavations at Remennecourt. Metz, Strasbourg, and Stuttgart have also furnished specimens. In Switzerland they have been found at Granges, Canton de Vaud. In Germany, at Schwarzacht, near Echternach, and particularly in the Roman camp at Dalheim. In England, at Stony Stratford; Spring-Head, in Kent; and in London

As remarked, these articles are nearly always discovered on the sites of Roman buildings, contiguous to Roman stations, or with Roman *reliquæ*. Not unfre-

---

[1] *Schmidt.* Recueil d'Antiq. trouvé à *A*venches, Culon, etc. Berlin, 1780.

quently the three models are collected on the same site, and at the same depth, and with them have also been found the usual Gallo- or Romano-Celtic horse-shoes. Antiquarians have been greatly puzzled how to designate them; for some time they were stands or supports for lamps; afterwards they were stirrups; and then they figure as temporary shoes or sandals for horses with diseased or hoof-worn feet; as slippers that the Romans have strapped on their horses' limbs at night after long journeys; and as real defences for ordinary work—a step in advance of the sock with its metal sole; and lastly, as busandals, or bullock-slippers.

As the subject is one of more than ordinary interest, on account of the various hypotheses raised, and from the fact that these articles are now becoming somewhat common in museums, where they are duly labelled ' Hipposandals,' we will glance at the description and probable uses of some of them at least.

Dalheim affords a good instance of a locality in which all three forms have been discovered, accompanied by Roman remains of every description, as well as the ordinary nailed horse-shoe. In the first report from Professor Namur,[1] amongst other relics, he mentions having dug up several ordinary horse-shoes, and beside them were five *pathological shoes.* The latter are described as having their base oval, with a hole in the middle, and on each side towards the front a clip $2\frac{3}{4}$ inches high, ending in a hook-like process. Behind was a prolongation, also terminating in a hook. These strange articles were sub-

[1] Public. de la Soc. pour le Recher. des Monumens Luxembourg, vol. vii.

mitted to veterinary surgeon Fischer, of Cessingen, in 1851, who, on examining them, gave it as his opinion that they were 'hippopodes pathologiques,' intended to protect and cure hoofs too much worn, through default of shoeing.[1] This supposed sandal and its mode of attachment were delineated as in the accompanying figures (figs. 112, 113). In 1852-3, the excavations being

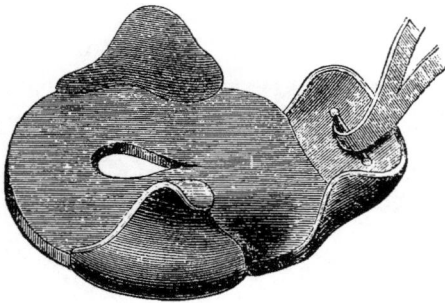 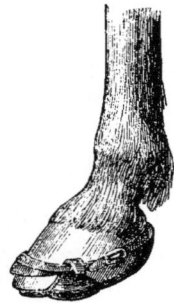

fig 112   fig. 113

continued, with many articles belonging to the Roman period were found one ordinary shoe and several of the so-called pathological *fers*. One of these belonged to the first description, but no horse's foot, so far as I am aware, was attempted to be fitted into it (fig. 114).[2]

In 1854-5, it is again reported that a new form of hipposandal had been discovered, accompanied by another belonging to the second category.[3] Allusion is made to the

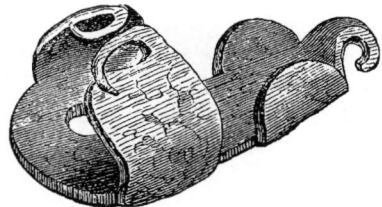

fig. 114

lusion is made to the former discoveries : 'Besides some ordinary shoes, there

[1] *Journal Vétérinaire de Belgique*, p. 30, 1853.
[2] Op. cit. vol. ix.   [3] Op. cit. vol. xi.

have been found others which are distinguished by a singular form, and which we may designate hippo-sandals or "hippopodes pathologiques." The base of these shoes is oval in shape, and in some there is an opening in the middle. On each side, and near the front part, there is a clip (*rebord*) furnished with a round ear, and another *rebord* at the heel is terminated by a hook turned towards the ground. These shoes (*fers*) were attached by means of straps, which passed through the two ears and under the hook behind. It appears that it was made use of when the hoof was diseased or worn by journeying, par-ticularly in mountainous countries. Such at least is the opinion of distinguished veterinary surgeons who have examined these shoes.' M. Namur then quotes the evi-dence of Fischer, who alludes to the writer in the 'United Service Gazette' we have already noticed, in saying: 'These shoes present much resemblance with the ancient shoes of Lycia,' &c.: showing how error is perpetuated and spread. We have no evidence to prove that horse-shoes were ever worn in Lycia; the resemblance of the Triquetra on a Lycian coin, to a shoe, was merely the fancy of a writer full of surmises and conjectures.

Namur continues: 'The use of shoes and straps (*fers à courroies*) is evidently much anterior to that of the nailed shoes.' Then reference is made to the new dis-covery. 'The excavations at Dalheim in 1854-5 have furnished two additional specimens. One, with clips, differs from those I have described, in that there is no hook behind. There is only a *rebord* pierced with two holes, in which are two oxidized nails with flat heads (fig. 115). The other specimen differs most essentially from the form generally known. It has also a base of an oval form, without an opening in the middle. The two lateral clips towards the anterior part, instead of being separate and terminated by ears, are brought together and united into a point which

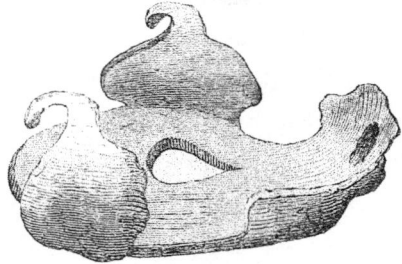

fig. 115

is bent towards the front in a hook or ear projecting above the anterior convex border of the shoe. This form appears altogether new, and M. Fischer has never seen one like it in the veterinary schools of Alfort, or elsewhere' (fig. 116). Professor Defays, of Brussels, has rehabilitated fig. 112, and attached it to a horse's limb. It will be observed that the fastening for the strap at the heel is rather awkwardly

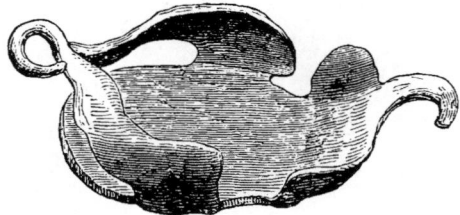

fig 116

placed, and so arranged that no horse could walk with it.

Fischer,' in describing those of the first and second class, previously discovered, remarks that they were not attached by means of nails, but by straps or cords. When the *fer* was found to be adapted to the size of a particular foot, the prolongation at the heel (supposed to be previously on a level with the body of the 'sandal') was then bent upwards in conformity with the dimensions

' Journal de Méd. Vétérinaire, 1853.

20

and shape of the hoof. 'Je pense qu'ils étaient employés comme fers pathologiques destinés à garantir et à guérir les pieds déjà usés par une trop grande course, et auxquels il etait alors impossible d'adapter des fers à clous.' This camp of Dalheim alone furnished twelve of these slippers.

An example of what we may term the second description was found in the Hill of Sacrifices, at Granges, in Switzerland, where ordinary shoes had been excavated. They were four in number, according to M. Troyon, who asserted that they were found on the feet of a horse or mule. They are thus noticed by veterinary surgeon Bíeler, though no mention is made as to whether he or M. Troyon, or any other persons worthy of credit, were present when the remains were exhumed. 'There was found near Granges, Canton de Vaud, in the midst of Roman ruins, the skeleton of a horse or mule, the four feet of which were garnished with iron boots. These articles, now in the museums of Avenches and Bel-Air, were the *soleæ ferreæ* spoken of by the ancients. They are composed of a plate of iron destined to be applied under the foot, round at the toe, and following the shape of the hoof, but narrowing towards the middle of the quarters in such a way as to allow a portion of the heels to rest on the ground; then they widen a little towards the posterior part, which is provided with an appendage or branch, with a hook raised at a right angle in the soleæ of the fore feet, but less elevated in those of the hind. In front, at each corner of the toe, a strong clip (*pinçon*), about $1\frac{1}{2}$ inch high, carries a buckle or hook at its summit. These three buckles were quite sufficient to fix the *solea* in a

firm manner, and it is scarcely possible that anything in-
tervened between it and the hoof, for no traces of holes or
rivets were perceived. The presence of straps leads to the
supposition that these soleæ were applied during work only,
and that they were removed when the animal entered its
stable. Without this precaution, the straps, already dangerous by the wear to which they might subject the skin
of the pastern, could not fail to be yet more pernicious if
left continually tightened around the feet. It is remarkable that the clips are only at the corners of the toes, and
that the iron sole should become narrowed at the part
which corresponds to the quarters; was this to prevent
slipping? Or did the Romans understand that the heels
were elastic? It is very possible that their spirit of observation taught them something respecting this. The
presence of these four *soleæ* on the feet of the same horse,
sufficiently indicates that they were not used for maladies
alone, as has been surmised, but habitually" (fig. 117).

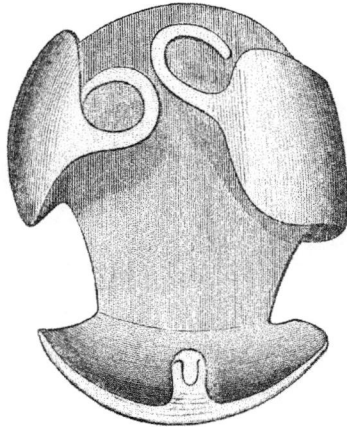

fig. 117

' Journal de Méd. Vét. de Lyon, p. 241, 1857.
20 *

The instrument found at Chateau Beauregard, Hautes-

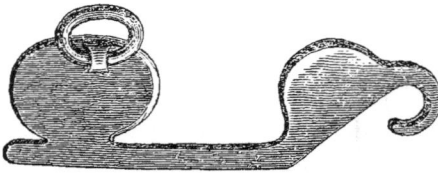

fig. 118

Pyrénées, and now in the ⎓Cluny Museum, ⸌belongs to the first class (figs. 118, 119), and is shown here in profile, as well as upper face. One of those discovered at Vieil-Evreux is also figured (fig. 120), and agrees with fig. 115 found at Dalheim. Of a more peculiar shape, but yet evidently intended for the same purpose, are two of the number recovered at Remen necourt, and delineat

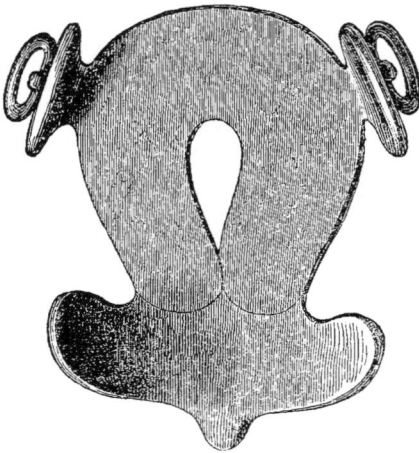

fig. 119

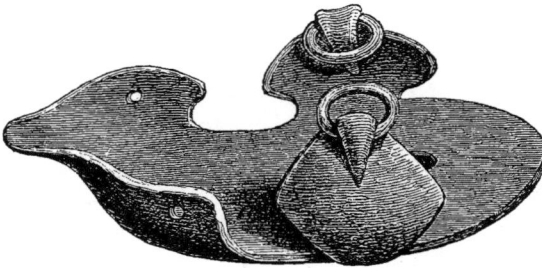

fig 120

ed by M. de Widrange, an antiquarian of Bar-le-Duc (figs. 121, 122). Figure 121 is remarkable for its possessing no rings or ears, or anything by which it could be attached to the hoof, supposing it to have been intended for such a purpose; and figure 122 is not much better adapted for a sandal.

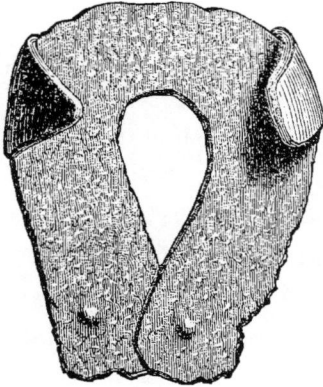

fig. 121

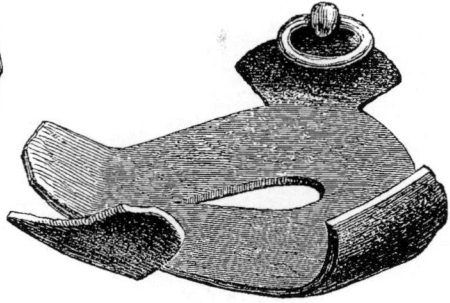

fig. 122

Professor Defays gives a drawing of another of this division, with an eye and ring posteriorly, two side clips without hooks, and the sole pierced by two round holes (fig. 123).

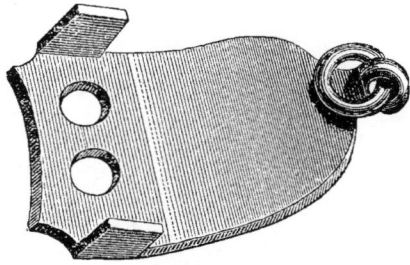

fig 123

Figures of the second type are as numerous if not more so, than those of the first; and they have also been found with them, and with nailed shoes, in various excavations on Roman and Frankish sites. The Museum of

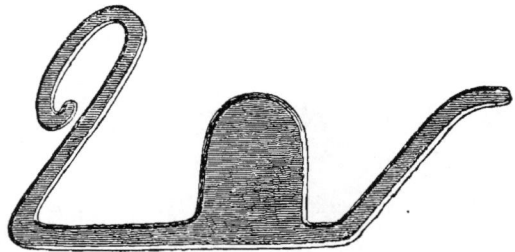

fig 124

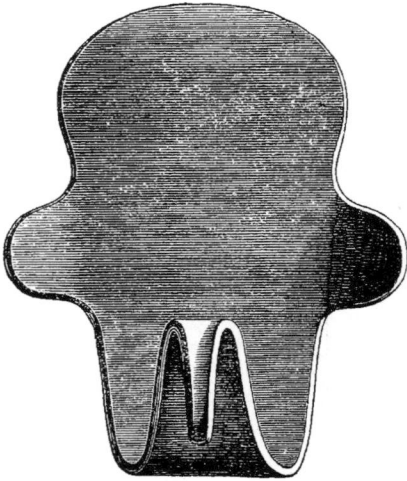

fig. 125

Cluny, France, ex-
hibits one as a hip-
posandal, and is here
shown in profile and
upper surface (figs.
124. 125); and a simi-
lar one, found at Scrupt
in 1846, is also delin-
eated (fig. 126). This,
M. de Widrange as-
sured the Abbé Cochet,
had been reported by
the   workman   who

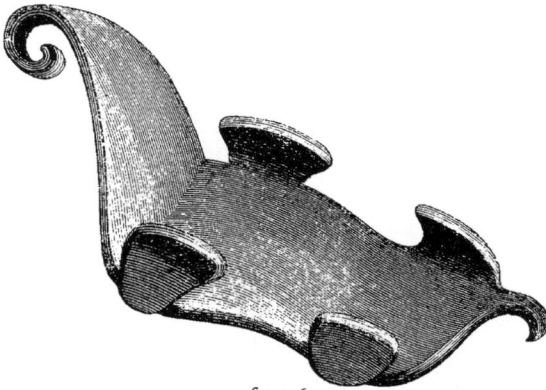

fig 126

found it, as yet attached to the limb of the animal by means
of straps that had been first passed round the pastern, then
through the eyelet in front, and buckled underneath the
hook behind. The Abbé, however, receives this inform_
ation with suspicion, and I think in this he is justified.[1]

[1] 'Je le déclare franchement, j'ai quelque peine à accepter cette as_
sertion, toute positive qu'elle paraît. La raison principale, c'est que M.
de Widranges n'a pas vu lui-même le fait qu'il raconte ; qu'il le tient

Figure 127 is a drawing of another of this class exhibited

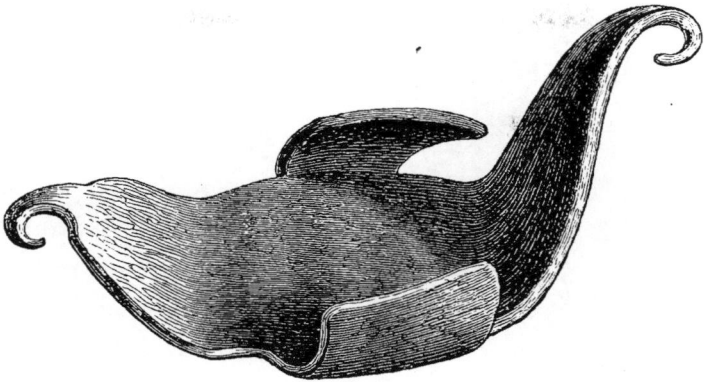

fig. 127

in the Museum of Besançon, which differs yet more in
shape, though, unlike the last, it has only a single clip on
each side.   M. Megnin,[1] who does not appear to have
noticed the existence of the class to be next described,
evidently believes the two kinds to have been employed
as *chaussures* for domestic animals.   'It is certain, indeed,
that these shoes could only have been worn by very slow-
paced pack animals, such as mules and oxen, and that the
name given to them by the Abbé Cochet, *hippo-sandals*,
is not suitable ; it ought to be *mulo-sandals* or *bu-sandals*.
This last designation was originated by M. Delacroix,[2]

d'ouvriers toujours disposés à en imposer ou à se faire illusion à eux-
mêmes, et enfin, parce que notre expérience nous a montré combien il
est difficile que le pied du cheval se soit suffisamment conservé pour
être aussi bien restitué, même par l'homme le plus compétent.   Quoi-
que M. de Widranges soit un fort honnête et trés-consciencieux arch-
éologue, je lui demanderai la permission de citer, sous sa seule re-
sponsabilité, les faits qui précédent, faits dont l'importance est d'autant
plus grand que jusqu'ici, en France, ils sont seuls de leur genre.'—
Le Tombeau de Childéric, p. 154.

[1] La Maréchalerie Française, p. 40.   Paris, 1867.

Mémoires de la Soc. d'Emulation du Doubs, 1864.

who has found iron *soleæ* which exactly fitted the foot

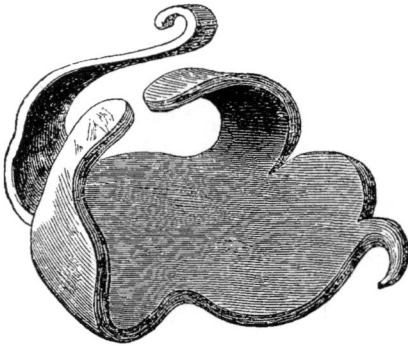

fig 128

of an ox, and even one that covered only one claw (figs. 128, 129); but it is none the less certain that some of the soleæ could be applied to the feet of mules.'

Specimens of the third model are not apparently so numerous. In addition to the one represented as found at Dalheim, an example is given of a still more peculiar article of this class found

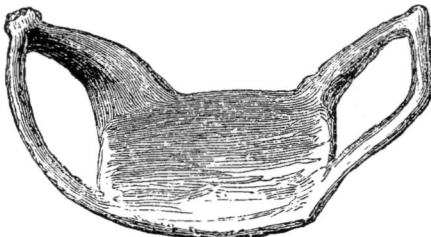

fig 129

at Abbaye Wood, Canton St Saens, France, in 1861; the Abbé Cochet designates it a 'hippo-sandal.'[1] It is remarkable for the two stud-like processes fixed to its lower surface, and for the slight

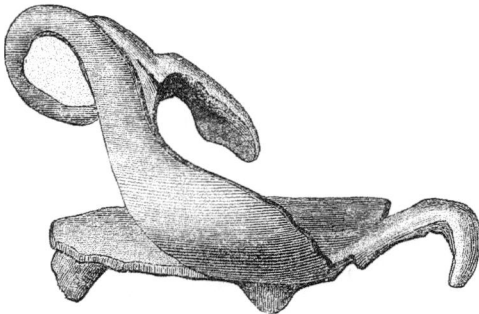

fig 130

inclination towards the front of its united branches, one of which has been partially destroyed by oxidation (fig. 130).

Another good specimen of the

[1] La Seine Inférieure, Hist. et Archæol. Paris, 1864.

third class is from an excavation in London, and is described by C. Roach Smith [1] It differs but little from the one found in the Roman camp at Dalheim, and is six inches in length (fig. 131).

The British Museum contains six of these mysterious instruments, one of them more curious than any yet discovered. It has only one real lateral

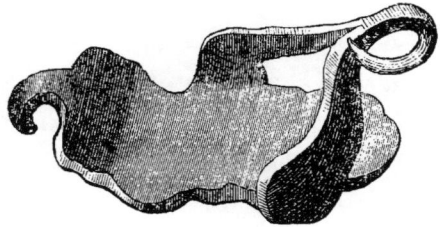

fig. 131

clip, the usual two being quite in front, where they are clumsily united to form a projecting hook. The sole is very narrow, and much oxidized on the ground surface, and the ordinary hook-like termination at the end is present (fig. 132).

The others belong to the three classes; one of the first has the side clips long and thin, and looking as if the hooks had been worn

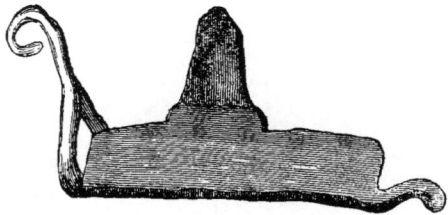

fig. 132

or rusted off, and the sole had been repaired by welding on a thin and narrow strip of iron in shape somewhat like a horse-shoe. The actual sole is six inches long, but the total length is six and three-quarters inches. The width across at the clips is four and three-quarters inches.

The others are somewhat different in length and

[1] Catalogue of the Museum of London Antiquities, p. 77, 1854. Collectanea Antiqua, vol. iii. p. 128.

width.   One from the Bridge of Reignac, belonging to
the second class, and presented by M. Picot to Sir J.
Lubbock, by whom it was given to the museum, measures six inches long, three and a half wide, and the
height of the front hook is two and three-quarters inches.
It is inscribed ' Fer de Cheval.'   Two of the specimens
exhibited have the flat strips of iron forming the clips
welded on to the sole, which in one of them is only two and
three-eighths inches wide.   To compensate for this want of
breadth, these project a little from each side before being
turned upwards at an acute angle.   The ground-surface,
as already mentioned, is notched or furrowed in various
directions.   The workmanship of all of them is very
rough and primitive, but the welding appears to be solid,
and the iron of excellent quality.   They are comparatively light, the sole plate being generally the heaviest
and strongest part.

Springhead, near Gravesend, Kent, so prolific in
antiquities belonging to the British, Roman, and subsequent periods, furnishes us with two specimens of the
first and second models.   These, through the obliging
kindness of Mr Sylvester, I have been allowed to inspect
very carefully.   Figure 133 has the oval or pear-shaped
sole with the wide opening in the middle.   One of the
side clips has been oxidized completely through, and
the other has been temporarily repaired; it is narrow,
and the height is three and seven-eighths inches.   The
point of the hook inclines inwards.   The sole is worn
and oxidized to a thin edge in front, and is thicker
behind towards the hook.   The specimen is little more
than an aggregation of rusty flakes; its length, not includ-

ing the hook at the extremity, is five and a half inches, and

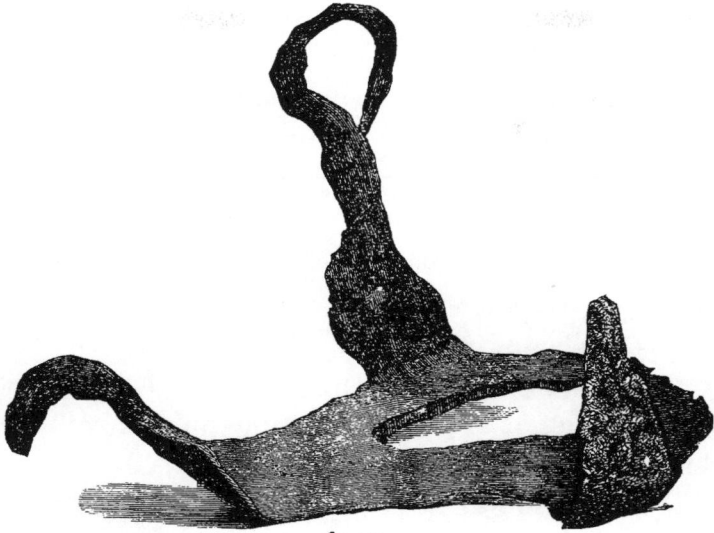

fig. 133

the width across the sole between the clips is four and a half inches; behind this part it contracts very considerably, and in bending slightly upwards expands a little.

Figure 134 is altogether a larger instrument. Its

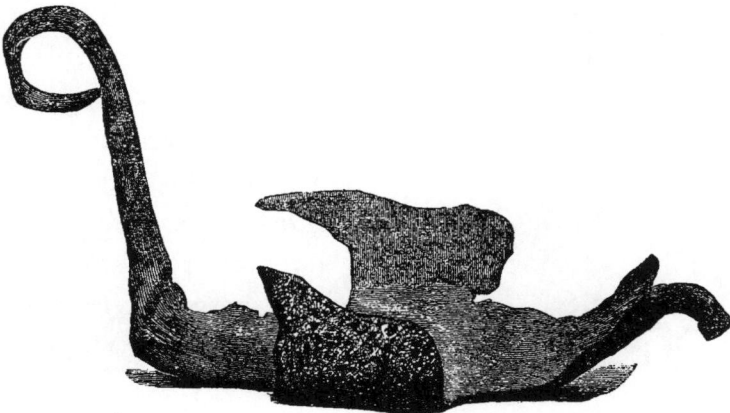

fig 134

length within the front and back hooks is six and a half

inches; the width between the side clips is four and a half inches, though the sole before and behind these is much narrower. This specimen is also much corroded, and the terminal hooks at the extremity of the side clips, if they ever were present, have disappeared. The face of the front hook is worn, as if it had been rubbed on the ground, or against some hard substance. The sole has transverse and longitudinal grooves. One side, as shown in this copy from a photograph, is much more worn than the other. The side clips are wide and have a slight twist inwards towards the front. One identical in shape with this was found in London, and is represented in the 'Archæological Journal' (vol. xi. p. 416). Another has been found at Langton, Wiltshire, and two discovered at Camerton are now in the museum of the Bristol Philosophical Institution.

Another example of the third type, resembling, in all its essential features, those found at Dalheim; Abbaye Wood, France; and in London, was picked up in the neighbourhood of Zazenhausen, near Stuttgart, among the roots of an old tree which was being removed. This was in a place where it appears the Romans had been really settled, for the remains of Roman baths, as well as

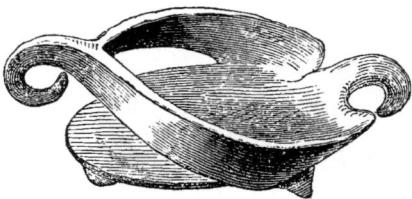

fig. 135

a number of arms and such-like articles of undoubted Roman origin, have been gathered there. It consists of a ground plate (fig. 135), corresponding, as Grosz[1] informs us, with the form of a horse's

[1] Op. cit. p. 13.

sole; into it is riveted three studs, or we might term them calks, about half-an-inch high, the foremost of which is placed in the middle of the toe of the plate, and the other two are placed on each side behind. From both sides of the back part springs a clasp or band as is usual in this type, about an inch broad, which inclines forwards and upwards, uniting in the middle, about two inches above the ground plate, to form a round eyelet or ring, through which Grosz supposed a thong was drawn. There is a hook for the same purpose at the rear of the plate, this veterinarian observes; though whether the article served as a so-called pathological shoe for diseased hoofs, as a temporary expedient when horses had lost a shoe, or whether destined for hoofs which were too much worn to be shod, he could not decide.

After an inspection of so many of these articles, which are apparently Roman, or belonging to the Roman period, the question arises, are they justly designated horse, mule, or bullock sandals? or have the Romans, or the people in whose territory they were found, ever employed them as a defence for the feet of their horses?

We have noticed that at one time they were supposed to be supports for lamps;[1] also *lychnuchi pensiles*, or hanging lamp-holders; the specimen found at Langton, Wiltshire, Sir S. Meyrick supposed to be a spur; then they were imagined to be ancient stirrups,[2] and now they are almost universally designated ' horse-sandals.' Professor Defays even contrives to adjust one to an animal's foot, though it must be rather uncomfortable about the heel;

---

[1] *Grivaud de la Vincelle.* Arts et Métiers des Anciens.
[2] *Cochet.* Le Tombeau de Childéric, p. 164, note.

and veterinary surgeon Bieler asserts they were in ordinary use; while others declare they were only employed
as temporary shoes, to be applied when the hoofs were too
much worn or the feet diseased.   Baron Ziegesar, of Berg,
after reading the report of M. Namur regarding the Dalheim discoveries, wrote to the President of the Archæological Society of Luxembourg, informing him that, in his
opinion, the *sabots*, or hippo-sandals, were intended to be
put on the horses' feet at night during a halt, and that
they were never used for marching.[1]   It is, indeed, difficult to understand why defences should be required when
the animals were at rest, and the hoofs not exposed to
attrition, and why they should be left off at the very time
they were likely to be needed.   If difficult to be retained
on the hoofs during the day, they would not be less so
at night when the horses would be lying down and getting
up frequently, and the uncouth projections behind, before,
and on each side of the feet, would be certain to entangle
the animals wearing them, and either cause these clumsy
contrivances to be torn off, or expose the horses and their
riders to serious accidents.

Mr Roach Smith, at first incredulous as to this application of these articles, appears to have become convinced
of its correctness by discovering that in Holland horses
yet wear sandals.   'At the present day in Holland it is
usual to bind long flat iron shoes to the horses' feet.   They
are fastened with a strap of leather, and are somewhat in
the form of an ordinary horse-shoe, but much longer and
wider; and, did we not know they are commonly used,

[1] Pub. de la Soc. *A*rch. de Luxembourg, vol. xii. p. 163.

would seem almost as unsuitable as the iron shoes under
consideration. Singular as the shape of these iron implements certainly is, we shall probably not be wrong in
explaining them as veritable iron horse-shoes, such as
Catullus refers to; and it is worthy of notice that at
Springhead, where some were dug up at the same time
and place, horse-shoes of the modern fashion were also
found, as well as other objects in iron.'[1] To what extent
they may be worn by the Dutch horses I do not know;
but from the shape of them, which that gentleman has
kindly permitted me to copy from an interesting but
unpublished work[2] (fig. 136), it will be seen that they are
very different to the Roman
productions, and not at all
intended for every-day wear.
They are only used, I presume, for travelling on deep
snow, or on marshy land where
there is danger of sinking, and
never on firm ground. I have
seen similar snow or bog shoes
used on horses in the Highlands of Scotland in removing peat. In this respect, as
well as in their form, they resemble the snow shoes of the
North-American hunters and

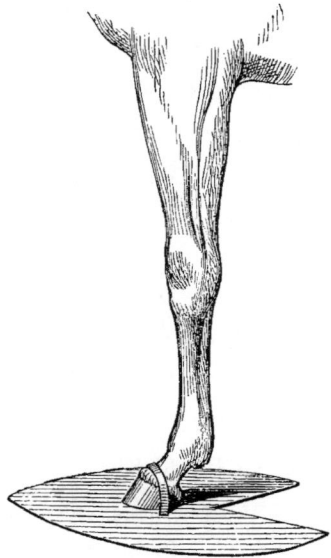

fig. 136

the Scandinavians. The so-called hippo-sandals could

[1] *C. R. Smith.* Illustrations of Roman London, p. 146.
[2] Letters from Holland.

never serve such a purpose, as they would no more preserve the animal wearing them from sinking than the shoe
of the present day.

Other authorities have not only decided that these
antique contrivances were fastened on the feet of solipeds
during the time of the Romans, but that they were in
use until a comparatively recent age. Baron de Bonstetten remarks : ' The employment of horse-shoes of this
form (modern) was only introduced by the Romans at a
late period; those we see at Rome and in the " Museo
Borbonico " at Naples are a kind of shoes (*souliers*) which
were attached by straps to the horse's feet, as the " induere" of Pliny attests.' [1]   And the Abbé Cochet writes :
' I also know that when a very distinguished Belgian
archæologist, M. Hagemans, the author of " The Cabinet
d'Amateur," was at Milan in 1858, he saw in the collection of the Chevalier Ubaldo an iron hippo-sandal in
magnificent preservation, and which did not appear to
him to be very old. Prince Biondelli, a learned Milanese
archæologist, who accompanied him, assured him that this
horse *sabot* ought to belong to the 10th or 11th century.
The Italian antiquary was also of opinion that the employment of shoes without nails was in vogue up to a late
period of the middle ages.' [2]

With all due deference to the deservedly high reputation of the many authorities who have inspected and
pronounced these iron utensils ' sandals,' after carefully
examining and measuring them, and perusing the evidence
brought forward to support that opinion, I cannot but conclude that the general opinion is an erroneous one, and for

[1] Recueil d'Antiquitiés Suisses, p. 30.   [2] Op. cit. p. 163.

the following reasons : 1. These objects have not, so far as I am aware, been found in any country at a period which we might designate ' pre-Roman '—that is, in any region where the Romans have not been, nor before their invasion of the regions in which these articles have been discovered. 2. They have been found most frequently, I think, in places where the simple ordinary nail-shoe has been met with, and either with it, or so situated as to show they belonged to, and were in use at, the same period. 3. The evidence now collected would appear to indicate that shoeing with narrow plates and nails was largely practised in several countries, even before the arrival of the Romans; and also that in all probability the Romans themselves shod their horses in the ordinary manner at the same time that these strange-looking fabrications were in use for some purpose or other. The advantages of shoeing by means of nails must have been very striking to the Romans when they first became acquainted with it; so much so, that we should indeed think them extremely stupid if they did not avail themselves of it, and still had recourse to this unlikely contrivance. Cognizant of the art of defending the hoof by a thin narrow plate of iron, pierced with six holes, and which could be made in a few minutes, and firmly secured to the hoofs in as brief a space of time, it cannot for a moment be conceded that they would either allow their horses to travel unshod until they were foot-sore, and then apply this complicated sandal, with a sole much harder than the ground, to the bruised surface; or work their horses continually with shoes which must have tasked the abilities of their blacksmiths to fabricate in less than an hour, and have required more than three or four times the quantity of iron that the Gallic or British shoe did. Though not an equestrian nation, we must give the Romans credit for common sense. As for their working their horses all day without any foot-cover, and applying these at night when they were not required, the idea is perfectly absurd. This is admitting that these articles were really intended to be attached to horses' feet; and that, though nail-shoeing was well known, and its efficacy and simplicity were recognized, the Romans, or the people among whom they were living, persisted in expending four times the weight of iron, twenty times the amount of labour, and a dozen times the quantity of charcoal.

But I cannot believe that these 'hippo-sandals' were ever made for such a purpose. Extremely few horses, if any, could travel with those of the first class on roads, in ascending or descending steep places, nor yet move at any speed. The projecting fastening behind, and the inside clip, as well as the insecurity and situation of the attachment, and the weight of the iron, all forbid this supposition.

For the second and third classes, I need only say that horses could neither travel nor yet stand in them. With far more reason might we expect two or three ranks of soldiers to walk, run, and manœuvre in *close order* with Canadian snow-shoes on their feet, than to see a horse walk, trot, and gallop with these so-called sandals. The majority of the second class could not be put on the hoofs, to begin with; and none of the third class could, by any possibility, serve such a purpose. A glance at the shape of these will show this to be the fact.

Besides, not one of those I have examined, though many

appear to have been subjected to wear in other respects, show any marks of *hoof wear ;* that is, still granting that they could be fastened to the extremity of the limb. It is well known that a horse's shoes, after being a short time subjected to use on hard ground, become rounded over at the toe, where the greatest amount of wear occurs ; also that the foot-surface, even with the shoe firmly nailed to the wall, becomes worn and channeled where any play or friction takes place. This is well seen in an old horse-shoe. No such evidences appear on the best-preserved of these so-called sandals. On the contrary, the upper surface of the sole is entirely free from traces of friction of any kind, and the under or ground-surface is usually most worn towards the middle, the extremities being sharp rather than rounded over. There is not the faintest trace of their having been worn at all by horses. No nation ever offered any contrivance so unsuited to the object to be attained as these so-called hippo-sandals, if we suppose them to have been intended for horses' feet. There is nothing at all reasonable in the supposition ; and in this opinion I find I am supported by MM. Delacroix and Quiquerez, antiquarians who have had abundant op-portunities of studying this matter, and have availed themselves of them. M. Quiquerez writes : ' The many excavations made by us in the Roman villas, camps, and castles of the Bernese Jura have never afforded us any of these *calceæ ferreæ,* or *hippo-sandals,* with which people would like to shoe the feet of Roman horses. But we have seen plenty of these articles, without being able to comprehend how a horse, starting at a gallop on an uneven road, could, for an instant even, carry such a *chaussure*. Always, however, out of respect for the opinion of others, we have never cast a doubt on the use of the socks for the Roman horses, because their employment for this purpose may have been one of those unfortunate essays of their military chiefs. Elsewhere in Switzerland, so few of these strap-shoes (*fers à courroies*) have been found, that it appears probable such a mode of shoeing, if it did exist, was for but a brief period. On the contrary, it is our conviction that long before the arrival of the Romans among the Gauls, the Sequaniæ, Helvetiæ, and Rouraks, in the vicinity of the Jura mountains, shod their horses as we now do. The almost total absence of *calceæ ferreæ* in our districts confirms this opinion ; which is, it is true, in disaccord with that of some archæologists, who only introduce nail-shoeing in the Roman armies towards the 10th century of our era, and as an importation by the nations of the North.'[1]

And M. Delacroix, when describing the shoes found in Besançon, makes a similar protest against these articles being designated hippo-sandals. 'Modern science, in the face of ancient authors mentioning horse-shoes, thinks it ought to consider as such the objects whose use is as yet unknown, which are found in ancient roadways, and to which it has been imagined to give the name of *hippo-sandals*. The figure of some *hippo-sandals* might, justly or unjustly, have authorized such an explanation of their use ; the collection of a tolerably large number of these articles, however, dispels the illusion. There are in the Archæological Museum of Besançon *hippo-sandals* provided with long hooks before and behind, and even on

[1] Mem. de la Soc. d'Emulation du Doubs, p. 132, 1863.

the sides. A horse furnished with such a *chaussure* could not walk four steps without mutilating himself and falling. What is more, we have *hippo-sandals* the two flanks of which are united above, and which could never make a shoe for a horse, even if the animal were standing still. . . . . When we see the same ground containing hippo-sandals and nailed shoes, it must be evident that the first were not destined for the feet of horses. It has been said that at least they might be employed for horses' feet in a bad condition; but besides the impossibility of using many of them for any such purpose, and which is obvious enough, we have discovered in our excavations a shoe intended for a diseased foot, one of the branches of which has been enlarged to an extraordinary degree, so as to cover one-half of the sole.'

Veterinary surgeon Duplessis, of the French artillery, likewise announces his disapproval of the name and the use given to these contrivances. Referring to the opinions of the Abbé Cochet and M. Megnin, he says: 'These gentlemen justly deny the possibility of these strangely formed bits of irons ever having been placed under horses' feet. I am of their opinion, for everything is opposed to such an admission. The lightness and freedom required for rapid paces would prevent their employment in this way, as well as the impossibility of fixing on a round flat foot a heavy ill-balanced machine like this. The example afforded by all the human foot-covers would show them (the Romans) that it was at least indispensable that it should resemble in shape the plantar surface of the foot.'[1]

[1] Journal de Méd. Vét. Militaire, vol. iv. p. 163.

M. Delacroix,[1] since the publication of his opinion adverse to these instruments being horse-sandals, has suddenly come to the conclusion that they are ox-sandals. 'The number of these articles in the Besançon Museum has actually increased to thirty. They affect various shapes, but yet retain a single and common feature—that of an iron plate worn beneath by friction. This character was so striking, that, among others, one of our able confrères who superintends the archæological museum of the town, was looking out every day for some proof as to the use of these *hippo-sandals*. One of these objects was at last brought to him, having two wings bent over towards each other (fig. 128), in an acute arch, and exactly representing the foot of an ox to which it had been moulded by the hammer and wear. There could be no doubt about it; M. Vuilleret had in his hands a shoe adapted for the bovine species; he had solved the problem. I carried this article to the farriers' shops in the suburbs, where oxen are usually shod, although after a different fashion   " This," said a workman at the first glance, " is a bullock's shoe." " This object," the farmers present generally assented, " could not be worn by an ox at work or at pasture ; it would confine their movements too much. But if a convoy of oxen or cows was sent along the roads, it might be of the greatest utility ; for there is always in a travelling drove animals whose feet are wounded, and for whom it is necessary to have recourse to temporary shoeing." This last explanation put us on the alert in comprehending the diversity in shape of the specimens in the museum ; and M. Vuilleret was not

[1] Mem. de la Soc. d'Emulation du Doubs, p. 143, 1864.

long in showing us shoes made for the single claw of the ox (fig. 129), and yet belonging to this class of pretended *hippo-sandals* . . . . . whose name it behoves us to rectify . it should be BU-SANDAL.' It appears to have been forgotten that a bisulcus or cloven-footed animal cannot travel easily with its digits restrained by a solid plate with two iron bands compressing them on each side. And we may ask if the experiment was tried of making oxen walk for a mile or two with any of these Besançon specimens? None of those I have examined would fit the foot of an ox, and there is no reason to suppose that they were ever used for that purpose by the Romans. I have already noted that tips of iron, conjectured to have armed the feet of cattle, were recently found at Pompeii. Until I have inspected these articles, or seen drawings of them, I cannot decide as to their having been so employed, though I think it improbable, as Cato the Censor (B.C. 160) speaks of the application of liquid pitch to the under surface of the hoofs of oxen to preserve them from wear, as is now done in the East with the feet of elephants and camels: ' Boves ne pedes subterant, priusquam in viam quoquam ages, pice liquidam cornua infima unguito.' [1]

It will then, I think, be admitted that these strange-looking iron plates are not horse, mule, or ox sandals, and that they could not be employed as such. The form and situation of the clips and hooks alone forbid such a sup-position, and the Romans would indeed deserve to be classed among the most clumsy of all contrivers if they ever attempted to put such a garniture on their horses', mules', or oxen's feet, even supposing they were ignorant

[1] De Re Rustica, cap. 72.

of nail-shoeing, which at the time these were made it appears they were not.

If not supports for lamps, ancient stirrups, sandals for sound or diseased feet, or iron socks for wearing at night while the horses were resting, what then are they? The first one I saw in the British Museum—belonging to the second class—suggested its probable use. Was it not a skid or drag (*sabot* or *enrayeur*) to put under the wheel of a carriage to moderate its descent on steep places? This appeared to me a very likely supposition. It is well known that the Romans employed such instruments for their vehicles, and they are often mentioned in their real, as well as in a figurative, sense, by the designation of 'sufflamen.' For instance, Juvenal, in the 1st century, in his eighth satire (148), writes:

Ipse rotam astringit multo sufflamine Consul.

And in his sixteenth satire (50) he also alludes to it:

Nec res atteritur longo sufflamine litis.

Seneca, also in the 1st century, speaks of the 'rota sufflaminanda;' and Prudentius in the fourth century (Psych. 417), notices it:

Tardat sufflamine currum.

Gruter, in his collection of Ancient Inscriptions (1803) gives the following reference to it: 'Fontium aquarumque cœlestium ex montibus delabentium torrenti sufflamen his muris fossaque opposuit, et ad plana perduxit.'

Ainsworth, in his Latin Dictionary, explains the meaning of the designation: Sufflamen. Sufflo, machinæ genus, quo in descendu vel procursu nimio tota solet sufflari, *i. e.*, retineri. And another classical dictionary explains it as 'lignum illud, quo per radios rotarum trajecto; *vel fer-reum instrumentum in modum soleæ formatum*, quo subter notæ unius canthum supposito, currus in declivibus locis nimio impetu ruentes cohibentur : illud Itali *stanga*, hoc *scarpa* vocant.

There can be no doubt, then, as to the Romans possessing such an instrument to facilitate the travelling of their carriages ; but I do not remember any mention being made as to their discovery anywhere ; and in all likelihood we have them here. I am aware that in a sepulchral bas-relief found at Langres, representing, among other objects, a cart drawn by three horses, two chains are seen attached to the body of the carriage, and in front of the hind wheel, one with a ring, the other with a hook at the end to lock round the felloe between two of the spokes, and make a fetter for the wheel. So says Mr Rich ; but this kind of contrivance would, one is inclined to think, be of as limited application in the Romano-Gallic days as now. It is a most expensive way of staying the velocity of a carriage. The shape of the supposed sandals presents but little difference from that of the skid or wheel-shoe ot now-a-days, except, perhaps, in length.

The drawing of one of those attached to the waggons of the Military Train will make this manifest (fig. 137).

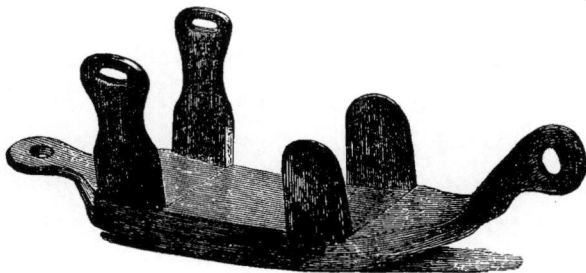

fig. 137

The resemblance to some of the 'sandals' of the first and second classes is very striking, particularly those figured by Professor Defays; that by M. Namur, found at Dalheim (fig. 114); that in the Cluny Museum; the one found at Serupt in 1846, and the specimen in the Besançon Museum. Some allowance must be made for the very large diameter of the modern wheels, which necessitates a longer *shoe* (though the London carriages offer a great many varieties as to form and length in these articles), but the sole of the one here represented measures about three inches across between the clips—the width of several of the sandals. The Roman wheels of small diameter and coarse workmanship would vary much in the thickness of the felloes and width of the hoops, which will readily account for the irregular width of many of these so-called sandals, and also, perhaps, for their difference in shape. The increased thickness of sole in the modern 'sufflamen' is rendered necessary by the much greater weight of the waggons and the loads they are intended to carry; but the abundance of material, and the facility with which our Vulcans can forge large masses of iron, makes this of little consequence, compared with the difficulties the blacksmiths of eighteen centuries ago had to contend with. It will be observed that this *wheel-sandal* has an eyelet at each end, like the horse-sandal of the second and third classes, for the attachment of a chain which fastens it to the body of the vehicle. One of them is higher than the other, and is the one to which the chain is usually attached; its elevation is intended to throw the stress of wear on the middle of the sole, exactly as it is in the *soleæ ferreæ*. The two clips on each side are intended to give greater security to the lodgment of the wheel, though, for that matter, with a smaller wheel, one central clip on each side, as in the first-class sandal, would suffice, especially if the sole diminished in width, as it does in that, towards the hook, which would wedge the wheel in more tightly. The longitudinal aperture at the upper end of each of the posterior clips is intended for the admission of a leather strap, which, passing across the wheel as it lies in the skid, prevents its jumping out when traversing broken ground. The hooks on each side of the first and second class sandals reveal a similar intention, and the union of the lateral clips in the third class may be also attributed to an attempt at simplicity in this direction. The analogy between the Roman sandal found at Dalheim (fig. 114) and this modern specimen is very marked ; so much so, indeed, that their being intended for the same purpose can scarcely be doubted ; one thing is certain, that no horse could journey a yard with the Military-Train specimen ; and we have yet to learn that the horses of Gaul, Germany, or Britain, during the Roman period, could travel in any other fashion than the horses of our own days. I have tried the two articles found at Springhead on several horses, but out of the number of many-sized hoofs experimented on, I could not find one to fit either of the hippo-sandals. The resemblance of the larger specimen to a skid struck several casual observers, who were not at all aware of their history or the functions imputed to them. Among others, I may mention Col. Tilley, of the Royal Engineers, who exclaimed, the first glance he got of it in my hand, 'Hilloa ! what have you got there ?   An old skid ?'

I only make the suggestion that these articles may have been employed for this purpose, from finding myself unable to believe that they were worn by domesticated animals ; the third type is certainly opposed to my opinion, but then it may not have been put to the same use as the others.

CHAPTER VIII.

FROM the preceding inquiry, we are led to conclude that the Celts, or Gallo-Celts, were the people who most anciently employed nailed iron-shoes for their horses' feet; but we are yet left to determine the probable date of this invention—an investigation surrounded with many difficulties.

It is recognized, however, by means of the proofs furnished by archæological and philological researches, that the different races of mankind which have succeeded one another in Europe have exhibited a constant progression, not only in physical development, but also in intelligence and in the aptitude to practise various industries and arts. The remains found in many regions exhibit this gradual advancement, until, from a state which appears that of savagedom, we arrive at a period when domestic animals are kept, and a knowledge of metallurgy is obvious. It is only, however, when we come to the epoch of the early migrations of the Aryan or Indo-Germanic races, that we find substantial traces of the employment of metals. The most important of these migrations, that of the Cimbri, who, with the Gauls, founded the Celtic race some eighteen hundred years before our era, and introduced Druidism into Gaul, when it reached Europe knew no other metals than gold, copper, tin, and the combination of the last two—brass. A study of Sanscrit, the mother-tongue of all these Aryan peoples, shows this to have been the case. The working in iron, or the 'Iron Age,' even with some civilized peoples, did not occur until a comparatively recent time. Lucretius admits that gold and brass were known before iron:

Sed prius æris erat quam ferri cognitus usus.

As no other migration of any importance occurred until that of the hordes who destroyed the Roman empire, and as we have seen that iron was worked by the Gauls long before the Christian era, it is between the period when the Gallo-Cimbri arrived, and the conquest of Gaul by

Julius Cæsar, that the utilization of iron may be placed. Archæologists are tolerably unanimous in fixing what has been designated the 'Stone Period,' at from five to seven thousand years; the 'Age of Bronze' at from three to four thousand years; and the 'Iron Age' at one thousand years before our era. This last period, though to many its commencement is shrouded in darkness, has been pretty accurately determined by Swiss geologists, who have based their calculations on the annual depositions produced by the torrent of Teniere, near Villeneuve, on the Lake of Geneva, and which cover the most ancient human habitations containing iron that have yet been explored.[1] These calculations have been further supported by the very interesting discovery made at Halstatt, in Austria, where more than nine hundred graves of the people who in old times laboured in the salt-mines there, were found. These contained, besides large clay vases, glass ornaments, cinctures, metal slings, swords, knives, lance-heads, and hatchets in bronze, similar to the objects met with in the pre-Roman, Helvetic, and Bisontine tombs. The same forms were reproduced in iron; so that it may be said this metal was abundant with these people. Taking into account the complete absence of lead and silver among these articles,—metals which were largely employed during the reign of Philip of Macedonia, four hundred years before the Christian era,—M. Fournet estimates that the people who rest in the tombs of Halstatt lived at the commencement of the iron age, very likely between B.C. 1000 and 500. Its duration is marked by well-known historical events, and

[1] *Fournet.* Le Mineur.

it only ends with the gradual spread of Christian civilization.

Numerous traces of iron-mining in these distant ages yet exist in the Swiss and Jura Alps, Burgundy, and the Pyrenees. In the latter mountains, the refuse of these mines yet remain as when formed. The so-called *cras siers*, or ancient depôts of iron scoriæ, are found in the vicinity of Digoin; they abound near Perigueux, at Royan (Drôme), Pont-Gibaud (Auvergne), between Hyères and Toulon, and on Mount Cenis, at 1800 mètres elevation. There were then forests where to-day there are glaciers. On the rich strata of Thortes and Beauregard (Côte d'Or), M. Guillebot de Merville noted the existence of seventy or eighty fragments of scoriæ of Gallo-Roman iron, the age of which is perfectly characterized by the peculiar tiles and the *débris* of every kind accompanying them.[1]

The remains of the Celtic furnaces M. Quiquerez discovered in the Jura are identical with, though much smaller than, the Catalan furnaces now at work in Ariége, Carinthia, and Dalecarlia.

In Carinthia, this is the primitive mode, according to Malot, by which the iron is extracted from the ore: As soon as a sufficient quantity of live coal has been accumulated in the pit, portions of very pure mineral are spread over it, then a layer of coal, then mineral, layer after layer, until it is judged that the ore is sufficiently reduced, when the fire is extinguished, and some scraps of iron are found among the cinders. In Dalecarlia, the method is the same, only the pit is larger and encircled by a circular stone wall.[2]

[1] *Fournet.* Op. cit.   [2] *Gmelin.* Metallurgie du Fer.

The Celts in Britain must also, long before the arrival of Cæsar, have smelted quantities of iron, wherewith to make their arms and utensils. Instead of money, they even used pieces of brass or iron reduced to certain weights.[1]

Traces of ancient iron-works are numerous in many parts of Britain; and, from appearances, this metal was smelted as above. Roman remains occur very frequently among the slag or cinders; but it is not unlikely the primitive inhabitants worked these mines before the arrival of the Romans.

Brennus and his Gaulish army at the capture of Rome, and the Helvetians at the conquest of Switzerland, were armed with iron swords, while the Romans yet wielded weapons of bronze. The Cimbri, defeated by Marius two hundred years before the birth of our Saviour, were covered with steel cuirasses.

'The arms of the Helvetians who took possession of Switzerland,' says M. Fournet, 'were identical with those worn by Brennus's soldiers during the occupation of Rome. They had long iron sabres, without point, and with very large handles; their lances had blades twenty inches long.' 'The Cimbric cavaliers who came from the Pont-Euxine to invade Gaul, about the time of the arrival of the Phoceans, wore steel cuirasses when they were defeated by Marius.' 'The iron of Norica, as well as that of Celtiberia, was in great esteem with the Romans for swords.'

---

[1] *Cæsar.* Bell. Gall. lib. v. cap. 10. 'Utuntur aut ære aut tallis ferreis ad certum pondus examinatis pro nummo.'

'If, then,' says M. Megnin,[1] 'we place the invention of horse-shoeing about the fifth or sixth century before our era—that is, at the period when Druidism was most flourishing—we only follow the indications furnished by the Celtic roads, and we remain within very probable limits. The Druids, taught the structure of the horse's foot by the numerous sacrifices they made of this animal, accustomed to the manipulation of metals, and their intelligence continually cultivated by study, were marvellously disposed to be the inventors of shoeing by nails. When we also look at the rational form they gave to their work—how wisely they placed the nail-holes, and how skilfully they made the nail-heads to form so many catches to assist travelling in rocky and mountainous regions—one cannot but be astonished at the perfection which the sacred smiths had attained in defending and assisting nature two thousand years ago.'

'The Druids,' writes Galtruch,[2] 'encouraged the study of anatomy; but they carried it on to such an excess, and so much beyond all reason and humanity, that one of them, called Herophilus, is said to have read lectures on the bodies of more than 700 living men, to show therein the secrets and wonders of the human fabric.'

The discoveries in the tombs of Alesia and in the vicinity of Besançon, furnish us with such undoubted testimony to the antiquity of shoeing, that a high authority in France, who had assisted in these researches, declared, 'after these evidences I have no fear in asserting that from the time of the conquest of Gaul by the Romans,

[1] Op. cit. p. 31.   [2] Poetical History.

many Celtic peoples, at any rate all the Gauls, knew the art of horse-shoeing.'[1]

Legends are generally good evidence, says Mr Wright,[2] of the great antiquity of the monuments to which they relate; and there is a curious legend connected with this art, which lends additional force to the facts already enumerated, and is besides so general over a large part of Europe, and is of so great an age, that it looks as if it had belonged to the days of Druidism, and the infancy of horse-shoeing. This is the legend of Wayland Smith.

The Vulcanian art was, we are told, so admired by the Greeks, that Xanthus, the smith, caused it to be inscribed upon his statue, that he was born of iron (σιδηροφυης, *ferrogenitus*);[3] and over their forges they had a prophylactic against envy, in the form of a phallus hung round with bells.[4] The anvil, hammer, and tongs, and Vulcan's cap wreathed with laurel, is not unfrequently met with on classical monuments, as the annexed illustration from Montfauçon will show (fig. 138). But the northern nations always associated something mysterious with the functions and character of their Vulcan, whether in the fabrication of arms or in shoeing their horses: reminding one of the secret arts of the Druids and their weird-like haunts. What

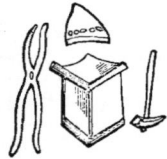

fig 138

makes the remembrance more vivid is, that the abode of this cunning, but awesome, personage, was always sup

---

[1] Moniteur Universel, 1862.
[2] The Celt, the Roman, and the Saxon.
[3] Pollux, vii. 24.   [4] Βασκανια. ibid. vii. 24, x. 31.

posed to be in a cave, cairn, or cromlech, such as that on the promontory of Alesia.

The early Saxons believed that a cromlech in Berkshire was a workshop of the mythic smith; the monument at Ashbury, in the Vale of White Horse, was called 'Weland's Smiththan,' or smithy, which in time became corrupted to Wayland Smith's cave. The great defeat given by Alfred to the Danish invaders, is said, by Mr Gough, to have taken place near Ashdown, in Berkshire. The burial-place of Baereg, the Danish chief, who was slain in this fight, is distinguished by a parcel of stones, less than a mile from the hill, set on edge, enclosing a piece of ground somewhat raised. On the east side of the southern extremity, stand three squarish flat stones, of about four or five feet over either way, supporting a fourth, and now called by the vulgar, Wayland Smith, from an idle tradition about an invisible smith replacing lost horse-shoes there.[1] 'The popular belief still clings to this wild legend,' adds Sir Walter Scott, 'which, connected as it is with the site of a Danish (?) sepulchre, may have arisen from some legend concerning the northern Duergars, who resided in the rocks, and were cunning workers in steel and iron. It was believed that Wayland Smith's fee was sixpence, and that, unlike other workmen, he was offended if more was offered. This monument must be very ancient, for it has been kindly pointed out to me that it is referred to in an ancient Saxon charter, as a landmark.'[2]

With regard to placing a piece of money on the

---

[1] *Camden.* Britannia, vol. i. p. 221. Edit. *Gough.*

[2] *Scott.* Kenilworth. Note B.

stone, we find it is still a practice among the peasantry at Colombiers, in France, for young girls who want husbands, to climb upon the cromlech called the Pierre-levée, place there a piece of money, and then jump down. At Guerande, with the same object, they deposit in the crevices of a Celtic monument bits of rose-coloured wool tied with tinsel.[1]

'Cromlech,' however, really means Druid's altar. The Celtic mythology, amongst others, had Esus or *Crom*, who was the creator of the world, and was represented by a circle of stones, an emblem of the infinite. From this name was derived 'Cromlech' or Crom-lekh.[2] Mr Davies thinks that the spaces under the cromlechs were used as the places where aspirants to the office of Druid were imprisoned during, or previous to, their initiation into the mysteries of this religion. 'This opinion,' says Mr Roberts,[3] 'seems to be confirmed by the name of a cell near the Ridgeway and the White Horse, in Uffington parish. It is called Wayland Smith, a corruption, I presume, of a Welsh name "Gwely," or "Wely-anesmwyth," that is, the uneasy bed. I know of no more probable origin of the name, and this explanation bears with it a signification of no small moment, as to the use to which it was probably applied. In Cardiganshire (Wales) there is a kind of cist-vaen called "Gwely Taliesin," which no doubt was intended for a similar purpose.'

Mallet,[4] we know, asserts that the tradition relating to

---

[1] *Wright.* The Celt, the Roman, and the Saxon.
[2] *H. Martin.* Hist. de France, vol. iii. p. 58.
[3] Popular *A*ntiquities of Wales, p. 45.
[4] Northern *A*ntiquities. Note.

this mysterious blacksmith is of Northern origin.   In Scandinavian mythology, the Völundar-Koiða recounts the tragic adventures of Völundr, who was the Dædalus of the North, and one of its mythical heroes.   The same high authority shows that the root of the word, which is Anglo-Saxon, is *Wealand, Welond,* or *Weland,* in German *Wielant,* and is the *Velint* of the Vilkina-Saga, is derived from the Norse *Vel,* skill, art, craft, or cunning, and the old German *Wielan,* Anglo-Saxon *Welan,* to fabricate, the participle of which would be *Wielant* and *Weland.* The word, therefore, according to Mr Mallet, denotes a skilful artificer, in which sense it is still employed by the people of Iceland, who say ' *Hann er völundr à jarn,*' ' He is a famous smith or workman in iron ; ' and a labyrinth with them is a Wayland house.

' It is in the Icelandic Sagas,' remarks Depping and Michel,[1] ' that Veland is the subject of long romantic fictions, and the story regarding him forms one of the oldest fragments of this poetical literature.   It has been attempted to trace the romance to a historical period,— to the reign of King Nidung, who appears to have lived in Sweden in the 6th century of our era, and who is reported to have been the protector of the smith.   But there is nothing historical in this, and if on the one hand such has been claimed for it, on the other hand it is as likely to belong to Scandinavian mythology.'

We must not forget that the Teutonic word ' Welsh,' ' Wilisc,' or ' Wælisc,' was the term for stranger or foreigner, and that France was called by the old and mediæval Germans ' Das Welsche lant ; ' while the

[1] Le Forgeron Veland. Paris, 1833

designation 'Wälsch' was applied in its primitive sense by the Saxons to the Britons. 'Wilisc' is often met with in the Anglo-Saxon laws, and denotes the Welsh. Might not the Druid blacksmith be designated by the ancient Germans, as the foreign or strange-land smith—Welsch-lant-Schmid ? The slight change in the pronunciation might readily occur in a short period.

It may be mentioned, however, that Langley Mortier[1] concludes that the name 'Gallia' was derived from *Wal*, happy, and *Land*, country: 'Walland' being the designation given to their territory by the Gauls.

This mysterious smith, it would appear, was no other than the traditionary armourer and farrier of the Celts and Gauls, as well as of the German and Northern nations 'The sacred blacksmith, such as Wayland,' remarks M. Castan, 'not only fashioned the weapons, but he also shod the horses of the heroes.'[2]

At Winchester, or Silchester, we are told in the 'Morte d'Arthur,' was a large stone, and 'in the myddes therof was lyk an anvyld of steel a ffote of hyght, and therein stake a fayre sword,' which only the heir to the sovereignty of Britain could draw; a feat performed by Arthur.[3] This romance-invested prince was King of the Silures, an ancient British tribe inhabiting the modern counties of Hereford, Radnor, Brecknock, and Glamorgan, and fought most heroically against the Saxons, Scots, and Picts, after the departure of the Romans. The

[1] Etymologies Gauloises.   [2] Les Tombelles Celtiques d'Alaise.

[3] With the Mongols, the anvil of Genghis Khan is still preserved on Mount Darkan. It is made of a particular metal called 'Bouryn, says the tradition, which has the properties of iron and copper, being at once hard and flexible.—*Timkowski.* Op. cit., vol. i. p. 173.

sword found with the anvil of steel, he afterwards wielded with terrible effect against his enemies ; it was named ' caledvwlch' (the hard cleft), or ' caliburn' (well-tempered or massive).[1] This weapon was no doubt fabricated by Weland.

In the metres composed by King Alfred on the ' Consolations of Boethius,' the learned monarch asks,

> Who then can tell, wise Weland's (ꝥelanðeȝ) bones
> Where now they rest so long ?
> Beneath what heap of earth and stones
> Their prison is made strong ?

A direct testimony to the great age of this tradition. And in the Anglo-Saxon poem on Beowulf, that chief, before going to battle, requests that there should be sent to Higelac

> My garments of battle.
> The best that my bosom bears,
> The richest of my clothes,
> The remains of the Hred-lan,
> The work of Weland.

In some fragments of an old Anglo-Saxon manuscript, published by Professor Stephens, we find this ancient worker in metals and shoer of horses mentioned in a complimentary manner as a maker of sharp swords. ' The Wieland (ꝥelanð) work will fail no man, who kenneth to wield biting Mimming.' This, we may be sure, was another of his celebrated blades.

In a French poem, conjectured to be of the 7th century, Weyland is supposed to be mentioned for the first time, when it is said that the cuirass made by Veland could not defend the hero Randolph from death.

[1] The Chronicle of Tysilio.

Gautier de Vascastein, in the legend 'De Prima Expeditione Attilæ regis Hunorum, in Gallias,' is said to have carried arms fabricated by Veland.

A chronicle of the 12th century relates that Count William of Angoulême received the cognomen of ' Taille fer,' in consequence of his sword, which had been made by ' Walander,' having cut in two a warrior covered with armour.[1] The name of the sword was ' durissima.' This Count William was the renowned minstrel Taillefer, who struck the first blow at the battle of Hastings, and who is described by his countryman Wace, in the following century, as having dashed on horseback into the ranks of the Saxons to meet a glorious death, while singing of

> De Karlemaigne et de Rollant,
> E d'Oliver, et des Vassals,
> C'y morurent en Roncesvals.

It is related of Geoffroy Plantagenet, Count of Anjou, 'Adultimum allatus est ei, ensis thesauro regio ab antiquo ibidem signatus, in quo fabricando fabrorum superlatum *Galanus* multa opera et studio desudavit.'[2]

In an English romance of the 14th century, it is said, in reference to a sword, 'Of all swerdes it is king, and Weland it wrought.' Godefroy of Strasbourg, in his poem of 'Tristan and Isolde,' speaks of the smith as ' Vilint.'

In Scandinavia, the strange personage is well known, and the legends concerning him differ but little from

---

[1] *Adhemar.* Chronic MS.

[2] Hist. Gaufredi Ducis Norman. Recueil des Hist. de France. See also *C. Depping.* De la Tradition Populaire sur l'Armurier ou Forgeron Veland. Mem. de la Soc. des Antiquaires de France.

those of other countries.[1]   His fame as a remarkably competent shoer of horses is not less than his reputation as a forger of swords.   In England, as we have already seen, the popular notion gave him credit for secrecy and despatch in arming the hoofs of animals belonging to less courageous owners who ventured near his mystic abode. The pedantic Erasmus Holiday, in 'Kenilworth,' sums up his proficiency in this respect, when alluding to the strange apprenticeship Wayland served to Doctor Doboobie, whom it was supposed the Evil One had flown away with.   The *faber ferrarius* is thus spoken of: 'This knave, whether from the inspiration of the devil, or from early education, shoes horses better than e'er a man betwixt us and Iceland; and so he gives up his practice on the bipeds, the two-legged and unfledged species called mankind, and betakes him entirely to shoeing of horses.'

In certain provinces of France at the present day, when a horse travels freely, they say, 'This horse goes as if he had been shod by "Vaillant."'[2]   As a proof that the smith with the Gauls, as with the Germans, shod the horses, while he fashioned and tempered the arms of the warriors, it has been observed, that not only do the shoes, weapons, and armour of an early period bear evident traces of fabrication by the same hands, but that they also carry a veritable maker's name struck upon each alike.[3]

Gay, in his 'Trivia,' refers to the weird occupation of this traditionary artisan,—this symbolical personification

[1] Saga Bibliotek, vol. ii.   Kjobenham, 1816.
[2] *De Sourdeval.*   Journal de Haras, 1862.
[3] *Megnin.*   Op. cit.

of the mystery attending the working of metals, particularly of iron, in primeval times:

> ' Far in the lane a lonely hut he found,
> No tenant ventured on the unwholesome ground ;
> Here smokes his forge, he bares his sinewy arm,
> And early strokes the sounding anvil warm ;
> *A*round his shop the steely sparkles flew,
> As for the steed he shaped the bending shoe.'

In Germany the same traditions are found, and have
been handed down from the remotest times. The
brothers Grimm have collected some of these from oral
tradition; the following was found in the neighbourhood of Münster. 'In the Detterberg, about three hours
from Münster, in old times, lived a wild man named
Grinken Schmidt (Grinken the smith), who lived underground in a deep cave, which is now covered with weeds
and briars ; but the spot may yet be seen. He had his
forge in this pit, and his workmanship was so solid and so
extremely perfect that it lasted for ever. No man could
open his locks without the keys. There is now on the
church-door of Nienberg, a lock made by him, that the
thieves and housebreakers have never been able to force.
When there was a wedding about to be celebrated, it was
customary for the country people to go to Grinken and
borrow a spit ; but in return for the loan, they had always
to give him a beefsteak. One day a peasant appeared
before his cave, and said, "Grinken Schmidt, give me a
spit." "You shall not have a spit if you do not give me
a steak," says Grinken. "Then you will not have a steak ;
so keep your spit," replied the peasant. Grinken, as
furious as possible, thereupon said, "Take care that I do
not take one from you by force" The peasant left the

mountain, and returned home.   He then saw, on enter
ing his stable, that his best horse had a gash in its thigh:
this provided the stake for Grinken Schmidt.'[1]

It is curious to note the different notions entertained
with regard to the sons of Vulcan—the protégés of Saint
Eloy.   In some countries they are looked upon with
strange dread; while in others, their handicraft confers on
them dignity and special privileges.   In Norway, handicraftsmen were known at a very remote period, and were
divided into classes; the smith was the most reputable individual, and associated or was on an equality with the
freemen.   Among the Gauls and the Welsh we have seen
they held high office; but it is questionable if, at first,
they did so to the same degree among the Anglo-Saxons.
The Druids felt the decline of their influence, and experienced the persecutions of the Teutonic invaders;
their rites had to be carried on in the greatest secrecy
and fear, and their business was transacted in a hidden
manner, while their utmost caution was required to elude
observation.   King Lear's idea of *shoeing a troop of
horse with felt*[2] may have been derived from the extreme
circumspection the Druidical priests, towards the de-
crease of their power, were compelled to adopt; and the
spread of Christianity, so burdened with gross superstitions, no doubt invested the traces of these rites with
everything of a repulsive and extraordinary nature.
Hence, perhaps, the tradition of Wayland Smith.

Even at a later day, blacksmiths, who, from the im-

[1] Deutsche Mythologie.

[2] 'It were a delicate stratagem, to shoe
A troop of horse with felt.'   Act iv., scene 6.

portance of their occupation, were very numerous in some parts of England, were not exempt from Christian (?) priestly malediction. The ancient town of Alauna (now Alcester), in Warwickshire, was at an early period famed for its smiths and its forges. Saint Egwin, Capgrave tells us,[1] reported that the inhabitants of this town were an arrogant and luxurious race, and were chiefly workers in iron. The founder of Evesham preached to them, to save them from eternal perdition; but the grimy blacksmiths were either too busy to listen, or cared but little to hear the miracle-working saint. So that, as he imagined, when he attempted to speak, in contempt of his doctrine, they thumped with their hammers upon the anvils, and made a great noise. Then this good man, full of love and mercy for his species, addressed a prayer to Heaven that the workers in iron might be destroyed:—' Contra artem fabrilem castri illius dominum imprecatus est.' And the town was immediately destroyed: ' Et ecce subito reædificato usque in hodierum diem in constructione novarum domorum in fundamentis antiqua ædificia reperiuntur. Nunquam enim postea in loco illo aliquis artem fabrilem recte exercuit, nec aliquis eam exercere volens ibi vigere potuit.'

But Saint Egwin appears to have been an exception to the priests of his age; for many of them were skilled workers in metals, and even shoers of hoofs; and they would have been far more likely to give the anvil-ringing burn-the-winds of Alcester, a hint for some new feat in metallurgy, than dooming them and their glowing forges to destruction.

[1] Nova Legenda *Angliæ*. The Celt, the Roman, and the Saxon, p. 139.

In Ireland, so long the stronghold of everything Celtic, the monks appear to have been clever workmen, and to have excelled in smithery. In Andamannus' Life of St Columba, a holy man who lived in the 6th century, there is mention made of one Columbus, a noted *faber ferrarius*, who dwelt in the centre of Ireland (*mediterranea scotiæ*). The notice of him is contained in a chapter 'Concerning an Apparition of Angels which a man of God had seen bearing to Heaven a certain soul, by name Columbus, a "fabri ferrarii," who was known by the cognomen of Coilriginus.' St Columba, who had fixed his abode in the island of Iona, hearing of the death of his colleague, gathered his priests around him and said: 'Columbus Coilriginus the smith (*faber ferrarius*) hath not laboured in vain, for he hath reached eternal happiness and life by the work of his hands (*propria manum laboratione*), and now his soul is being borne by angels to the celestial country. For whatever he acquired by the practice of his trade he spent in works of charity.' [1] From the mention of this monk's occupation and the immortality he derived from it, we may suppose him to be the COLUM ZOBA (Colum the Smith) commemorated in the calendars on June 7th. We also find that St Patrick (4th century) had three smiths, who duly appear in the same Irish calendar. [2] St Dega, Bishop of Iniscaindega (now Iniskeen, Monaghan), derived his name of Dayg (*hoc enim nomen Scotica lingua magnam flammam sonat*) from his employment in making 'plurima de ferro et ære de auro atque argento utensilia

---

[1] Vita Sancti Columbæ. Auctore Andamnano. Lib. iii. cap. 9. Dublin, 1857.

[2] *O' Donovan. Annals of the Four Masters.*

ad usum ecclesiæ'[1] His day in the calendar is the 18th of August.

Smithcraft was no doubt as important an occupation among the Anglo-Saxons as among the Gauls or Celts. Under the designation of 'isern-smithas,'—the Gothic or old German appellation introduced into England by the Anglo-Saxons, the grimy workman is frequently mentioned in their records, and he appears, in time, to have been held in nearly as high honour as his congener at the ancient British court. Verstegan, referring to those who derived their surnames from their occupations, speaks of the origin of Smith :—

> ' From whence came Smith, all be he knight or squire,
> But from the smith that forgeth at the fire ' '

Aldhelm[2] is eloquent in describing the 'convenience of the anvil, the rigid hardness of the beating hammer, and the tenacity of the glowing tongs;' and remarks that 'the gem-bearing belts and diadems of kings, and the various instruments of glory, were made from the tools of iron.'

In Elfric's colloquy, the smith says, in alluding to the multiplicity of objects he could make· 'Whence the share to the ploughman, or the goad, but for my art? Whence to the fisherman an angle, or to the shoe-wyrhta (shoemaker) an awl, or to the sempstress a needle, but for my art?' And to this the other replies: 'Those in thy smithery only give iron fire-sparks, the noise of beating hammers, and blowing bellows.'[3]

---

[1] Act. SS. August. vol. iii. p. 659.
[2] *Aldhelm.* De Laud. Virg. 298.
[3] MSS. Tiberias, A. 3.

We have selected two representations of the Anglo-Saxon Vulcan from ancient manuscripts in the Cottonian library. The first (fig. 139) represents this worthy working at an anvil, which, it is proper to note, has no beak or horn. The hammer he wields is not unlike those in use at the present day. In the compartment adjoining him, but

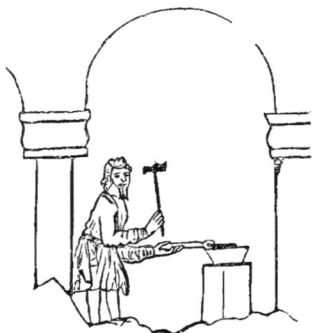

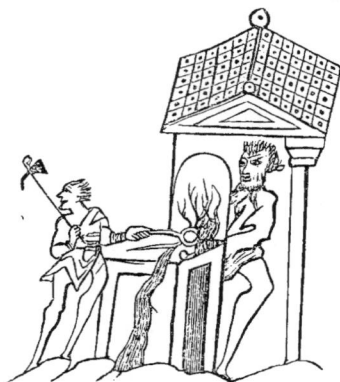

fig 139   fig 140

which is not shown here, was a harper, a combination that reminds us of the Welsh king's court, or the multiple functions assumed by some of the Anglo-Saxon priests, who were musicians, blacksmiths, goldsmiths, and other handicraftsmen combined. The second figure (fig. 140) shows the 'isern-smithas' at work in a less ostentatious manner, and at a hearth like those of our own time. His apron is of the most meagre dimensions, and his naked legs must often have been tickled by the burning sparks. His hammer is curious, and may have been used in battering the heads of enemies as well as bars of iron; for, according to Fabricius, 'the ancient Saxons had their shields suspended by chains, their horsemen used *long iron sledge-hammers*, and their armour was heavy.' Behind the iron plate that screens the fire is seen the gigantic *aide,* who appears to be engaged in blowing the bellows. He, too, is gaunt and unprotected about the lower limbs, though his brawny arms and hairy chest bespeak a man eminently fitted to perform the more physical portion of the labour. On the hearth, and partly concealed by the blazing fire, lies a piece of iron-work which looks not unlike the calkin of a horse-shoe.

These are the earliest representations of the Anglo-Saxon farrier I can find, and they are certainly curious.

In the royal household of the king's palace, we dis cover a number of officers similar in rank and functions to those we have already indicated as attending the Court of British sovereigns or chiefs: these are the 'hors thegn,' or master of the horse, the 'ambiht-smith,' and the 'hors wealh.' The latter has been already noticed. The rank of the Court smith may be inferred from what is mentioned in the laws of the Anglo-Saxon king, Athelbirht (6th century): 'If the king's ambiht-smith slay a man, let him pay a half leod-geld (or *wer-geld,* compensation-money).' This was one-half the amount paid by ordinary individuals, and shows that this iron-worker was one of the privileged 'ministeriales' of the Crown.

In the laws of King Ine (7th and 8th centuries), we observe that the smith was still an important individual, and also attached himself to a lower class than the great nobles and kings. 'If a gesithcund-man (a somewhat similar rank to the *leudes* of the Franks and Visigoths) go away, then may he have his reeve (steward) with him, and his " smith," and his child's fosterer.'

In the *Saxon Chronicle,* the song on King Edgar's

death designates the Anglo-Saxons as 'the illustrious smiths of war!' The Dooms-day Book, though composed in the reign of the first Norman king of England, may be said, for our present purpose, to be Saxon: it often alludes to workers in iron. For instance, we find that in the City of Hereford there were six smiths, who paid one penny each for his forge, and who made one hundred and twenty pieces of iron from the king's ore. To each of them threepence was paid as a custom, and they were freed from all other services. It would appear that the iron-mines of England were well worked in Saxon times. Iron-ore was obtained in several counties, and there were furnaces for smelting. The mines of Gloucestershire, in particular, are alluded to by Giraldus Cambrensis as producing an abundance of this valuable metal; and there is every reason for supposing that these mines were wrought by the Saxons, as they had been by their predecessors, the Romans.[1]

The Anglo-Saxon monks were, as already hinted, like the Druid priests, skilful workers in iron, and the Venerable Bede describes one of these people as well skilled in smithcraft. Speaking of Easterwin, Abbot of Weremouth, he says: 'This abbot, being a strong man, and of a humble disposition, used to assist his monks in their rural labours, sometimes guiding the plough by its stilt or handle, sometimes winnowing corn, and sometimes forging instruments of husbandry with a hammer upon the anvil.'[2]

King Edgar even enacted that the clergy should

[1] Pictorial History of England, Book ii. chap. 6.
[2] Hist. *A*bbat. Weremath., p. 296.

pursue this and other crafts : 'We command that every priest, to increase knowledge, diligently learn some handi craft.' [1]

The famed St Dunstan, the most proficient man of his age, and who lived in the 10th century, among his other accomplishments, was a cunning worker in metals, and particularly iron.

Glastonbury Abbey, where Arthur, the last of the British kings, had been buried, was, on the admission of the future abbot, principally filled by Celts or Scots from Ireland, who were at that time the most learned men. This abbey was famous throughout all the land for the ability of its monks, and a British population dwelt in the surrounding country. The usual austerities of a monastic life did not suffice for Dunstan in his earlier years, but, like a Druid, he gave himself up to a solitary existence, practising his skill in secret. He built a kind of Wayland Smith's cave by the side of the sacred edifice, in which he enclosed himself. This cell or hole was only 5 feet in length and $2\frac{1}{2}$ in width, and it barely rose 4 feet above the ground. The earth was excavated just enough to enable him to stand upright, though he could never lie down. His biographer (Osberne) was so puzzled with this strange re-treat that he knew not what to call it. Cells were commonly dug in an eminence or raised from the earth, but this was the earth itself excavated. Its only wall was its door, which covered the whole, and in this was a small aperture to admit light and air. In this sepulchre he abode, denying himself rest as well as needful food, fasting to the point of starva-tion, and constantly working at his forge when not engaged

[1] *Wilkins.* Ibid. p. 83.

in prayer. The hammer was always sounding, except when silenced by his orisons; and here he imagined himself assailed by the Evil One. On a certain night all the neighbourhood was alarmed by the most terrific howlings, which seemed to issue from his den. In the morning the people flocked to him to inquire the cause. He told them that the devil had intruded his head into his window to tempt him while he was heating his iron-work; that he had seized him by the nose with his red-hot tongs; and that the noise was Satan's roaring at the pain![1]

The simple people are stated to have venerated the recluse for his amazing exploits with the enemy of mankind; and indeed he appears to have been as expert in fabricating tales as horse-shoes or other iron-work.

That priests of the highest rank on the continent at a very early period shod horses, tradition abundantly testifies. Saint Eloy or Eloi, who lived in France in the 7th century, during the reign of Clotaire II., is frequently spoken of as a goldsmith;[2] but in mediæval delineations he is most commonly represented shoeing solipeds. We have alluded to him elsewhere as a rather popular saint among horsemen during the Middle Ages. He has been the patron of the horse-shoer in nearly every country in Europe, and

[1] *S. Turner, F. Palgrave.* Hist. Anglo-Saxons. This fable concerning the attacks of his Satanic Majesty on the crafty Dunstan, is paralleled by that sustained by St Benedict in the 6th century. That worthy was tempted by the devil, who appears to have been particularly addicted to trifle with the feelings of the mediæval saints, in the form of a *mulomedicus:* 'ei antiquus hostis in mulomedici specie obviam factus est, cornu (to give the horses medicine) et tripedicam (an instrument to bind horses' feet) ferens,' etc.—*Vita St Benedicti,* Muratori, Scrip. Rer. Ital., vol. iv. p. 223.

[2] *Michelet.* Histoire de France, vol. i. p. 243, 1852.

was the protector of animals not only in England, France, Italy, and Burgundy, but even in Germany we find that St Job and St Eloy were invoked in the incantations against the maladies of horses.

One of the most curious representations of the patron saint of the farriers is that given in the frontispiece to this work. The original was a distemper painting, discovered on the north side of the eastern pier, between the nave and north transept of St Michael's church, Highworth, Wiltshire, during very recent restorations. This painting was unfortunately destroyed during the alterations, but not before a drawing of it was obtained. A copy of this, for which I am indebted to the Rev. Mr Bowden, the rector of the church, shows a chapel-like building, with forge apparently outside. To the left is the blazing fire, with the bellows behind, and hung round with shoes which have clumsy calkins, and only four nail-holes each; while near it is perhaps a trough containing a lot of tongs. St Eloy, in his full array of church vestments, stands behind a peculiar anvil holding a shoeing hammer in his right hand, on the back of which is a curious mark, while the other has evidently grasped the leg of a horse, whose hoof rests on the anvil, and to this the Saint attaches the shoe. At the foot is seen the Evil One, who never appears to have been absent from the company of these holy men.

The painting might be ascribed to the 13th or 14th century, and had sustained rough treatment at some time; parts of it having been rubbed off. A marble tablet, dated A.D. 1650, had been fastened over the centre of it.

In the Library of Zurich, Switzerland, there is a painting belonging to the 14th or 15th century, representing St Antony of Padua and St Sebastian, with a farrier between them shoeing a vicious horse, one foot of which rests in his hand, perhaps in consequence of some magical spell induced by a witch who is present, and whose nose the farrier pinches in an enormous pair of tongs, as a punishment for her witchcraft.

Travelling from the Anglo-Saxon period to other lands and recent times, we come to Abyssinia, where the trade of blacksmith is hereditary, and considered as more or less disgraceful, from the fact that blacksmiths are, with very rare exceptions, believed to be all sorcerers, and are opprobriously called 'Bouda.' They are supposed to have the power of turning themselves into hyænas, and sometimes into other animals; as being, in fact, either tormented by or allied with evil spirits, like the Middle-Age saints.

'I remember a story of some little girls, who, having been out in the forest to gather sticks, came running back breathless with fright; and being asked what was the cause, they answered that a blacksmith had met them, and entering into conversation with him, they at length began to joke him about whether, as had been asserted, he could really turn himself into a hyæna. The man, they declared, made no reply, but taking some ashes, which he had with him tied up in the corner of his cloth, sprinkled them over his shoulders, and, to their horror and alarm, they began almost immediately to perceive that the metamorphosis was actually taking place, and that the blacksmith's skin was assuming the hair and colour of the hyæna, while his limbs and head took the shape of that animal. When the change was complete he grinned and laughed at them, and then retired into the neighbouring thickets. They had remained, as it were, rooted to the place from sheer fright, but the moment the hideous creature withdrew, they made the best of their way home. ∴ . . . Few people will venture to offend a blacksmith, fearing the effects of his resentment.'[1]

Burton says: 'It has been observed that the blacksmith has ever been looked upon with awe by barbarians, on the 'same principle that made Vulcan a deity. In Abyssinia all artisans are Budah, sorcerers, especially the blacksmith, and he is a social outcast as among the Somal; even in El Hejaz, a land, unlike Yemen, opposed to distinctions amongst Moslems, the Khalawigah, who work in metal, are considered vile. Throughout the rest of El Islam the blacksmith is respected as treading in the path of David, the father of the craft.'[2]

Barth writes: 'All over the Tawárek country, the "enhad" (smith) is much respected, and the confraternity is most numerous. An "enhad" is generally the prime minister of every little chief. The Arabs in Timbuktu call these blacksmiths "mállem," which may give an idea of their high rank and respected character.'[3]

With the Arabs, farriers are held in great esteem, and enjoy extensive and invaluable privileges, in consequence of the benefits 'their art confers on the indispensable complement of the Arab—his horse. The smith lives

---

[1] *Mansfield Parkyns.* Life in *A*byssinia, vol. ii. p. 144.
[2] First Footsteps in East *A*frica, p. 33.
[3] Travels in *A*frica.

in a tent set apart from the tribe, called the 'master's douar;' he pays no contributions, and when grain is bought, he gets a share without payment; neither is he called upon to offer shelter to any one; so that he is exempted from what in many cases is imposed upon all— hospitality. The constant toil demanded by his calling, the unavoidable accidents to which he is liable through the urgent wants of his brethren night and day, and the sleepless nights he has to undergo, entitle him to certain gifts called 'master's dues.'

On their return from the purchase of grain, every tent makes him an allowance of wheat and barley, and a quantity of butter. In the spring he gets the fleece of a ewe; and if a camel is killed for eating, he gets the part between the withers and tail. When dividing plunder, no matter whether or not he has taken part in the expedition, he gets his share, usually a sheep or a camel, and this is called the horseman's ewe. The most important privilege accorded to him, however, and which shows more than anything else the high esteem in which his art is held, is the gift of life on the field of battle. If a farrier is on horseback, with arms in his hands, he is as liable to be killed as any other horseman; but if he dismounts, kneels down, and imitates with the two corners of his burnous the movements of his bellows, he will be spared. This is only, however, when he has led an in- offensive life, and followed his art. 'A "lanæ" (one share of the plunder) is given to the farrier of the tribe, for he contributes his skill and labour to the success of the enterprise. To kill a farrier is deemed infamous. It is a deed that will recoil upon the guilty tribe, who will be pursued by a curse ever after.' So afraid are the Arabs of losing their farrier, that if he happens to grow rich, a quarrel is fastened upon him, and a portion of his wealth taken away to prevent his leaving the district. A farrier whose tribe has been plundered, seeks out the robbers, and on the simple proof of his trade, recovers his tent, tools, utensils, and horse-shoes.[1]

In Persia the traditions belonging to the craft are many and curious. One of these relates to Baduspan, who, very many centuries ago, possessed himself of the sovereignty of Ruyan and Rostemdar, a district of that country, and who was a descendant of that blacksmith so famous in the history of the East—Kawe by name. This valiant worker in iron overthrew the tyrant Sohak, and hoisted his leather apron for a flag; which distinguishing badge, adorned with pearls and jewels, glittered till the end of that monarchy, as the national standard.

After conquering the tyrant, Feridun, the legitimate heir to the throne, was duly proclaimed king by the magnanimous smith, Kawe. Feridun's mother had taken refuge in the forests soon after his birth, and had fed the child with the milk of a buffalo cow, the head of which, sculptured on that monarch's mace, has become no less celebrated among the national insignia than the leather apron.[2]

In Java, and throughout the Eastern Archipelago, the workers in iron hold very high rank, and in ancient times were not unfrequently kings or princes. In other countries, it has often been the boast of monarchs and

---

[1] *E. Daumas.* Les Chevaux du Sahara.
[2] *C. Von Hammer.* Histoire des Assassins, p. 230. Paris, 1833.

great chiefs that they could handle the tools of the smith. Longfellow declares that—

‘ Since the birth of time, throughout all ages and nations,
Has the craft of the smith been held in repute by the people.’

In speaking of Basil the blacksmith,

‘ Who was a mighty man in the village, and honoured of all men ; ’

he intimates that even in the New World the traditional attributes of the grimy occupation had found a congenial home. There is something very pleasant in reading of the home-like scenes in ‘ Evangeline,’ where, in the far-off Acadie, the children of the village, hurrying away to Basil’s forge,

‘ Stood with wondering eyes to behold him
Take in his leathern lap the hoof of the horse as a plaything,
Nailing the shoe in its place ; while near him the tire of the cart-wheel
Lay like a fiery snake, coiled round in a circle of cinders.
Oft on autumnal eves, when without in the gathering darkness
Bursting with light seemed the smithy, through every cranny and crevice,
Warm by the forge within they watched the labouring bellows,
And as its panting ceased, and the sparks expired in the ashes,
Merrily laughed, and said they were nuns going into the chapel.’

There appears to be every reason to believe that the mysteries of Druidism, and those secret metallurgical rites anciently practised in the East, and known as the ‘ Samothracian Mysteries,’ were very closely allied. From a comparison of the texts of Strabo, Diodorus of Sicily, Herodotus, Clement of Alexandria, and others, who speak of the Dactyli, Cabiri, Curetes, Corybantes, and Telchines, as people who came from the far East to Phrygia and Crete, where they introduced the working of bronze and iron, and worshipped in Rhea and on Mounts Ida in Phrygia and Crete, but chiefly in Samothracia, M. Rossignol draws the following conclusions: ' In the collection of facts which spring from the same source, are woven together by regular deductions, and all tend to the same end, it is impossible to mistake the existence of a religious doctrine founded on the discovery and the first employment of metals, as that of Eleusis was on the introduction of the culture of wheat. Therefore we do not hesitate to believe, that by this comparison we have thrown light on the mysteries of metallurgy, hidden under the name of the Mysteries of Samothracia.'[1]

And Martin writes: ' The ancients have not mistaken the close relationship of these mysteries (of Druidism) with those of Samothracia, where the same symbol i found nearly entire. Gwyon is the Gijon of the Phœnicians, the Pelasgic Casmil; Koridwen is the grand goddess of the Cabiric rites of Thrace and Phrygia (Rhea). A very positive indication is to be found in the names of the Cabires—those cosmical genii from Western Asia, which exist scarcely changed in Irish poetry. The Gaëls no doubt carried these symbols with them from the West.'[2] Strabo lends his authority to this assertion in an unequivocal manner: ' In one of the sacred islands near the coast of Britain, are celebrated mysteries similar to those of Samothrace and Eleusis; these are the mysteries of Koridwen, to the observance of which the Druidesses appear to be more particularly devoted.'[3]

In the mysteries of Samothrace, the sacred order of the

Des Origines Religieuses de la Métallurgie.
[2] Hist. de France.   [3] *Strabo.*   Lib. iv. p. 190.

Cabiri were the artificers, and reserved to themselves the monopoly of working in metals; they made the arms, armour, and all other metallic articles, in great secrecy, as did the *ovates* among the Druids. The chief workmen of the Druids guarded the centre fire to which so much mysterious importance was attached.[1]

But, it may be asked, if the Gauls and the Germans, long before the Romans came in contact with them, shod their horses with iron plates nailed to the hoofs, why was a practice of so much utility, and indeed of necessity, not adopted by the Romans, and mentioned in their writings, when they became acquainted with these races? This, like so many others, is a difficult question to answer. Unless we admit that the *soleæ ferreæ* were the nail-shoes of the Teutons and Gauls, or that the *glantæ ferreæ* only once found in the Roman writings were attached by nails to the hoofs, we have nothing whatever in the way of written evidence, as before stated, to show that this device was resorted to by the Romans. The custom was, in all likelihood, prevalent in Gaul, Switzerland, Germany, and perhaps also in Britain, when invaded by the imperial armies, and it would appear that in time the Romans did resort to it. If we admit that the *soleæ*

---

[1] *Megnin.* Op. cit., p. 9.   'La nuit du 1er Novembre, les traditions Irlandaises rapportent que les druides se rassemblaient autour du " pere-feu" gardé par un *pontife-forgeron* et l'éteignaient. A ce signal, de proche en proche s'éteignaient tous les feux de l'île; partout regnait un silence de mort; la nature entière semblait plongée dans une nuit primitive. Tout à coup le feu jaillissait de nouveau de la montagne sainte, et des cris d'allégresse éclataient de toutes parts; la flamme empruntée au " pere-feu " courait, de foyer en foyer, d'un bout à l'autre de l'ile et ranimait partout la vie.' *Martin.* Op. cit., vol. i.

ferreæ were not like the modern shoes, then it might be surmised that with people professing Druidism—a religion represented by a caste who had a monopoly of working in iron, the requisite knowledge being only acquired after initiation, and which it was worse than sacrilege to divulge—would not be likely to yield their most sacred secrets to their conquerors, and put them on an equality with themselves. We know that the Romans were, for centuries, in contact with the Gauls, and yet had only weapons of bronze; and that while their plough was of the most primitive description, even in the time of Virgil, the Gauls had an implement approaching perfection; and so with other objects in metallurgy.

The Romans were, in several respects, slow to adopt or improve; and prejudice, especially towards the arts of a conquered and a *barbarous* people, may have operated strongly with regard to shoeing. After a time they appear to have practised it, but to a limited extent; and only (to judge from the evidence at present before us) in those countries where it was already in use on their arrival did they attempt it. But why was it not mentioned by their historians or hippiatrists? When we find these writers anxiously describing the evils resulting to the hoofs from travelling, it might be expected that so simple, and yet so bold, a means of preventing them would have obtained notice. This omission, however, need not cause us so much surprise when we learn that sometimes great undertakings were overlooked, forgotten, or left unrecorded by the Roman historians. The Caledonian Wall, for example, was a most important work, entailing a vast amount of labour, and built by the Romans themselves, yet only one of their writers makes the faintest allusion to its erection.[1]

As already observed, the climate of the North, where hoofs are soft, roads rugged, and moisture prevails, may have had much to do with the invention of shoeing among the Celts, and compelled the Romans to resort to it when they left their sunny southern climate, where hoofs are hard, and their wonderful paved *strata*.

If the relics found in the battle-field of Alesia belong to the final struggle between Julius Cæsar and the Gauls, then the Romans must have been cognizant of this means of defending horses' feet at a comparatively early period. Beger[2] has figured a curious bronze medal (fig. 141), which

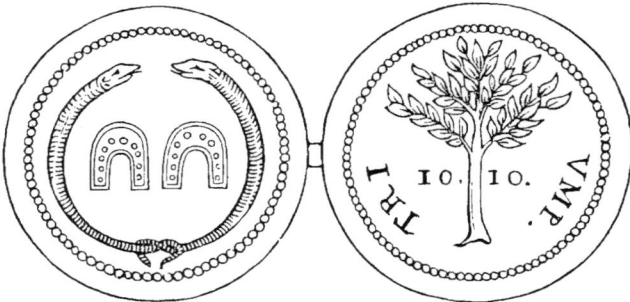

fig. 141

he classes among those of Julius Cæsar, though he heads them 'Numismata Incerta;' and this uncertainty deprives it of much of the great interest it might possess with regard to the subject of our treatise. On the obverse of this medal appear two snakes with their tails entwined, and in the middle of the circle they form are two objects resembling one of the German shoes found by Linden-

---

[1] *Wilson.* Prehistoric *A*nnals of Scotland, vol. ii. p. 39.

[2] Numismata Romanorum, vol. ii. p. 597.

schmidt at Gaufelfingen. These may be horse-shoes;
they have each eight holes, disposed three on each side
and two at the toe; and the extremities have an appearance as if there were calkins, though the engraver has
unfortunately forgotten to copy them accurately; but
altogether their form and the disposition of the holes is
peculiar, and certainly not like the shoes of the earlier
periods. On the reverse of the medal is a laurel-tree,
with the letters I O on each side of the trunk, and the
legend TRIVMP (triumph). Nothing is known as to
the history of this curious relic, or where it was discovered;
but as it was in the collection of the Elector of Brandenburg, it may be of Germano-Roman origin, in which case
we may then conclude that the objects resembling shoes are
really intended to represent them, and may be compared
with the specimen from the Gaufelfingen tumulus.

It may be added, however, that Beger[1] seems to have
been much baffled by the medal, and could come to no
conclusion as to its import. 'Quid autem serpentes
caudis connexio? quid calces equorum? nisi cum Patino
bellum prudentia gestum intelligas, non explicavero.'
Eckhel, in his 'Doctrina Nummorum Veterum,' asserts
that he has also seen this money, on which is impressed
the 'two shoes placed between two serpents with interlaced
tails.' He observed it in several collections, and thought
it an evident allusion to the success of a race-horse in the
circus. One or two of these coins were in the museum
of the late M. Blacas.

M. Nickard, who appears determined not to admit
that horses were shod with the ancients, has been as much

[1] Thesaur. Elect. Brandenburg, vol. iii. p. 597.

troubled with these specimens as other numismatists and archæologists, and is inclined to think that what we have designated horse-shoes are intended to represent fetters (*entraves*) for slaves, supporting this opinion by several references to the practice of manacling these unfortunate creatures. He does not, however, attempt to describe the fetters, or account for the presence of holes in these supposed examples.

As I have just said, I am willing to believe that they are horse-shoes, and that Eckhel is not far from the truth in ascribing the origin of the coin to victories in the hippodrome.

As tending to confirm this opinion, it is worthy of note that quite recently, in a German work on farriery,[1] a tail-piece to one of the chapters shows a serpent encircling a well-arranged and characteristic group of objects (fig. 142), consisting of a horse-shoe (modern German pattern), nails, hammer, pincers, buffer, rasp, and 'boutoir' or 'hufmesser.'

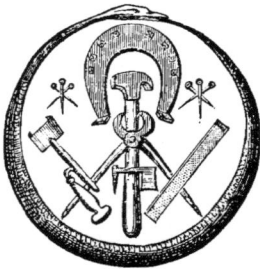

fig. 142

It must not be forgotten that the serpent is the emblem of the metempsychosis and eternal renovation of Oriental mythology, and held a prominent place among the superstitions of the Druids. The egg of that creature was looked upon by them as a most potent talisman, and Pliny[2] describes how these articles were

[1] Lehr- und Handbuch der Hufbeschlagskunst. Von J. T. Grosz. 3rd edition. Stuttgart, 1861.

[2] Hist. Naturalis. Lib. xxix. cap. 44.

procured. The Druids wore them round their necks richly set, and sold them at a very high price. They appear, nevertheless, to have been nothing more than the shells of echini or 'sea-eggs.'

At a very early date we discover another evidence of the high antiquity of shoeing among the Celtic and cognate races, in the frequent occurrence of a name to designate those who had charge of horses, and who had to attend to their shoeing. In French, German, and early British writers, instead of ἱππίατρος and *mulomedicus*, employed in classical times to denote the veterinary surgeon, there is used the designation 'mariscalcus,' 'manescalcus,' 'marescallus,' ' mareschallus,' and finally ' mareschal ;' all, as Verstegan asserts, derived from the German word ' march' —*horse*. ' In the ancient Teutonicke,' he says, '*mare* had sometime the signification that horse now hath, and so served for the appelation of that whole kind, to wit, both male and female, and gelding, and so all went in general by the name of horse. *Scalc*, in our ancient language, signifieth a kind of servant, as the name of *scalco* (though a Teutonicke denomination) in Italy yet doth. *Marscalc* (or marschal) was with our ancestors, as with the ancient Germans, *curator equorum*, one who had charge of horses. The French, who (as we in England) very honourably esteeme of this name of office, doe give unto some nobleman that bare it the title of Grand Maréschal de France. And yet notwithstanding they doe no otherwise terme the smith that cureth and shueth horses than by the name of *mareschal*.' [1] Lobineau [2] says

---

[1] Restitution of Decayed Intelligence in Titles of Honour. 1635.
[2] Hist. de Bretagne.

it is formed from the Breton word signifying 'horse;' but as the Britons, expelled from this country in the 5th century, took refuge there, giving it their name, and as the Bas-Bretons yet speak a dialect of the Celtic, this only lends additional proof as to the origin of the term.   Pausanias, in his 'Phocians,' intimates that the term *march* is ancient Gaulish.

The first part of the word 'maréschal' is evidently Celtic, and the second, *schal,* Teutonic; the designation being therefore composed of a Celtic and Teutonic root, it does not appear to date earlier than the fixation of the Francs on the soil of Gaul, and their renunciation of vagabond habits, and in this way characterizes the amalgamation of the two people.   The history of the first *maréschal* mentioned in the early chronicles, supports this opinion.   This individual, whose name was Leudaste, was a Gaulish slave belonging to the island of Ré, who at a later period of his life became a great dignitary. Markowefe, the wife of Haribert (A.D. 556), confided the charge of her best horses to him; and among the domestics of the royal household he was enrolled by the title of 'Mariskalk.'[1]   Encouraged by his success, he did not remain satisfied with this title, which gave him the highest rank among the *fiscalin* serfs, but aspired to have the entire control of the royal stud, and to gain the position of *comes stabuli,* or constable, a dignity the barbarous kings, with many other things, had introduced at the imperial court. At the death of the queen, he so cultivated the growing esteem of King Haribert, as to distance all competitors and gain his object. After enjoying for a year or two

[1] *Greg. Turon.*   Hist. France, vol. ii. p. 261.

the superior rank he held in the domesticity of the palace, this fortunate son of a serf vine-grower in the island of Ré, who had run away several times to escape slavery, and had one of his ears cut off in consequence, was made Count of Tours, one of the most considerable cities in the kingdom ruled by Haribert.[1]

The compound word, then, was originally used, it appears, to signify a groom or horse attendant;[2] afterwards, as the importance of the office increased, it was applied to a man who had charge of twelve horses, as exemplified in the following extract from an ancient German law:[3] ' Si mariscalus, qui super XII caballos est, occiditur.'

Subsequently, and particularly in the time of the Merovingians, the individual who had under his charge all the ' mareskalks ' was designated by the title of ' Comes Marestalli ' or ' Stabulorum ;'[4] probably in imitation of the ' contostaulos ' of the Byzantine empire.[5]   The posi-

---

[1] *Megnin.* Op. Cit., pp. 30, 63.

[2] *See* Leges Salic. *Walter.* Corp. Jur. German., vol. i. p. 22.

[3] *Anton.* Geschichte der Deutschen Landwirthschaft, vol. ii. p. 298.

[4] *A. Thierry.* Récits de Tems Merovingiens, vol. ii. p. 198.

[5] The fondness for display in the matter of horses and stables manifested by the Byzantine Emperors, and which was quickly imitated by the Goths and Franks, gave a great impulse to veterinary science.   In the reign of Constantine Porphyrogenitus, the Master of the Horse was one of the first dignitaries of the court, and was styled χόμης τοῦ σταβοῦ. ' Magnus contostaulos comes stabuli, Gallis connétable, nomen conflatum ex contos seu conto comes, et staulos stabulum, σταυλος seu σταυλον ex latino stabulum detortum.   Habebant quoque veteres Franci comitem stabuli, ut videre est in epist. 3. Hincmari, c. 16, quem vulgus corrupte appellabat constabulum, ut est apud Regionem, l. 2, et apud Tyrium passim legere est constabularis.'—*Codini.*

tion, however, was as yet one of no great honour; for we find that the *wehr-geld*, or 'blood-money,' of the mareschal in the Salic, German, and Burgundian laws, was only forty sous-d'or, a lower price than that fixed for a Roman tributary, which was sixty sous. The murderer of a Frankish noble had to pay six hundred sous, and for a common Frank two hundred. A Roman or Gallo-Roman's life was valued at one hundred sous. The *sous-d'or* was equal to about fifteen francs present money.

With the more universal adoption of nail-shoeing, the horse was rapidly becoming a very important animal in civilization at the commencement of the middle ages, and by far the most essential portion of a chevalier's property. The 'comes marestalli' was, therefore, as we might expect, a very distinguished personage, and held high rank. We have already seen that with the Celts in Wales, the groom of the rein occupied a dignified position as well as the smith; and the maréschal in France was no less in favour, as we have had occasion to notice; for after the time of Charlemagne, he had not only the care of all the horses of kings or princes, but was appointed to superior commands in the army, ranking finally as one of the most exalted personages at Court.

There was nothing degrading in a nobleman shoeing horses during the era of chivalry; and the maréschal, in the 10th and 11th centuries, was on a footing of equality with the chamberlain, falconer, and other officers who formed the establishment of the chevalier or prince. In the suite of a great noble there was an *écuyer de corps*, the highest in rank; then an *écuyer de chambre*, or chamberlain; an *écuyer de table*, or carver; an *écuyer d'écurie*, or *maréchal;* an *écuyer* of song; and one falconer, etc. The *écuyer* of a poor chevalier had to perform the duties of four or five; for it was not enough to understand birds, dogs, and horses—to know how to handle a lance, battle-axe, and sword—to get over a fence or a ditch—to climb well in an assault—to speak with politeness to ladies and princes—to dress and undress his master—to wait upon him at table—to parry the blows aimed at him in a *mélée* —but, in addition, he should know something of medicine, and be capable of dressing wounds. He should also be able to *shoe a horse,* and repair with the hammer broken armour, or with the needle mend a hole in a mantle. These varied acquirements were all necessary to make up the accomplished *écuyer* (or squire), who might after-wards aspire to the honours of chivalry, and flatter himself to be worthy of them.[1]

The Cartulary of Besançon furnishes some curious details relative to the establishment kept up by Arch-bishop Hughes I., in the 10th century: 'The grand officers of the Archbishop, all of whom possessed fortified hotels in the town, were nine in number. These were the chamberlain (*camerarius*), the master of the house-hold (*sénéchal,* or *dapifer*), the butler (*pincerna*), the pantler (*panetarius*), the maréchal (*marescalus*), the forester (*forestarius*), the purse-bearer (*monetarius*), the " vicomte " (*vicomes*), the mayor (*major* or *villicus*) The maréchal held the superintendence of the Arch bishop's stables and the command of his men-at-arms (*maréchaussée*). Those innkeepers who desired to be established in the street La Lue, could only do so after

[1] *A. Callet.* Dictionnaire Encyclopédique. *Art.* Ecuyer.

paying him the tribute of a cask of wine; and all the workers in metal who sought to open shops in Besançon had to pay him a tax of as much as five sous.   When the Archbishops of Besançon, or their assistant-bishops, entered the town for the first time, the maréchal escorted them, and afterwards claimed the horses or mules they had ridden, as also the cup with which they had made their first repast.   When it happened that the emperor came, the same right was exercised, *but only on the condition that the maréchal had previously garnished with his own hands the hoofs of the monarch's steed with four silver shoes!'* [1]

The Normans, on their arrival in France, were, like the Saxons and the Franks, far behind the Celts and Gauls in equitation or their management of the horse.   On their reaching Neustria, Wace, the troubadour of the 12th century, sings :

> N'étoient mie chevaliers
> N'ils ne saroient chevalchier
> Tot à pié portoient lor armes.

And Rollo the 'Walker,' as the chroniclers tell us, never rode.[2]   Yet they soon conformed to the customs of the people among whom they settled, and in a hundred and fifty years after disembarking from their ships, they had established the finest studs of horses in France.   So that we need not be surprised that the Norman princes should also have instituted the office of 'March-shall,' to super-

---

[1] Mem. Soc. d'Emulation. Besançon, p. 379, 1859.

[2] *E. Houel.* Hist. du Cheval. *Snurlson.* Heimskringla. The Saga in this work says he received the *sobriquet* in consequence of his enormous size; no horse could be found to carry him, so he was compelled to walk.

intend their extensive stables in various parts of Normandy, but particularly at Rouen and Caen. This office sometimes became hereditary, and frequently gave a title of nobility to families—among these may be mentioned the 'Maréchal de Venoix.' To the fief of Venoix, near Caen, was attached the duty of managing the stables of the Duke of Normandy, and everything relating to them: as the gathering of the forage from the fine prairies of Caen, Venoix, and Louvigny, for the use of the Duke's horses. Through holding this office, the owner of the fief was designated ' Maréchal de Venoix,' or ' Maréchal of the Prairie.' [1]

Among the noble families of France who derived their origin from this Norman source, we find Laferrière and Ferrière; and these yet bear on their scutcheon eight horse-shoes.[2] The King of France, as also the nobles, his vassals, had among his officers a maréchal, who, under the ' connétable,' officiated as master of the horse, superintendent of the shoers, and as veterinary surgeon. Father Anselmo,[3] speaking of the duties of the constable, gives an example:

The king pays to the cavaliers the value of the horses they have lost in war, and for all those killed or disabled on service; the constable ought to value, through his maréchal, the war-horses belonging to him and his companions and all the people of his hôtel, and such price as the maréchal may fix, the king should allow.'

The first French maréchal to the king who commenced to elevate the dignity of his office in a military

---

[1] *E. Houel.* Op. cit., p. 178. *Megnin,* p. 75.
[2] Le Nobiliaire de Normandie.
[3] Histoire de la Maison Royale de France.

point of view, was Albéric Clément, lord of Metz, in Gâ-tinais. He accompanied King Philip Augustus to the Holy Land, and distinguished himself at the siege of Acre, where he was killed at an assault conducted by William the Breton and Rigord, in 1191. He had on many occasions led the advanced guard into battle,[1] and it was he who inaugurated the brilliant series of French marshals. His son, though very young, was, in recognition of the father's services, made maréchal, and in 1225 commenced his duties, which, though military in their character, were yet made to include the management of the king's horses, and everything pertaining to them.[2] It is not, however, until the 15th century that we find the maréchal separating himself from horses and stables, and occupying a position second only to that of the sovereign.

In relation to shoeing, the designation, elsewhere than in France, is of very frequent occurrence. In the reign of James II., King of Aragon (13th century), in appointing a maréchal, it is ordained: 'Which Marescallus shall be near our person when we journey, furnished with nails and shoes, and other necessaries.'[3] In the Hist. Dalphini, for the year 1340, in defining the duties of this person, it is stated: 'Also the said Marescallus, every morning and late at night, is to see that the horses are properly groomed, . . and also to ascertain that they are well shod.'

---

[1] *Guillaume le Breton.* Vie de Philippe *A*uguste:

> Fit subito tetra castris irruptio nocte
> Quippe marescallus festinum duxerat agmen.

[2] *Père Anselme.* Hist. de la Maison Royale de France. Paris, 1730.

[3] Leges Jacobi ii. Reg. Majoric. vol. iii.

It is also found in the Charta Buzelinum (P. 528) for the year 1034; in the 'Statutis Ordinis de Sempringham' (P. 743); in 'Institu. Cap. Gener. Cisteric (cap. 36); and in Foris Bigorre (art. 40).[1]

After the arrival of the Normans in England, and who in all probability brought it with them, the designation or title is a common one; the maréchal or smith being often typified by hammers, tongs, anvils, and horse-shoes, and marshall or marescallus became a common name. For instance, in the 'Annales Cambriæ,' for the 11th century, it is recorded, 'Willielmus Marescallus factus est comes Penbrochiæ.'

We also notice that Walter Marshall, seventh Earl of Pembroke, who died in the Keep of Gooderich Castle, in 1246, had for his seal a horse-shoe, and a nail within its branches. This seal is of interest to us in not only show-ing the origin of the name, but as affording a good idea of the shoes and nails in use at this period (fig. 143).

In the curious work entitled 'Fleta,' written in the reign of Edward I., the 'Marescalcia' and 'Marescallo' are specially alluded to. For example, in speaking of the 'Hospitio Regis,' it is written: Item eleemosynar' janitorem,

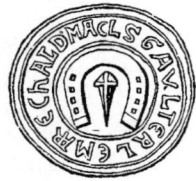

fig. 143

servientem ad custod' summar', et carectarum deputatum, et clericum de Marescalcia cum Marescallo, *ferratore equorum*, qui quidem clericus de expensis fœni et avenæ, literæ *ferrure equorum* et harnes' pro equis, et carectis, ac de vadiis servientum, scutiferorum, clericorum, et garcionem respondebit cujus interest scire de hiis qui

[1] *Du Cange. Glossarium ad Scriptores Mediæ et Infime Latinitatis.*

de novo erunt admisi ad vad' Reg. quam de extravaganti-
bus,' etc. And again, ' Marescalli autem de supervenien-
tibus debent inferiori Marescallo testimonium perhibere.'[1]
The functions of this dignitary are thus defined : ' Officium
autem Marescalli est præbendam contra præpositum talli-
are, et numerum equorum Senescallo hospitii in compoto
diei qualibet nocte computare, at ipse in rotulo suo numerum equorum possit inverere, specifiando nomina super-
venientium de eorum adventu, et morâ. 2. Item furfur
à præposito per talliam recipere, cum vide necesse habue-
rit, et inde Señ compotum reddere, ut fiat de furfure, sicat
de avena. 3. Item contra præpositum de *ferris et clavis*
ab eo receptis talliam recipere, *tam de numero ferrorum,*
quàm de eorum custibus, et ubi ea allocaverit Sen' de-
monstrare ; *nec sine sua licentia alienos equos vide licebit
ferrare.* Item fœnum et literam equis deliberare.'[2]

In London, during the reign of Edward I., we not
only find the designation of ' Mareschal' in every-day
use, but also a regulation defining the prices to be charged
by him for his labour and materials ; from which we
learn, that for putting on a common shoe with six nails,
$1\frac{1}{2}d$. was to be paid ; with eight nails, $2d$. ; and for removing the same, $\frac{1}{2}d$. For putting a shoe on a courser,
$2\frac{1}{2}d$. ; on a war-horse, $3d$. ; and for removing a shoe on
either, $1d$. This is notified in the Norman French of
the ' Liber Albus' of the London Guildhall, and is headed
as follows :

' DE MARESCALLIS, FABRIS, ET ARMURARIS.

' Qe Mareschals preignent pur fer de chival, de vi
clowes, i denier obole ; de viii clowes, ii deniers ; et pur

---

[1] Fleta, Lib. ii. cap. 14, p. 4.   [2] Ibid. cap. 74.

remover dicel, obole; et pur fer de courser, ii deniers obole; et pur fer de destrer, iii deniers; et pur removere un diceux, i denier.'

From Letter-Book G, dated from A.D. 1353 to A.D. 1375, and preserved in the Records of the City of London, we make the following extract:

'Item, qe Mareschal preignent pur ferure des chivalx, cest assavoir, pur fer de viii clowes, ii deniers; et de meyns, i denier obole; et pur remover, obole.'

That the designation was general wherever the Normans had established themselves in England, is proved by the accompanying drawing (fig. 144) from the brass matrix of a curious seal now in the possession of Mrs Wooler, of Darlington, and which was found at Piersbridge, near that town. A farrier displays a horse-shoe, heavy and clumsy, and pierced with six almost square holes, as well as a shoe-

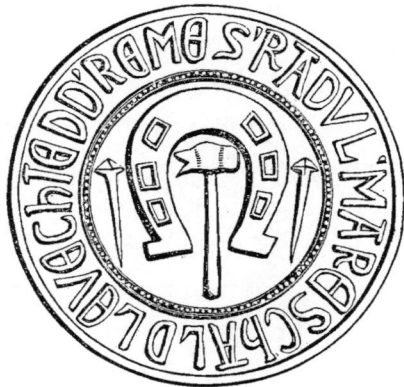

fig 144

ing hammer and two nails as a badge of his craft the legend around them being S. Radul, Maréchal d' l'Evechie d' Dureme—which signifies that it was the seal of Ralph, farrier to the bishopric of Durham.

The word mareschal remained in vogue in England long after the Norman French had ceased to be the popular or Court language, though it generally gave place to 'farrier,' 'ferrier,' or 'ferrator,' a designation which had also been in use for very many centuries, and was derived, no doubt, from the 'faber ferrarius,' who not only worked generally in iron, but also shod the horses. In old French records it is not uncommon to find *ferrier* and *maréschal* employed to designate the shoer.

In the list of the slain at the battle of Bannockburn, fought between the English and Scottish armies on 25th June, 1318, in which the first was defeated and the national independence of Scotland established, we find on the English side, among the knights and knight bannerets, the name of William Le Mareschal, and among the prisoners in the hands of the Scots, the knight Anselm de Mareschal and Thomas de Ferrers.[1] These individuals, however, may not have been in any way connected, but by name, with the shoers of horses.

It is curious, notwithstanding, to find the two designations combined so late as the 16th century, and applied to the healer of equine maladies. For instance, in an account of Queen Elizabeth's expenses from 1559 to 1569, there is an entry for 'Curinge and Dressinge of the Queen's Horses;' and among other sums disbursed by 'John Tamworthe, Esquire, one of Her Majesties grooms,' and which were to be refunded to him, it is written : 'Also he is allowed for money paide to Martin Hollyman, *Marshall Ferrer*, and others, for curinge and dressinge of the Queen's Majesties coursers, horses, and geldings, at divers tymes, within the tyme of this accompt, as in the said book doth appere, £65 10s. 4d.'[2]

[1] *Trivet's A*nnals. Hall's edit. vol. ii. p. 14. Oxford, 1712.
[2] *J. Nichols.* The Progresses and Public Processions of Queen Elizabeth, vol. i. p. 269. London, 1823.

The designation of 'Farrier' or 'Ferrator' is very ancient, and may have been in general use before the introduction of the Norman one. For instance, in the reign of Alexander II. of Scotland, at the commencement of the 13th century, a family named Ferrier lived in Tranent, in Haddingtonshire, whose seal of arms was appended to an alienation of some lands in that locality to the family of Seton, and on this seal was a shield charged with three horse-shoes.[1]

It is somewhat surprising to find the mareschal as an officer of importance in the household of the ancient Celtic, or rather Hebridean, chiefs in the Western Isles of Scotland. Every family had two of these functionaries, who, in their language, were called 'Marischal Tach,' both of whom had an hereditary right to their office in writing, and each had a town and land for his service. Some of these rights Martin has seen fairly written on good parchment.[2]

For the year 1240, the Ferrator is mentioned as being it would appear, on an equal footing with the cook: 'Besides these there were two offices of the same kind, namely, the office of cook and that of "Ferratoris;" the liberty of exercising these lies with the citizens and the clergy.'[3] And in the Miracles of St Ambrosius it occurs: 'D. Gescæ uxor Fei Ferratoris de populo S. Martini.'[4] 'Fabros' is sometimes substituted for 'ferrator,' as, for example, in a charter of Henry V. of England (1413),[5]

[1] The Scottish Nation, vol. ii. Edinburgh, 1868.
[2] *Martin.* Western Isles. [3] Hist. Dalphin. vol. i. p. 142.
[4] Chronic. Senoniense, lib. iii. *Martin*, p. 205.
[5] *Rymer's* Fœdera, vol. ix. p. 250.

where it is said: 'Thou knowest that we have assigned thee as many horse-shoes and nails as may be necessary for the shoeing of the horses of our stables in our present travelling, with *Fabros et ferrum*, and all other necessaries required for the office of shoeing (*ferruræ*).' In connection with the various designations for the farrier in use during the Middle Ages, we also find a diversity of names for the horse-shoes, not the least frequent of these being 'ferratura.' So early as 1184, in Charta Lucii III.[1] it is enacted: 'Pro se et duobus scuteriis et tribus equi taturis fenum et avenam habeat, et candelas, et *Ferraturas* equorum de curia ipsa percipiat.' In another charter for the year 1252, it also occurs, 'Una Ferratura equi.'

The general name, however, was *ferrum* or *ferrus*. In the 'Regestum Constabulariæ Burdegal' (fol. 106) the former is expressed: ' Dixit se teneri facere D. Regi Sex Ferra nova equi cum suis clavis in mutatione Domini;' and the latter in the Acta St Raynerii Pisani (vol. iii.. Junii, p. 432), 'Ferrati enim equi qui illuc equitabant, sine aliquo ferro in pedibus regrediebantur, et qui suos *Ferros* reservabant, optimos habere pedes perhibebantur.' This affords us some evidence as to the insecure manner in which the shoes were attached to the foot at this period, as well as the wise conclusion arrived at, that those hoofs which longest retained their armour were generally the best. With regard to the word 'maréchal,' it is still the only designation for the farrier in France; but to distinguish between the shoer of horses and the highest dignitary in the land—though both originally were one—

---

[1] Miræus, vol. iii.　Diplom. Belgic. p. 1189.

the word *ferrant* is added to the title of the former (*Maréchal ferrant*).

Some strange superstitions are allied with horse-shoes and horse-shoeing, but chiefly with the shoes. It is im possible to fix the age of many of these curious fancies, but they appear to belong to the remotest antiquity—to be coeval, indeed, with the early mysteries, and to have held their ground long after these had disappeared, descending from one age to another, until they have even reached our own day. Finding a horse-shoe, and nailing it to a door or other place in order to keep away witches or ill-luck, is one of those frailties of the human mind not alone confined to the West, but ranging over a large extent of the earth's surface.

Burnes,[1] in travelling through Central Asia, remarks: 'Passing a gate of the city, I observed it studded with horse-shoes, which are as superstitious emblems in this country as in remote Scotland. A farrier had no customers: a saint to whom he applied recommended his nailing a pair of horse-shoes to a gate of the city. He afterwards prospered, and the farriers of Peshawur have since propitiated the same saint by a similar expedient, in which they place implicit reliance.'

Aubrey[2] tells us that in his time 'it is very common to nail horse-shoes over the thresholds of doors, which is to hinder the power of witches that enter into the house. Most houses of the West-end of London

[1] Travels into Bokhara, vol. ii. p. 87.
[2] Miscellanies; on *A*pparitions, Magic, Charms, &c. London, p. 148, 1696.

have the horse-shoe on the threshold. It should be a horse-shoe that one finds.' He adds : ' In the Bermudas they used to put an iron into the fire when a witch comes in. Mars is enemy to Saturn ' ' Under the porch of Stainfield church, in Suffolk, I saw,' he mentions, ' a tile with a horse-shoe upon it, placed there for this purpose, though one would imagine that holy-water would alone have been sufficient. I am told there are many similar instances.'

Ramsey[1] speaks of nailing shoes on the witches' doors and thresholds to keep them in ; and Mr Francis Douce, in his manuscript notes, says : ' The practice of nailing horse-shoes resembles that of driving nails into the walls of cottages among the Romans, which they believed to be an antidote against the plague : for this purpose L. Manlius (A.U.C. 390) was named Dictator,—to drive the nail.'

We have already noticed the singular custom for many centuries prevailing at Oakham, in Rutlandshire. In Monmouth-street, London, Brand,[2] in 1797, saw many shoes nailed to the thresholds of doors ; and Henry Ellis, in 1813, counted no less than seventeen in that street fixed against the door-steps.

The fair, but frail, ladies of Amsterdam, in 1687, believed that a horse-shoe which had either been found or stolen, and placed on the chimney-hearth, would bring good luck to their houses.[3]

There is a curious and somewhat remarkable old German saying in reference to a damsel who has met with a

---

[1] Elminthologia, p. 76.   [2] Popular *Antiquities*
[3] Putanisme d'Amsterdam.

misfortune—'Ein Mädchen dass ein *Hufeisen* verloren
hat.' The origin of this strange application of the word
is unknown; but the mishap may have been compared to
a horse stumbling and losing its shoe.[1]

In Germany horse-shoes are stuck up in all the
'Schmiedeherbergen,' or 'Gasthäusern' (smiths' pub-
lic-houses), and are called the 'arms of the guild' (*Zunft-
gilde*).

Holiday, in his comedy of the 'Marriage of the Arts,'
among other good wishes introduced, gives one to the
effect 'that the horse-shoe may never be pulled from your
threshold.'

To nail a horse-shoe, which has been cast on the road,
over the door of any house, barn, or stable, is an effectual
means of preventing the entrance of witches in Cornwall
and the West of England to this day.[2] I have recently
met with instances of this custom in Kent.

Butler,[3] in his unrivalled 'Hudibras,' says of his con-
jurer that he could

> ' Chase evil spirits away by dint
> Of cickle, *horse-shoe*, hollow flint.'

Misson[4] mentions the popularity of this custom in
England, and its being intended as a defence from witches:
' Ayant souvent remarqué un fer de cheval cloué au seuils
des portes (chez les gens de petite étoffe), j'ai demandé a
plusieurs ce que cela vouloit dire? On m'a répondu
diverses choses différentes, mais la plus générale réponse
a été, que ces fers se mettoient pour empêcher les sorciers

---

[1] Notes and Queries, vol. v. p. 391.
[2] Romances of the West of England. Second Series, p. 240.
[3] Canto iii. pt. 2, line 291.   [4] Travels in England, p. 192.

d'entrer. Ils rient en disant cela, mais ils ne le disent pourtant pas tout-à-fait en riant; car ils croyent qu'il y a là-dedans, ou du moins qu'il peut y avoir quelque vertu secrète: et s'ils n'avoient pas cette opinion, ils ne s'amuseroient pas à clouer ce fer à leur porte.'

And Guy, in his fable of the Old Woman and her Cats, makes her complain that

> ' crowds of boys
> Worry me with eternal noise ;
> Straws laid across my path retard,
> The horse-shoes nail'd (each threshold guard).'

It was considered a lucky omen to find a horse-shoe on the road; for one obtained in this way was far more potent against the ill-natured old ladies than one procured otherwise. Scott [1] alludes to the virtues of the hoof-armour in this respect, when he causes Summertrees to rail Crosbie with, ' Your wife's a witch, man ; you should nail a horse-shoe on your chamber-door '

Only a few years ago, when the wealthy banker, Coutts, went to reside at Holly Lodge, two old horse-shoes were fixed on the upper step of the marble flight of stairs.

Specimens will be shown of two horse-shoes—one of the 13th, the other of the 16th, century—which had been fastened to the church door of Saint-Saturnin, in France.

It used to be the custom in Devonshire and Cornwall, to nail to the great west doors of churches these old articles to keep off the malicious witches, one of whose special amusements it was

> ' To untie the winds and make them fight
> Against the churches.'

---

[1] Red *Gauntlet*, chap. v.

Church doors appear to have been rather favourite depôts for horse-shoes. On that of the church at Halcombe, Devonshire, were formerly four shoes, said to be those taken from a horse ridden some distance into the sea by one of the Carews, for a wager.

The odd custom even appears to have extended itself from the church to the precincts of the grave; for Lin denschmidt found horse-shoes in the tombs of Gaufel fingen, and could not account for their presence there.

At Schwarzenstein, about half-a-league from Rastenburg, Prussia, two large horse-shoes, says tradition, were to be seen hanging to the church walls, and this is their antiquated history: 'Not far from the church dwelt a tavern-keeper, who, in selling beer to the people, did not give them just measure. The devil came upon him unawares one night, and, before mine host could give the alarm, he was carried off to the village forge. His Satanic Majesty with difficulty wakened up the smith, and said to him, "Master, shoe my horse!" The astonished Vulcan, who was justly suspected of being in partnership with the publican in his fraudulent transactions, knew not what to do; but as soon as he drew near the beer-seller whispered in his ear, "Partner, don't be in a hurry, but work slowly." The smith, who had taken him for a horse, was greatly terrified when he heard the familiar voice, and the fright caused him to tremble in every limb; consequently the operation of shoeing was greatly retarded, and in the interval the cock crew. The devil was then obliged to take to flight; but the inn-keeper was very ill, and did not recover for a long time after.' If the devil were to shoe all the inn-keepers who give short measure, runs the moral of the tradition, iron would soon be beyond price![1]

There was to be seen at Ellrich, in Germany, in days long gone by, four horse-shoes, of immense size, nailed to the door of the old church. They astonished everybody; and since the church was destroyed, they have been carefully preserved in the curate's dwelling. In very ancient times, Count Ernest rode one Sunday morning from Klettenberg to Ellrich, in order to contend, glass in hand, with the most intrepid tippler, for a chain of gold. He met a great number of rivals, and defeated them all; and having put the chain round his neck, he was returning, as conqueror, through this little town to Klettenberg. As he crossed the principal thoroughfare, he heard the vespers chanted in the church of Saint Nicholas: drunk as he was, he made up his mind to enter the sacred building. So he rode in, through and over the people, up to the very altar; but scarcely had his horse put its feet on the steps to clear them, than all at once its four shoes were torn off, and it fell with its rider, both stiff dead on the floor. The shoes have been preserved for ages as a memorial of this event.[2]

Even the loss of shoes from the hoofs appears to have given rise in the middle ages to as great an amount of superstition, as the virtues ascribed to their discovery. So late as the 16th century we find the accomplished diplomatist, brave soldier, and skilled poet, Du Bartas, blaming the humble little plant, moon-wort (*Botrychium lunaria*), for drawing the iron coverings from the horses' feet.

[1] *Prætorius.* Weltbeschreib. vol. ii. *Grimm.* Deutsche Mythologie.   [2] *Otmar and Grimm.* Deutsche Mythologie.

' And horse that, feeding on the grassy hills,
 Tread upon moon-wort with their hollow heeles;
 Though lately shod, at night goe bare-foot home,
 Their master musing where their shooes become.
 O moon-wort! tell us where thou hid'st the smith,
 Hammer, and pincers, thou unshoo'st them with?
 *A*las! what lock or iron engine is't
 That can thy subtile secret strength resist,
 Sith the best farrier cannot set a shoo
 So sure, but thou (so shortly) canst undoo?'

Longfellow speaks

' Of the marvellous powers of four-leaved clover and horse-shoes

as a superstition among the primitive settlers in Acadie, now Nova Scotia. And we have quoted M. Megnin's opinion that the apex of the ensign of a Roman cohort, figured on Trajan's column, was surmounted by a hoof-iron. If this be really a horse-shoe, it not only demonstrates that the custom of shoeing was known to the Romans, but that the strange virtues superstitiously attached to that object had already been credited by them; as it would also appear to have been by the Arabs in Mahomet's time.

CHAPTER IX.

SHOEING IN ENGLAND AFTER THE NORMAN CONQUEST. EUSTATHIUS. REVIVAL OF VETERINARY SCIENCE. JORDANUS RUFFUS. PETRUS DE CRESCENTIUS. LAURENTIUS RUSIUS. SHOD OXEN. SHOEING FORGES. COUNTING THE HORSE-SHOES AND HOB-NAILS. LIBER QUO-TIDIANUS. THE DEXTRARIUS AND HOBBY. HAWKING. STRATAGEM OF REVERSING SHOES. ROBERT BRUCE AND DUKE CHRISTOPHER OF WURTEMBERG. VALUE OF SHOES AND NAILS FOR HORSES IN ENGLAND IN THE 13TH AND 14TH CENTURIES. COAL. THE RE-VOLT OF THE DUKE OF LANCASTER. TUTBURY CASTLE AND THE RIVER DOVE. CURIOUS DISCOVERY OF TREASURE AND HORSE-SHOES. FROISSART. WARS OF KINGS EDWARD II. AND III. GLOU-CESTER CORPORATION SEAL. STATUS OF THE FARRIER. DIFFERENT BREEDS OF HORSES. GROOVED IMPORTED SHOES. THE DAYS OF CHIVALRY. FAMILY COATS OF ARMS. LOMBARDY AND FLEM-ISH HORSES. THE CHATELAINE OF WARRENNE. HAMERICOURT. FARRIERY IN SCOTLAND. AN UNJUST LAW. STATUTES OF EDWARD VI. HENRY VIII. AND SHOEING WITH FELT. CURIOUS CUSTOMS AND EXTRAVAGANCE. GOLD AND SILVER SHOES. FARRIERS. CÆSAR FIASCHI. DIVERSITY OF SHOES. GERMAN WRITERS. CARLO RUINI.

AFTER the Norman invasion of England, the shoeing of horses, and indeed everything relating to that noble animal, received much attention. Instead of being an obscure art, and apparently but rarely resorted to among the Anglo-Saxons, the Norman knights brought with them from the continent their maréchals of high rank, and their esteem for chivalry, which, without horses, could scarcely have existed. The advantages arising from the employment of horsemen had been amply demonstrated to them at the battle of Hastings, where their victory was mainly due to the well-equipped cavalry force they carried from Normandy. We have seen that in France shoeing was extensively practised at this time, and was, indeed, an inevitable necessity, from the custom introduced of cumbering men and horses with heavy weapons, and encasing them in massive armour. At Hastings, even the steeds were rendered proof against the attacks of the Anglo Saxons by an impenetrable covering. Roger de Hoven den, writing of this period, says, 'Cepit Rex Angliæ 100 milites, et septies viginti equos coopertos ferro, et servientes equites, et pedites multo.'[1]

So that in England the practice of shoeing horses with iron shoes attached to the hoofs by nails, was, after the settlement of the Normans, completely established and general. The form of shoe introduced by them was, perhaps, more artistic than that of the earlier periods, and the same as that in use in France; being usually furnished with calkins, heavy, larger in size than those found before their arrival, and having three, or more rarely four, nail-holes on each side. These nail-holes were nearly square, and wider at the top or ground-surface than the bottom or foot-face. The heads of the nails were also square, to fit the holes, and projected more or less from the surface of the shoe. The points of the nails, when driven through the hoof, were cut off, and only enough of the nail left to double over and form a clench or clinch.[2] Examples of

[1] *A*nnal. p. 444.
[2] This term would appear to be neither of Greek, Latin, nor French origin, but derived from the *A*nglo-Saxon *Glh-lenched*, twisted, gradually

these shoes are to be found in the seals of Walter Marshall, and Ralph of Durham, already figured. Some years ago, at the formation of the London, Chatham, and Dover railway, in a cutting near Meopham, Kent, a shoe of this description (fig. 145) was disinterred. It is very

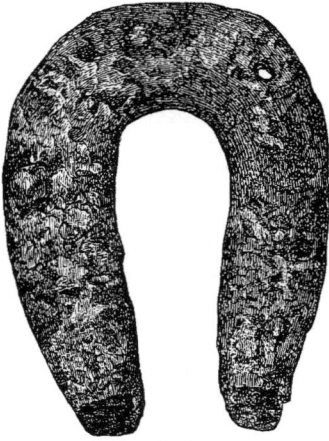

fig 145

heavy, large, and shaped as if for the foot of a mule. The nail-head yet remaining has been somewhat worn, yet enough is left to exhibit its peculiar square shape. The shoe appears to have been pulled off, as it is much twisted. The toe looks as if it had been slightly bent or ' curved' up, like the present French shoe, and there are four nails

on each side. The calkins are solid, thick, and high, and altogether it is a clumsy shoe ; measuring, as it does, $4\frac{1}{2}$ inches across the quarters, $5\frac{5}{8}$ inches long, and $1\frac{1}{8}$ inch wide in cover ; and though much oxidized, weighing $18\frac{1}{4}$

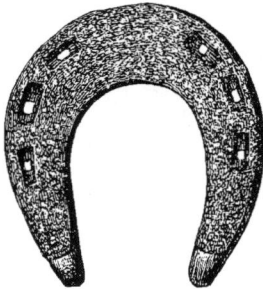

fig. 146

ounces !

Another specimen is here shown from the excavations at Besançon, and which is supposed by M. Megnin to belong to the middle ages [1] (fig. 146). And a curious example of the shod horse, in which the nailheads and calkins are very con-

becoming *glenced, clenced,* and *clenched.* The word has been in use from a very remote period in the history of this craft in Britain.

[1] Hist. Ferrure, p. 26.

spicuous, is now also copied from a French manuscript of the Apocalypse, written in the 13th century. The prominence given to the armature on the horse's hoofs shows how important it was deemed (fig. 147). Another

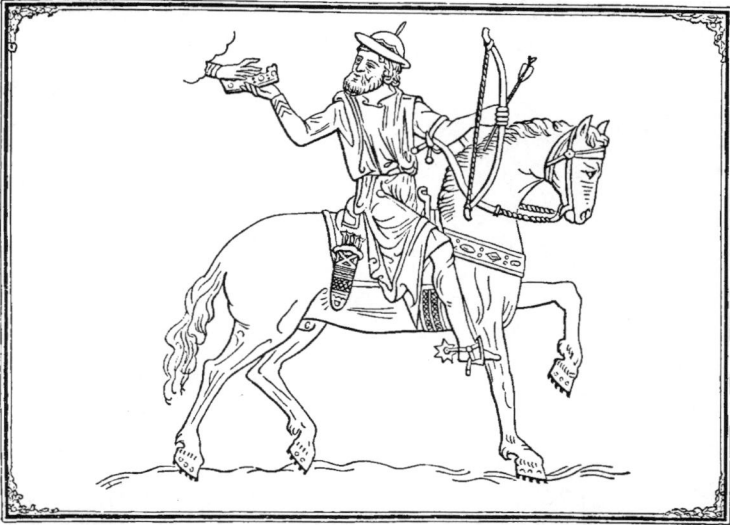

fig. 147

delineation will be found in a rare pamphlet printed in 1485, entitled 'Jacobi publici Florentini. Oratoris Institutio.'

In nearly all the manuscripts of this period, in which horses figure, their hoofs are represented as shod. We will give some additional examples of these presently.

Writers more frequently mention shoeing. Eustathius, who wrote a commentary on Homer, in the 12th century, is the first to mention the Greek horses of antiquity as shod, a statement we conclude to be erroneous, but which shows that Eustathius was well acquainted with the art. With the revival of learning, what may be designated veterinary medicine was again attracting attention, and the writers who previously treated of this branch of science, and were altogether silent regarding shoeing, now speak of it and its requirements.

Foremost among these was the Calabrian, Jordanus Ruffus, Master of the Horse (*Comes Marestalli*) to the great Frederick, who lived in the 13th century. This hippiatrist appears to have held high rank at Frederick's Court, for in one manuscript he signs his testament, ' Ego Jordanus, magnus justitiarius Ruffus de Calabria imperialis Marescallus major interfui his et subscribi feci.' In the Harleian Codex of the British Museum is a manuscript in the Sicilian language, beginning, ' Izi cominza la libra di manischalchia compostu da lu Maestro Giordano Russo di Galicia, mariscalo del imperatore Federica.' Another codex is in the Damiani library at Venice, a Latin translation of which begins, ' Incipit liber manescalchiæ. Nui Messeri Jordan Russu de Calabria volimo insignari achelli chi avinu a nutricari cavalli secundu chi avimu imparatu nela manestalla de lu imperaturi Federicu chi avimu provatu e avimu complita qusta opira nelu nomu di deu, e di Santu Aloi.' The patron saint of farriers was thus, it appears, invoked to countenance his labours.

The only good edition to which I have had access, is that published at Bologna in 1561, with the title, ' Il dottisimo libro non più Stampato delle Malscalzie del Cavallo, del Signor Giordano Rusto, Calaurese.' The work is curious, but by no means despicable; and his brief remarks on shoeing are sensible enough. After mentioning that it is useful to wash out the horse's mouth and rub it with powdered salt, particularly if the animal does not drink willingly; he recommends that the hoofs be shod with shoes of a convenient weight, round, and adapted to the shape of the feet. The shoe to be light, and narrow towards the extremity of the branches, as in proportion to the narrowness of the shoe at the heels would the horse's hoofs become hard and strong. The thicker the shoes of the young horse, so the more liability was there to the hoofs becoming weak and soft; and so long as horses continued to be shod in their youth, so would the hoofs become large and hard.[1]

Veterinary medicine at this stage in the revival of the arts and sciences was almost, if not entirely, Italian, and the best and most original writers on it were natives of Italy. After Ruffus, the principal author on the diseases and management of the domestic animals at this period is Petrus de Crescentiis, of Bologna, a philosopher, lawyer, physician, and traveller.[2] His work, written when he was seventy years of age (1307), had an immense success, treating, as it did, of every branch of agriculture; and

---

[1] 'Ancora è utile al cavallo lavarghi spesso la bocca con umo buono, et fregargliela con il sal pesto: et facédo cosi, il cavallo beverà piu volontieri, et facciasi ferrat con ferri di peso convenevoli, et che sieno rotondi, tanto che s'adatti à l'unghia di piedi. Il ferro deve esser leggieri, et stretto nella sua estremita; imperoche quanto sono piu stretti di dietro, le unghie del cavallo, tanto sono piu dure, e forti. Et sappi, che quanto piu spesso si ferra il caval giovane, tanto piu fa divenir l'unghia debbile e molle; et però per il continuo suo andar ferrato nella giovanezza, le sue unghie diveramo dure, et grandi.'

[2] I have not been able to refer to the first Latin edition—'Opus Ruralium Commodorum,' printed in 1471; but of the ten editions afterwards published, I have selected for reference that of nearly a century later—'De Omnibus Agriculturæ partibus, etc., per longo rerum usu exercitatum Optimum et Philosophum Petrum Crescentiensem, principem rei publicæ Bononiensis,' etc. Basileæ, 1548.

though with respect to the maladies of the lower animals, he borrows largely from the Latin Scriptores Rei Rusticæ, and Jordanus Ruffus, yet he appears to have been an enlightened observer, and much less superstitious than the majority of medical men at that time. He describes several disorders the foot of the horse is liable to, and points out the difference between the hoofs of horses reared and employed in mountainous districts, and those bred in low-lying plains. When giving directions as to the management of the horse, he recommends that the shoes be round, light, and narrow, so that they might adhere firmly to the circumference of the feet. Thin shoes, he adds, render the horse agile, and to pare and lighten the hoofs makes them large and strong. When, however, new shoes are applied, and fastened on with either new or old nails, it is necessary the horse should rest, lest harm ensue.[1]

Perhaps among the most noted of the 14th-century hippiatrists, stands Laurentius Rusius (Ruzzius, Russo,

---

[1] The first and second sentences of this recommendation are from the edition I have mentioned: ' *Ferrari* debet equus ferris sibi convenientibus rotundis admodum ungulæ lenibus, et ungulis in circuitu strictis, et bene adherentibus, nam levitas *ferri* reddit equum agilem ad levandum pedes, et ipsius strictura ungulas majores et fortiores facit.'— Lib. ix. cap. 5.

Aldrovandus, who may have had access to a more complete edition, quotes this somewhat differently, and adds to the last sentence given above—' Crescentiensis monet ut soleæ sint leves, rotundæ, et strictæ, ita ut ungulis in circuitu bene adhæreant. Nam levitas (inquit) ferri reddit equum agilem ad levandum pedes et strictura ejus ungulas majores et fortiores facit. Cum autem novæ soleæ inducuntur, aut veteris novis clavis firmatæ aliquanti per equum quiescere patiemur, ne post recentem molestiam alia noxei objiciatur.'—Op. cit., p. 50.

Rusius, Ruzo, de Ruccis, Rusé, Rugino, Rosso, and Riso—for by all of these names is he designated in the many editions of his writings), a veterinary surgeon of Rome (as he styles himself), and a friend of Cardinal Napoleon de Ursinis, who lived in the 13th and 14th centuries. His observations on the maladies of the lower animals, though similar to those of Ruffus, are, for the time in which they were written, remarkably exact, and on shoeing, though brief, they are yet reasonable. 'It is necessary to shoe horses with good and proper shoes, shaped like the hoofs; the more the extremities of the shoe—the heels, are narrow and light, the more easily will the horse lift his feet; and the narrower the shoe is, so much more will the horn grow. It is also advantageous to know, that the oftener we shoe a young horse, so rapidly does the horn become thin and weak; and, on the contrary, to accustom it to travel without shoes while it is young, is to make the hoofs larger and stronger.' [1] In other chapters, the diseases of the foot, many of them arising from shoeing, are carefully described.

In the 11th century, I think we have the first written intimation that oxen were shod for travelling. Guibert de Nogent, a contemporary of Peter the Hermit, and who has so well and so eloquently described the almost morbid excitement attending the preaching of that worthy in favour of the Crusades and the rescue of Jerusalem, gives as an illustration, that of 'the rustic, *who shod his oxen like horses,* and placed his whole family on a cart; where it was amusing to hear the children, on the ap-

---

[1] La Mareschallerie de Laurens Ruse. Paris, 1563. Translated from the Latin edition published at Spire in 1486.

proach to any large town or castle, inquiring if that were Jerusalem.'[1]

This allusion is ·curious, inasmuch as it informs us that oxen were *shod*, and, as if something very remarkable, *like horses*. It is well known that oxen cannot travel far with the continuous oval-shaped horse-shoe; the armature for the foot must be in two portions, one for the outer margin of each claw. Guibert, however, may only have referred to the manner of nailing on an iron plate on cloven hoofs, as very unusual.

It is not until the 13th century that we find any positive record of special buildings for shoeing, and also for treating horses medically. In 1202 there are two entries for shoeing in a booth : ' Pro Travillis et pro circulis et pro vectura duorum ferratorum lx. s.' ' Pro merreno ad tres *Travallos ferratorum* et uno ferrati et pro duvis xliii. s.'[2] In a charter for about the year 1302, a place of this kind is also notified as a ' Travaillium.' ' In which street was placed a certain *travaillium* (workshop, from the French *travail*), for the use of the smith to shoe horses in, which was and had been called a travaillium, and was placed and allowed to be retained there by our command.'[3] And in England, in 1235, during the reign of Henry III.,

---

[1] *Novigent.* Opera, Lib. ii. cap. 6.

[2] *Du Cange.* D. Brussel, vol. ii. De Usu Feud., pp. 142, 155.

[3] Ibid. Tabul. Carnot. Trabs also adduces Borellus' testimony for the year 1267, as follows : ' Inquesta facta . . . ad sciendum utrum . spectat ad dom. Regem. Travalla equorum et stalla terræ defixa, quæ sustinentur super columnas solo adherentes, quæ cheminis et viis præstant impedimentum, propter hoc tollere. Probata est hæc consuetudo, videlicet quod potest tollere stalla aut scalla et Travalla terræ noviter defixa, præstantia viis impedimentum.'

Walter le Bruin or Brun, a farrier or maréchal, had a piece of land granted him in the Strand, in the parish of St Clement's Danes, London, whereon to erect a forge, on condition that he should render at the Exchequer, annually, for the same, a quit-rent of six horse-shoes, with the nails (62) thereunto belonging. This strange payment was made twice during the reign of Edward I., and, curiously enough, was continued so late as 1827 (and may be even now), at the swearing-in of the annually elected Sheriff of London and Middlesex, on the 30th September, to the representative of the Sovereign, for the said piece of ground, though it has long been city property. This was the origin of the odd custom of counting the horse-shoes and hob-nails.'[1]

From the daily expense book of the 28th year of Edward I.[2] (1299—1300), we learn that the pay of the smith was fourpence a day, and that horse-shoes were charged at ten shillings per hundred, and nails twenty-pence a thousand. Iron sold at fivepence per stone. In it also notice that the functions of the armourer and smith were divided, special workmen representing each of these crafts. In the same record we find an entry for divers instruments of farriery to shoe horses, which appear to have been sent to that monarch in the Holy Land: 'Diversa utensilia ferrator equorum qui missa fuerunt Regi in terra Sancta ut dicebatur.'

The draught-horse (*equus ad tractandum* or *carrectarum*) was as yet a somewhat rare animal, the state of

[1] *Madox.* Hist. Exchequer. *Allen.* History of London, vol. i. p. 76.

[2] Liber Quotidianus Contrarotulatoris Garderobe. London, 1787.

the roads seldom allowing the passage of wheeled carriages. The Court travelled on horseback, the ladies even being obliged to resort to this kind of conveyance. The 'equus dextrarius,' or war-horse, was in high favour, and kept only for state occasions or for battle; while the 'equus discopertus,' or hobelar, was used for quick travelling. The light cavalry soldiers, who rode these small horses or hobbies, were called hobelars. This convenient-sized creature was also that generally ridden in hawking and other sports of a like character, as it was hardier and more conveniently managed. All appear to have been regularly shod; and in the illuminated manuscripts of this period, the greatest pains is taken to represent the shoes and nails. This will be seen by referring to the annexed engraving (fig. 148), copied from the Louterell Psalter, perhaps one

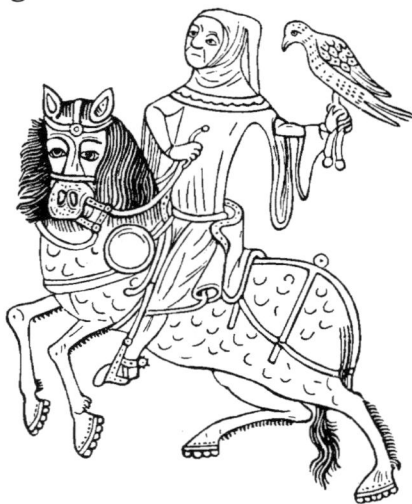

fig 148

of the finest manuscripts in existence, and now in the possession of the Weld family, Lulworth Castle, Dorsetshire. It is supposed to belong to the 14th century, and is a most valuable document for reference with regard to the domestic history of that period in England.[1]

The subject is a gentleman hawking, and mounted on

---

[1] A number of the illustrations, with descriptive notes, has been published in the Vetusta Monumenta, vol. vi.

one of these hobbies. The artist has exerted himself to show not only the shoes and nails, but in some of his illustrations he has even made manifest the latter in their passage through the hoof. The calkins and nail-heads are certainly very massive and clumsy-looking, though there can be no doubt they would afford a powerful hold of the ground. The presence of calkins had, besides, another advantage for those who were inclined to resort to a stratagem like that already described when speaking of Spain. When Robert Bruce returned to London with King Edward in 1302 (some accounts say 1305), his associate, Cumyn, treacherously betrayed him; but a secret friend gave him due notice of his danger by a present of a purse and a pair of spurs. This hint the Scottish champion was shrewd enough to understand, and made his escape, as Hollingshed [1] tells us, by 'causing a smith to shoo three horses for him, contrarilie with the *calking* [2] *forward,* that it should not be perceived which waie he had taken by the track of the horsses, for that the ground at that time was covered with snowe, he (Robert Bruce) departed out of London about midnight.'

Lest we forget to remember at the proper moment, it may be here stated, that a similar ruse was adopted by Duke Christopher of Würtemburg in 1530. When that nobleman fortunately freed himself by flight from the power of the Emperor Charles V., he reversed the position of his horse's shoes, and thus made his pursuers believe he was going in a contrary direction.

[1] Historie of Scotland. Year 1302.

[2] The word *calkin* or *calking* would appear to be derived from the Latin *calyx,* the heel, or *calcare,* to tread.

26

Iron horse-shoes were at this period, according to Mr Rogers,[1] sold by the hundred, and nails by the thousand, as at present. In 1265, we find the former articles selling at Dover 225 for 5*s.* 5¼*d.* per hundred, and nails at 1*s.* 3*d.* a thousand; whereas at Odiham, in Hampshire, 84 were purchased for 5*s.* 6½*d.*, and 1000 nails at 1*s.* 1*d.* These prices vary considerably, but in increasing proportion up to 1398, when we find 26 fore-shoes sell at Oxford for 16*s.* 8*d.*, and 22 hind-shoes at 12*s.* 6*d.*; while nails at the same place, in 1390, were 2*s.* 6*d.* per hundred.

In the accounts and annals of farms and estates during the 13th and 14th centuries, it is shown that the chief expenditure incurred in the keep of horses was the cost of shoeing. In the earlier part of this period, shoes were occasionally made, it appears, out of the iron purchased by the chief bailiff, and fashioned by the village smith. But shoes were nearly always bought ready-made, and in considerable quantities. They must, indeed, have been very slight, and little more than tips; the necessity for strong shoes, in the absence of hard or well-metalled roads, not being so urgent as now-a-days. It is possible, also, that the hoofs of horses have in our time become less solid, in consequence of the continual paring and mutilation which the modern system of shoeing involves. If we compare the price of iron by the hundred with the cost of shoes, says Mr Rogers, and remember also that the charge of working iron was generally almost equal to that of the material, we shall find that the mediæval horse-shoe

[1] History of *A*griculture and Prices in the 13th and 14th Centuries. Vol. ii. p. 328.

could not have possibly weighed more than half, and probably very often not more than the third of a pound. Traces are to be found of heavier shoes. Thus several of the entries in bailiffs' accounts, from 1265 to 1276 (unless we conclude that wrought iron was always dearer in the eastern counties, owing to the general enhancement of wages in a region then so favoured by manufacturing activity), seem to indicate stouter and heavier shoes than are ordinarily found. So marked is this difference on some occasions, that Mr Rogers was obliged to omit certain entries at very high prices from his calculations of the annual average, lest he should give a false impression as to the value of this ordinary manufacture in certain years. Thus, while particular shoes are returned from Ospringe in 1286, 1287, and 1288, at 3*s*. 4*d*. the hundred,—a rate which is very frequent in the 13th century,—others are quoted at 5*s*., 5*s*. 6*d*., and 8*s*. 6*d*., and are specially designated as ' great shoes.' These may have been like the specimen figured on page 392 *ante*. Similarly, the entries for the last year in which evidence is afforded, are shoes supplied for the saddle-horses of Merton College, and the price, it must be admitted, is very high. The Hornchurch return for the year 1396 is also excessive; but the purchase is made for the farm stud, and represents probably only that dearness which is found, even in those early days, in the vicinity of London. On the occasions when the kind of shoes are distinguished, a difference is generally made between the price of cart-horse and affer, or stott, shoes. The latter, Mr Rogers observes, were a breed of ponies used for the rougher kinds of husbandry, or for such work as that in which endurance and hardihood were more

26 *

needed than strength. Sometimes, however, as in 1297, cart-horse shoes were less than stott shoes. It is probable, too, that the strength of the shoe varied with the soil and the work. Thus at Gamlingay, in 1343, the shoes of the cart-horse were dearer than those needed for ploughing horses. The theory given above, that the shoes were light, is supported by the fact that at Farley, in the year 1320, ox-shoes are quoted at little less price than horse-shoes. The range of prices for shoes, indicated by Mr Rogers's researches, is equally suggestive with that of any other commodities. In the first ninety years shoes are dearest in 1311 — 1320, though the price is not materially enhanced. Afterwards they fall again, and would have fallen still more markedly, were it not for the immediate results of the Great Plague occurring at that period. This visitation produces its effects at one place only in the year 1348—this being Boxley, where the price is at once nearly four times that at which purchases were made in 1339 and 1340; but afterwards the effect is universal. Shoes customarily worth only a halfpenny before, are instantly and permanently a penny, and the price never falls again. For when we consider how steadily the need increased for these articles, how universal was the smith's labour, and how the relative value of the commodity was governed by causes over which the interference of the legislature could exercise only a very partial control—if, indeed, it could effect any real control at all—we should be prepared to anticipate the result which actually ensued, that the price was doubled. Even here, however, we may trace the same phenomenon, adds Mr Rogers, which has so often occurred. Prices are higher in the decade 1371 —

1380, and are lower afterwards. 'Were there sufficient evidence for the last ten years, the facts which I have been able to collect would, I am confident, have been varied in the averages, and the quotations in all likelihood would have to be put on the ten years at 8*s.*; instead of being, as I am constrained to return them, at the great price of 13*s.* 6½*d.* The causes to which the deficient information of the later part of the period must be ascribed, are : the change which takes place in the method of agriculture, and the change which the course of events had induced upon the condition of the smith. The reader will anticipate that the former cause consists in the fact, that the system of bailiff farming was gradually relinquished after the event of the plague. But accounts are not kept in so careful a manner. The dearth of hands had produced its effects on the inferior clergy, the scribes and accountants of the middle ages. Items which used to be carefully distinguished are lumped in one general sum—credited, for instance, to the bailiff, as the year's charge for shoeing. Services which used to be cheap and effectual, had now become dear and negligent ; and such symptoms were apparent in the economy of agriculture, as designated that a radical alteration in the method of tenure was impending. And there are also indications that oxen, according to Walter de Henley's advice, were superseding horses in farm-work. The other cause is the change which comes over the condition of the artisan. Hitherto it was very seldom that such persons dealt in finished goods. As a rule, they were hired to do work on materials purchased by their employer; and in some occupations, as in the building trades, this purchase of materials continues for centuries after the time before us. Thus, although at a very early time horse-shoes were bought by the hundred at fairs and market-towns, they were also fashioned out of the bar-iron bought annually by the bailiff for the use of the farm. This revolution in the relations of employer and artisan was effected, of course, not only by the fact that the latter obtained better terms for his labour, but because he had become possessed of capital, was able to lay by a portion of his gains, and could therefore work for a future market.' 'Any person,' says the Professor, 'who studies, even superficially, a farm account at the beginning, and another at the end of the 14th century, must obtain indications of the change which has taken place in the habits and in the condition of the labouring classes. So, out of the gains which were thus amassed, temptations to spend coming but little in the way of the mediæval labourer, those estates were pur-chased on which the yeomanry of the 15th century lived in comfort.'

'Equally characteristic is the history of the price of horse-shoe nails. These articles were purchased at the same times and places with the shoes. Knowing what horse-shoe nails must have been, we can readily judge from the price at which they were purchased, what was the size of other nails. These nails, bought by the thousand, were made, it is probable, with broad heads, *the grooved shoe being, considering the price of iron and the lightness of the plate, an invention of later times.* But the nail must have been of length sufficient to pass through so much of the hoof as would serve to keep it tightly on, and it must have been of such temper as to insure its toughness and endurance. To judge by the price, the horse-shoe nail must have contained two-thirds more iron than the lath-nail, and about half as much as the broad nail. The price of these nails rises and falls evenly with that of horse-shoes. During the first ninety years, they are dearest in the years 1311-20, and though the price declines slightly after this time, it does not revert to the cheap rates of the thirteenth century. After the plague, the rise is instant and permanent, the rate being doubled, and remaining high, the dearest time being, as before, the decade 1371—1380. Evidence for the last ten years is wanting, but judging by the exactness with which the price of these articles follows that of horse-shoes, we might certainly affirm that if the latter stood at from 8s. 4d. to 8s. the hundred, the former would be about 2s. 6d. the thousand. The general rise on the average of the last forty years is not, indeed, quite so large as that of horse-shoes, though it is upwards of 100 per cent.; but it will be remembered that the rate of horse-shoes for the last ten years is excessive, and the evidence insufficient.'

The annexed illustration, from the Louterell Psalter, represents a waggon-team ascending a terribly steep hill, the horses' feet being shown as well armed with shoes and large-headed nails (fig. 149, next page). This drawing is of great interest in many respects, but particularly as displaying the mode of harnessing and driving draught horses at this period, as well as the construction of the waggons.

In the reign of Richard II. (1377-99), from a bailiff's account of a manor in Surrey, it appears that the fore-

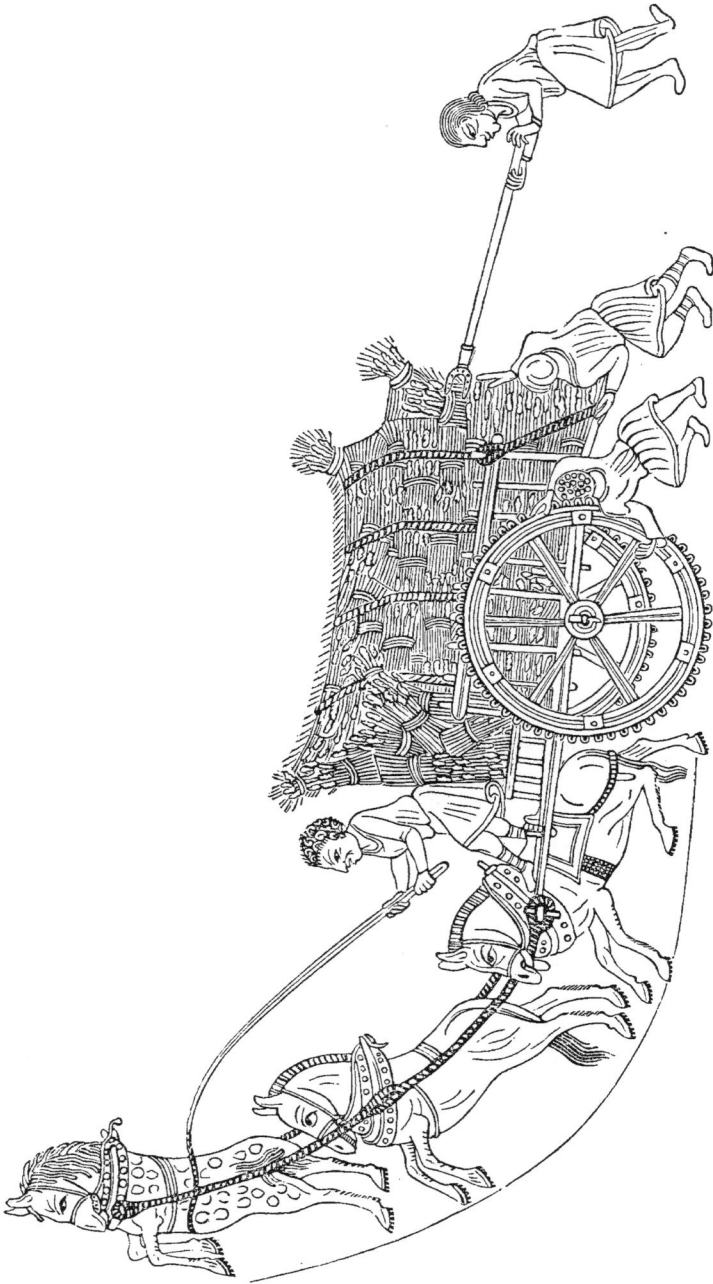

fig. 149

feet of oxen used in ploughing, and heifers or *stotts* in harrowing, were shod at threepence each.[1]

It is necessary here to remark, that Richardson[2] derives the word 'stott' from the Anglo-Saxon *stod-hors*, and as applied to oxen from the Swedish *stut*, Danish *stud*, a steer. The word has given rise to some discussion, it having been used for a very long time in Scotland as a designation for a steer, heifer, or bullock, and the notice in the above is thought by the antiquarian who quotes it, to mean heifer. Of this, however, there may be considerable doubt; as the term has been constantly applied in England to under-sized strong horses or cobs. In the 'Vision of Piers Plowman' (1362?) it occurs in this sense:

> Grace of his goodnesse, gaf
> Peers foure *stottes*.

And Chaucer, in his 'Canterbury Pilgrims,' says:

> This Reevè sat upon a right good *stot*,
> That was all pomelee (dappled) gray, and highte Scot.

Signifying, I think, that the word came from beyond the Tweed. Sir David Lyndsay also applies it to a horse. On a part of the border of the so-called Bayeux tapestry, representing the landing of William the Conqueror and the battle of Hastings, a piece of needlework by some ascribed to Saxon embroiderers, there is a representation of a man driving a horse attached to a harrow—one of the earliest instances we have of horses being used in field-labour; but which was a common enough custom in the time of Richard II.

[1] Archæologia, p. 284. London, 1817.
[2] Dictionary of the English Language. London, 1837.

Stow, for 1273, informs us that coal was not allowed to be burned in or near London, being ' prejudicial to human health,' and that smiths were even prohibited from its use, and obliged to burn wood. This may have materially influenced the cost of iron-work at this period. Chaucer, in the ' Canon Yeoman's ' tale, frequently speaks of coals being used by the alchemist.

A great degree of interest attaches to the next two drawings of shoes belonging to this period, from the fact that the actual specimens are closely related to an incident which somewhat prominently marks the otherwise eventful reign of Edward II., and are melancholy *souvenirs* of the downfall of a brave English nobleman.

We have already noticed the grants of land bestowed on Henry de Ferrarius by William the Conqueror, and mentioned that among these was Tutbury, an estate situated on the Staffordshire side of the river Dove, which there forms the boundary between that county and Derbyshire.

Standing on a commanding eminence of gypsum rock, which may have been selected as a stronghold by the ancient Britons and Romans, and on which there certainly stood a fortification during the Anglo-Saxon Heptarchy, but which was afterwards destroyed by the Danes, the castle of Tutbury was rebuilt on a much larger scale than before, by the Norman—farrier we had almost called him, and was a place of some importance in those days of family fortresses.

In 1269, this place, with his other possessions, was forfeited by Robert de Ferrers, Earl of Derby, and given by Edward I. to his brother Edmund, Earl of Lancaster,

who dying in 1297, left it to his son Thomas, the second
Earl of Lancaster, when the castle was still more beautified
and improved, and made a general residence. In a short
time, however, this nobleman embroiled himself with his
nephew, Edward II., the next sovereign; for, becoming dis-
gusted with the manner in which that monarch allowed
himself to be swayed by his successive favourites, Gaveston
and the two Spensers, and pitying the people who were the
victims of his rapacity, as well as instigated by his own
private wrongs, he, at the head of a number of barons,
first remonstrated with his king, and afterwards took up
arms in open rebellion. The consequence was a civil
war, which for some time was carried on vigorously by
both sides.

The king had advanced into the heart of the king
dom while the earl was in the north, and before the latter
could intercept it, the royal army had penetrated nearly
to Burton in Staffordshire. Here, by great exertion, the
earl had been able to arrive before Edward, and occupied
the town, situated on the western bank of the river Trent,
which is here very deep. Lancaster determined to make
a stand at this place, as it was the key to his castle of
Tutbury; the long, narrow, and crooked bridge across
the river being easy of defence, and so long as successfully held, preventing any approach, except in a round-
about way, to the important stronghold.

Though deserted by the barons who had at first re-
belled with him and had joined his standard, the earl might,
nevertheless, have offered good fight, but, unluckily for
him, a countryman had shown the king's army a ford
about five miles above Burton; so while one portion

menaced the town, another crossed the river and threatened the castle. The earl's position was now untenable, and he was obliged to fly to his apparently impregnable fortress.

Tutbury is only about five miles from Burton, so that Lancaster soon reached his home, though scarcely had he got across the drawbridge before the royal forces were at the gate. It was soon discovered that to attempt defence was impossible, and to come out on the Staffordshire side quite impracticable; while the river Dove, at that time greatly flooded and scarcely fordable, and over which there was no bridge, appeared to cut him completely off from Derbyshire, through which he might have passed to his castle of Pontefract, in Yorkshire. Thus hemmed in, nothing was left but surrender or hazardous flight across the Dove.

The latter alternative was adopted; and after leaving his baggage and military chest in charge of his treasurer Leicester, with directions to convey them in safety, and as quickly as possible, to Pontefract, he and his followers made the attempt, and, in spite of the high floods, succeeded in gaining the opposite bank in safety.

Such, however, was not the fortune of Leicester's charge—the military chest, which contained all the money the earl had been amassing to pay his retainers and discharge the current expenses of the disastrous war he had undertaken. This servant, following his master at night, did all he could to convey the treasure safely from the castle, but in the confusion of getting down the steep hill and across the swollen river in the dark, with a fugitive panic-stricken guard and terrified waggoners, the chest and its contents were lost in the Dove, and the unlucky treasurer, compelled to fly before daylight discovered him, never after had an opportunity of returning to attempt their recovery.

The earl himself, deserted by those on whom he depended, was soon after betrayed into the hands of his enemies, who conducted him to Pontefract, where, after suffering the greatest indignities, as is generally the case with fallen greatness, his head was struck off, towards the end of March or beginning of April, 1322.

The subsequent troubles appear to have caused the loss of this treasure to be forgotten, and probably of the few who witnessed its immersion in the Dove none ever returned to Tutbury; so that the poor earl's money, which perhaps might have saved him his head, had he chanced to possess it before his capture, was destined to remain in the bed of the river undisturbed, except by the rushing waters, for more than five hundred years, and would in all likelihood have continued so, but for a curious chance.

This happened in June, 1831. In the long interval that had elapsed, the Dove had been spanned by two bridges; corn and cotton mills were erected on its banks near this spot; and the stream had been troubled with all manner of weirs and dams, cuts and alterations, but without revealing the secret it contained. On the 1st of June, in that year, however, the proprietors of the cotton mills having commenced the operation of deepening the river, with the object of giving a greater fall of water to the wheel, the workmen found among the gravel, about three-score yards below the present bridge, a few small pieces of silver coin, of a description they had never seen before.

Sir Oswald Mosley, Bart.,[1] in referring to the history of this Earl of Lancaster, gives the following account of the finding of these coins: ' Mr Webb, the proprietor of the cotton mills at Tutbury, being desirous to obtain a greater fall for what is commonly termed the tail-water of the wheel which works the machinery of his mill, prolonged an embankment between the mill-stream and the river much farther below the bridge than it formerly extended; and as a part of his plan, it became requisite to remove a considerable quantity of gravel out of the bed of the river, from the end of his water-course as far up as the new bridge. While they were engaged in this operation, on Wednesday, the 1st of June, 1831, the workmen found several small pieces of silver coin about sixty yards below the bridge; as they proceeded up the river, they continued to find more; these were discovered lying about half-a-yard below the surface of the gravel, apparently as if they had been washed down from a higher source. On the following Tuesday the men left their work in the expectation of finding more coin, and they were not disappointed, for several thousands were obtained that day; as they advanced up the river they became more successful; and the next day, Wednesday, June the 8th, they discovered the grand deposit of coins from whence the others had been washed, about thirty yards below the present bridge, and from four to five feet beneath the surface of the gravel. The coins were here so abundant, that one hundred and fifty were turned up in a single

[1] History of the Town and Houses of Tutbury.

shovelful of gravel, and nearly five thousand of them were collected by two of the individuals thus employed on that day; they were sold to the bystanders at six, seven, eight, or eight shillings and sixpence per hundred; but the next day a less quantity was procured, and the prices of them advanced accordingly. The bulk of the coins were found in a space of about three yards square, near the Derbyshire bank of the river. Upwards of three hundred individuals might have been seen engaged in this search at one time, and the idle and inquisitive were attracted from all quarters to the spot. Quarrels and disturbances naturally enough ensued, and the interference of the neighbouring magistrates became necessary.

'At length the officers of the Crown asserted the king's right to all coin which might subsequently be found in the bed of the river, since the soil thereof belonged to his Majesty in right of his duchy of Lancaster.'

The consequence was, that all persons were prohibited from collecting coin except those appointed by the Chancellor of the duchy, who, on behalf of the Crown, instituted a search on the 28th of June that lasted until the 1st of July. In this brief period more than 1500 additional coins were found, and then the excavation from which they were principally extracted was filled up and levelled over. The total number of coins thus found is supposed to have been, upon the most moderate computation, no less than 100,000.

Often those who found one of these pieces had much difficulty in detaching it from the gravel in which it had become imbedded. Having been for so long a period lying amid the soil which once formed the bed of the stream, and on which the water had gradually deposited stratum upon stratum of sand and pebbles, the mass had become a hard substance, scarcely yielding in solidity to stone itself, in which coin after coin appeared to form some of the original component parts. Pieces of iron from the waggon or chest had also, in the process of oxidation, become pulpy, and still firmer bound and increased the strange conglomerate.

The earl's chest appears to have contained some curious and varied specimens of the currency then in use. Besides a number of sterlings of the Empire, Brabant, Lorraine, and Hainault, and the Scotch coins of Alexander II., John Baliol, and Robert Bruce, there was found a complete English series of those of the first Edward (fig. 150),

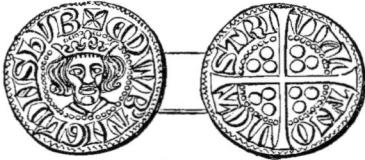

fig. 150

who, at various times, had his money struck at several towns in England, Scotland, and Ireland. There were also specimens of all the prelatical coins of Edward I., Edward II., as well as many of Henry III.,—both of his first and second coinage,—and a few of the most early of Edward II. On the whole, a finer museum of English, Scotch, and Irish coins was never before, under any circumstances, thrown open to the inspection of the antiquary and historian. Yet it seems very surprising that the English coins found should, with only one exception, have been of the same small size and value. This exception was a very beautiful coin of silver, about the size of half-a-crown, and of the reign of Edward I. Nor is it less surprising that the chest should have contained no jewellery or other valuable articles, one ring alone being found in the river, which was probably lost by some one of the earl's officers in fording. It was rudely chased, and bore within the circle the motto 'Spreta vivant.'[1]

Fortunately for our subject, a mass of this ferro - argentine conglomerate was purchased from the finder, and is now in the possession of Llewellynn Jewitt, Esq., of Winster Hall, near Matlock, Derbyshire. In this is most wonder-

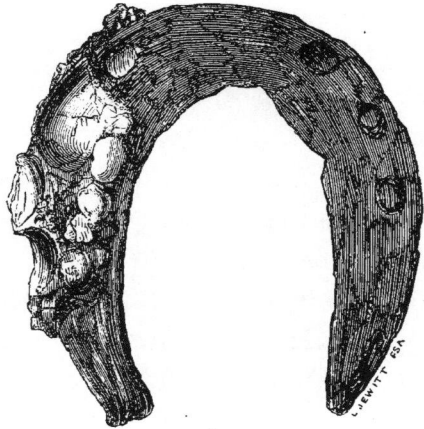

fig. 151

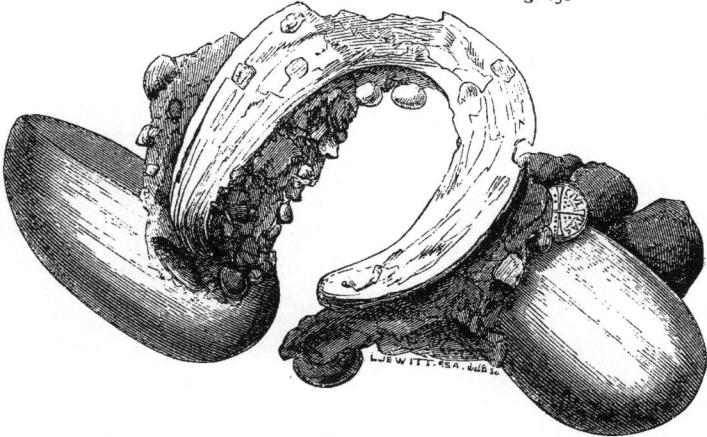

fig. 152

fully imbedded several horse-shoes of the shape here delineated, and which have been most kindly drawn and engraved for me by that gentleman, as although they were the most perfect specimens, they were yet too friable to travel safely for my inspection (fig. 151, 152).

[1] Penny Magazine. No. 166, p. 430.

27

In all probability, on the eventful night on which the treasure was lost, the waggon and horses conveying it were also left to perish in the Dove.

From the examination I have been able to make of the other shoes, it appears that the horses were small. One specimen would, when perfect, have been about $4\frac{1}{4}$ inches wide, and $4\frac{1}{2}$ long.   It had a small raised (not *rolled-over*) calkin on one side; only three nail-holes were visible on each branch, and the shoe altogether was very narrow and light, as if it had been worn by a saddle-horse.   The iron appeared to be fibrous and of excellent quality.   Another half-shoe was a trifle smaller, had three holes on each side, and the calkin was formed by doubling over the end of the thin branch, as in the Chedworth and Gillingham specimens.   Completely encased in a compact slab of rusty-coloured conglomerate, a portion of which has been removed, is one more example that may have been a little larger, though it is still a small shoe, and would fit a horse between 14 and 15 hands high; while a fragment of another, though about the same dimensions, had a little more cover or breadth, and probably was worn by one of the waggon-horses.

None of these show any traces of toe-clips; all have the even border of the present shoe, and their holes are the ordinary quadrilateral apertures with which we are now familiar; they have not been fullered or widely stamped for the nail-heads.   Both surfaces appear to have been plane; and altogether the shoes are not of a bad type, but one that, if the hoofs were not mutilated by paring, could do a horse but little harm.

In the interesting chronicles of Froissart, we find many

interesting details about shoeing. Describing the first attempted invasion of Scotland by Edward II., he gives us an instance of the importance this art was assuming, and what an amount of inconvenience might be apprehended when circumstances prevented its being attended to. When the army of that king had marched as far as New-castle-on-Tyne, the cavalry were in a miserable plight, and apparently ineffective. 'It never seased to rayne all the hoole weeke, whereby theyre saddels, pannels, and counter-syngles were all rottyn and broke, and most part of their horses hurt on their backs: nor they had not wherewith to *shoo* them that were unshodde.' When the troops reached Durham, however, they were obliged to rest there for two days, 'and the oste rounde about, for they coulde not all lodge within the cite, *and theyre horses were newe shoode,* and set out on theyre march to York.' [1]

In these chronicles, embracing as they do, the latter part of the reign of Edward II., and terminating with the coronation of Henry IV., there is repeated mention of shoeing, and particularly in the wars which England was then waging on the Continent. In the great army Edward III. carried into France in 1359,—the greatest, according to Froissart, that had ever left England, we find a completeness in equipment and material which is somewhat astonishing when we look at the present condition of our army and consider its fitness for a continental war, particularly in the matter of land transport. Our warrior king appears to have omitted nothing that could render success impossible. On arriving at Calais, he

[1] Chronicles, edit. 1812. Vol. i. p. 21.

'took the field with the largest army and best-appointed
train of baggage-waggons that had ever quitted England.
It was said there were upwards of 6000 carts and waggons, which had all been brought with him.'[1] Describing
the order of march, Froissart goes on to say that 'in the
rear of the king's battalion was the immense baggage-
train, which occupied two leagues in length : it consisted
of upwards of 5000 carriages, with a sufficiency of horses
to carry the provisions for the army, and those utensils
never before accustomed to be carried after an army — such
as hand-mills to grind their corn, ovens to bake their
bread, and a variety of other necessary articles.

There were also in this army of the King of England,
500 pioneers with spades and pickaxes, to level the roads
and cut down trees and hedges, for the more easily passing of the carriages. . . . . I must inform you that the
King of England and his rich lords were followed by carts
laden with tents, pavilions, mills, and *forges*, to grind their
corn and *make shoes for their horses*, and everything of
that sort which might be wanting.'[2] This appears to
have been the first occasion on which field forges for
shoeing horses accompanied an army, as well as ovens to
bake the soldiers' bread. The introducer of these, as well
as of artillery, appears to have even made an approach
towards the employment of pontoons not very unlike,
so far as material is concerned, those which are now being
brought into use in the Royal Engineers; for we read

[1] Chronicles of England, France, Spain, and the Adjoining Countries.
Edit. I. Johnes. Vol. ii. p. 469.   London, 1808.
   [2] Ibid.   Vol. ii. pp. 2, 3, 29.

that 'there were on these carts many vessels and small boats, made surprisingly well of boiled leather.'[1]

By a statute of 1350 (2, c. 4, 25 Edward III.), it appears that the farrier was yet designated in the Norman French, then fashionable in legal and court language, the 'Ferrour des Chivaux;' and with a number of other craftsmen, such as saddlers, spur-makers, armourers, &c., was regularly sworn-in before the justices to do and use his craft in a proper manner, and to confine himself to it.[2]

Gloucester has been alluded to on several occasions not only as a repository of antique horse-shoes, but also as a town celebrated for its iron trade from time immemorial —a circumstance due to its proximity to the mineral districts of the Forest of Dean.[3] The business of nail-making

---

[1] Ibid. p. 29.   [2] Statutes of the Realm, vol. i. p. 312.

[3] The Rev. S. Lysons, Honorary Canon of Gloucester Cathedral, has most kindly furnished me with the following particulars relative to Gloucester, its iron-trade, and its arms. ' Gloucester was celebrated for its smiths, being so near the mines of the Forest of Dean, which were worked both by the Romans and the Britons; coins of the former and tools of the latter having been found in them. The *Via Falrorum* of Roman Gloucester still retains the name of Long Smith Street. The chief employment of the town of Gloucester, before the reign of William the Conqueror, was making and forging of iron; and in the times of King Richard II. and Henry IV. it was famous for its iron manufacture. The ore was brought from Robin Wood's Hill, about two miles from the city, where it is said to have been found in great abundance. This town had anciently its proper signature. On an old seal of the time of King Edward III., which is still used for recognizances, on each side of the effigy is a horse-shoe; one horse-nail near it, and three below it, two and one; with the like number above it placed in the same order. It is said that King Richard III., when he made this a Mayor town, gave it his sword and cap of maintenance. The arms of the town was then " a sword erect, with a cap of mainten-

appears to have been carried on in it for a long time prior to the Norman conquest ; and local tradition has it that the royal farrier a rather important personage in his way, resided in that city. However this may be, it is certain that horse-shoes and nails must have been looked upon as important articles in the reign of King Edward III., and have held a prominent place in the crafts of the town, as the corporation seal of that epoch—for an impression of

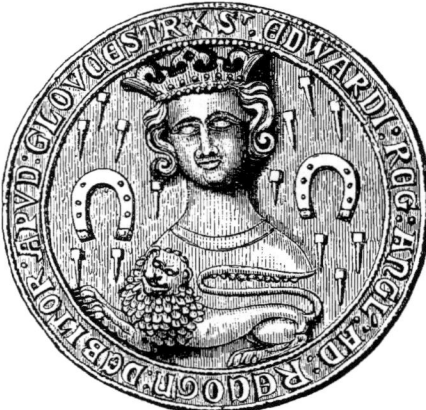

fig 153

which I am indebted to Mr Fryer, town-clerk of Gloucester—exhibits the royal effigy reared upon a lion couchant, and surrounded by a number of these emblems of farriery. The annexed drawing (fig. 153) represents this curious

memento of days passed away. It is the exact size of the ance on the point, on each side a horse-shoe, and three nails at length on the base."

'In the reign of Queen Elizabeth, the city used a seal which had in the middle a sword in bend, the pommel in base, between six horse-shoes and ten horse-nails. Christopher Barber, Garter Principal King-at-Arms in 1538, granted to the city the following arms : Vert, a pale or, a sword azure besanted the hilt and pommel gules ; upon the point a cap of maintenance purple, lined ermine ; upon the field two horse-shoes argent pierced sable, between six horse-nails in triangle. On a chief party per pale or and purple, a boar's head coupee argent ; in his mouth a quince apple gules between two roses. These elaborate arms have disappeared, and horse-shoes and nails are no longer a part of the armorial bearings of the city.'

seal, which bears the inscription, S. Edwardi: Reg: Angl: Ad: Recogn: Debitor: Apud: Gloucester:

Connected with this period, it may be noted that a few years ago a large number of shoes were collected on the farm of West Nisbet, Berwickshire, which is supposed to be the site of the battle of Nisbet Muir, fought in 1355, between the English and Scots. No description has been given of these relics, save that they were of an uncommonly small size;[1] and I have been unable to trace their whereabouts, though in all probability they were consigned to the metallurgical operations of the village blacksmith, and converted into defences for the hoofs of the larger and more peaceably designed steeds of the 19th century.

As has been repeatedly noticed, the shoes worn by horses appear to have varied greatly in size after the Norman conquest; a circumstance due, no doubt, to the introduction of larger breeds from the continent at different times. What these breeds of horses were it is difficult to say in some instances. From the size of the shoes previous to the conquest, we infer that the horses were small— from 12 to 14 hands high. The Normans had extensive breeding studs in Normandy, and no doubt improved their horses by crossing them with the Barb and Spanish races, and these would also be the breeds imported to England. For some time previous to his invasion, William had been buying the best horses of Spain, Gascony, and Auvergne,[2] and these, we may take for granted, accompanied him. The size of their hoofs would not, however, be much larger than those of the breeds already in

---

[1] *Trans. Socy. Scottish Antiquaries,* vol. iii.
[2] *Guill. Pictav.,* apud Scrip. Franc. xi. 181.

use in this country. During the reign of Henry II. (A.D. 1154) armour became very heavy both on horse and man, and the lance had grown so ponderous that it could only be used couched ; ' great horses ' were therefore required. These were probably the largest and strongest of the imported, but light races. In the 13th century, horses of greater size and power were eagerly purchased on the continent, where attention had been recently paid to rearing this kind of animal, and sent to England. They were rare, however, and a pair from Lombardy, in 1217, cost the enormous sum of £38 13s. 4d. In the rich pastures of the river Po, a race of ponderous *destriers* or *destrieros* had been formed, which, if they at all resembled those figured by the early sculptors on the monuments and statues of Condotieri, were nearly equal to our largest breed of dray-horses.[1] But these importations were so few in number, from the scarcity of the horses and their great expense, that they could make but little impression on the size of the common races in Eng land, and consequently would not alter, to any very appreciable degree, the dimensions of the shoes. King John imported 100 chosen stallions from Flanders, and these were probably of large bulk and stature for those days ; while King Edward II. purchased 30 Lombardy war-horses and 12 heavy draught-horses. Up to this period, I think we have only the small and medium-sized shoe, with, or but seldom without, calkins; and the rectangular, countersunk nail-holes, but destitute of a toe-clip to catch the hoof in front and prevent the shoe driving backwards. In the reign of the last-named monarch, who

---

[1] *Smith.* Naturalist's Library, p. 140.

was particularly partial to ambling horses, and introduced that unnatural pace, in order to teach them, the
fore-legs were trammeled or fastened together with bands
of yarn, or even with iron fetters [1] made by the farriers,
whereby the unfortunate creatures were compelled to
move in that shuffling oblique manner so much admired. Sometimes, to expedite the process, the hind-feet
were shod with shoes having a long sharp point at the
toe, which struck the back of the fore-leg, and thus
forced the animal to make a greater effort to move the
manacled limb out of the way. These variations in the
form of the shoe are not unfrequently met with in this
country and on the continent, at this and a subsequent
period. The most remarkable example we have met
with is one shown by Lafosse,[2] Jun., as attached to the
door of a chapel at Saint Severin, in France. It belongs
to the time of Philip the Fair (13th and 14th centuries), and

was supposed to have been
placed there by some farrier,
as a specimen of his workmanship. Its shape is ex-
tremely curious, and it appears
to have been intended to follow the whole natural outline
of the hoof—frog as well as
wall (fig. 154).

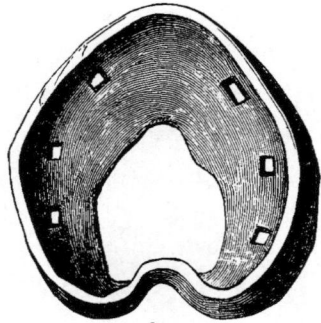

fig 154

It is not until a period bordering on the 14th or

---

[1] An iron fetter and chain which must, I think, have been used for
this purpose, was discovered, with horse-shoes, at Springhead, near
Gravesend, and is now in the possession of Mr Sylvester at that place.

[2] Cours d'Hippiatrique. Paris, 1798. *Megnin.* Op. cit. p. 62.

15th century, or perhaps much later, that we find evidences of the employment of the grooved or fullered shoe in England; and then we can only infer that it was imported from Germany and the Low Countries. This is somewhat remarkable, if we consider that this kind of plate is very ancient on the continent, M. Quiquerez tracing it back to the 5th century, and the Emperor Napoleon allotting it even to the era of the conquest of the Gauls by Julius Cæsar. We may entertain some doubt of the latter being correct however, as M. Megnin has examined these Alesia specimens, and found many, if not all, with the undulating border. Shoes, we have seen from Mr Rogers's History, were largely bought in England ready made, and by the hundred, and many of these may have been imported. In Mercer's History of Dunfermline, it is stated that in the 15th century, Flemish horse-shoes were in demand in Scotland: 'Flanders was the great mart in those times, and from Bruges chiefly, the Scots imported even *horse-shoes,* harness, saddles, bridles, cart-wheels,' &c.

All those found with the groove round their margin, so far as I can learn, have been of comparatively large size. One here represented (fig. 155) was found at Spring-

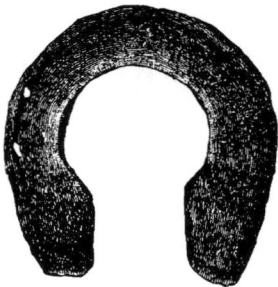

fig 155

head, near Gravesend (England). Its measurement indicates that it would fit a tolerably well-bred horse about $15\frac{1}{2}$ hands high, or a coarse-bred one of a less height. Its length is 5 inches, width $4\frac{7}{8}$ inches; the breadth is variable; at the toe and one of the quarters it is $1\frac{1}{4}$ inch, and at the heels as much as $1\frac{1}{2}$ inch. The groove is very near the outer circumference of the shoe, and contains four nail-holes on each side; these are oblong and small, and a portion of a nail yet remaining is not unlike our present nail. There is no toe or other clip, and the outer circumference of the shoe is thinner than the inner, in such a way that the ground surface is slightly convex, and that towards the foot, particularly at the heels, is concave. There are no calkins, and the shoe altogether is coarse and heavy. Though much worn and oxidized, it yet weighs nearly 12 ounces.

Another specimen, found in excavating for a sewer in Walworth road, London (fig. 156), in 1825, is very similar in shape and character. It was discovered at a depth of 10 feet, and from the fashion of a buckle procured with it, is assigned by Mr Syer Cuming[1] to the first half of the 17th century; though I am inclined to give it an earlier date. It is of large size, with

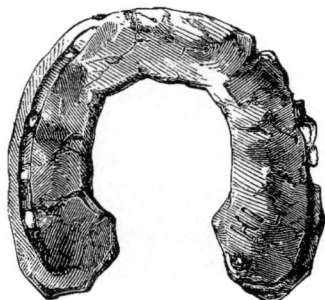

fig. 156

a wide surface grooved or fullered very near the margin, and apparently had eight nail-holes. The heels were furnished with thin calkins, and near one of them occurs the letters H I. A shoe of the same kind was dug from a depth of 12 or 14 feet, in making a sewer in Kennington Lane, London. From their scarcity, they do not appear to have been in very great repute, and are found along with the square-holed shoe.

The period of Edward III. and his gallant son, the

[1] *Journal of the Archæological Association,* vol. vi.

Black Prince, was the most glorious, perhaps, in the annals of chivalry.   Then, gentlemen scorned the idea of fighting otherwise than on horseback, and the universal motto of the knighthood of Europe was 'Tout l'amor, tout à l'honor;' then the squire, during his final period of probation, groomed, trained, and shod his own horses; practised leaping, running, and mounting on horseback, clad in all his armour, and resolutely attacked the quintain; and the most menial offices were raised to an honourable degree by the dignity of the person who performed them.   But of all the services rendered by the squire to the knight, the most important were naturally those which were connected directly or indirectly with the grand object of the lives of both, war.   'When the knight mounted his horse, the squires of his body held his stirrup; and other squires carried the various pieces of his armour, such as the brassards, the gauntlets, the helmet, and the buckler, on the road behind him.   With regard to the cuirass, or hauberk, the knight was no less careful of its preservation than the Greek and Roman soldiers were of their bucklers.   Other squires bore the pennon, the lance, and the sword.   When only on a journey, the knight rode a short-tailed, ambling-paced horse—a palfrey or a courser; and the war-horses were led by the squires, who by always leading them in their right hand, obtained for them the name of "dextriers." The war-horse was delivered to the knight on the appearance of an enemy, or when he was about entering the field of battle: this was what they called "mounting the great horse."'

When travelling, the squire carried his master's hel

met resting upon the pommel of his saddle ; and when preparing for fight, this helmet and all the other parts of his arms, offensive and defensive, were given him by the different squires, who had them in their keeping ; all evincing equal eagerness in assisting him to arm. By this means they were taught the art of arming themselves on a future day, and with the despatch and caution necessary for the protection of their persons. It demanded much skill and ability to place together and fasten the joints of the cuirass, and the other pieces of armour ; to fit and lace the helmet upon the head with correctness ; and to nail and rivet carefully the visor or ventail.[1] The burgesses and yeomen, who were not by the rules of chivalry permitted to enter the lists as combatants at jousts and tournaments, nor to appear mounted, used in England to tilt on foot against a large wooden shield on which a horse-shoe was painted.[2] In a manuscript in the Bodleian Library (No. 264, and dated 1344), there are delineations of both the fixed and movable quintain, upon each of which is a large horse-shoe remarkable for its equal breadth, the ends of the branches being turned out and somewhat upwards, and from their being pierced with nail-holes throughout their entire length. This is indeed the form of shoe which, in heraldry, according to Guillim, is borne by the families of Borlace, Cripps, Crispe, Ferrers, Randall, and Shoys well.[3]

The very heavy armour worn by man and horse at

---

[1] *L. de Sainte-Palaye.*   Mém. sur l'Ancienne Chevalerie. Paris, 1826.   [2] *Strutt.*   Sports and Pastimes, p. 117.
[3] *Syer Cuming.*   Op. cit.

this period, and even up to the 16th century, necessitated
the employment of horses more like our lumbering
draught breed than chargers, and these were first obtained
from Lombardy.   Their excellence is described by
Chaucer in the ' Squire's Tale':

> ' Great was the press that swarmèd to and fro,
> To gazen on this horse that standeth so ;
> For it so high was, and so broad and long,
> So well proportionèd for to be strong,
> Right as it were a steed of Lombardy :—
> Therewith so hoarsely and so quick of eye
> As it a gentle Polish courser were ;
> For certes from his tail unto his ear
> Nature nor Art could him not amend
> In no degree, as all the people ween'd.'

But the Flemish horse, the probable progenitor of our
heaviest breeds, was at an early period in high repute as
a war-horse, and adapted to carry the enormous loads
imposed upon him, when pace was not so much an object
as strength to bear weight and withstand the shock of an
encounter with couched lances.   These horses were oftentimes severely tested before final acceptance as fit for the
fray ; and strong large shoes, with projecting calkins and
nail-heads, were not only an indispensable necessity for
ordinary duty, but for the more important contests in the
field, where a good grip of the turf by the horse's feet
was as requisite as a firm seat on its back.   This is well
illustrated in the case of the redoubtable Châtelain of
Waremme, who, in 1325, was the leader of the Awans, a
powerful faction in Belgium.   He was a man of such
gigantic bulk, that, when he was encased in his armour,
it required the assistance of two strong esquires to lift him
into the saddle.   His friends. on the morning of a great

battle with an opposing faction—the Waroux—expressed
to him their fear that he was too heavily armed, but De
Waremme replied, 'Have no fear, for I swear to you, by
God and St George, that since it has required two men
to seat me on my good steed Moreal, it shall take at least
four to make me get off again.' And this was no idle
vaunt, as the events of the day proved.

Another gigantic warrior who fought for the Awans
was the Sire de Hemricourt. The strength of limb and
massiveness of frame of this man were such that, except
his stirrup-leathers broke, it was impossible to unhorse
him; and in confirmation of his prowess, the following
story is told: Being engaged as one of fifty knights
chosen to fight on the side of the King of Sicily, against
an equal party for the King of Arragon, a war-horse was
sent to him by the king to ride on the day of battle.
But Hemricourt, like the champion of Israel in the
choice of his weapons, would not trust his steed till he
had tried him. He therefore mounted, and, accompanied
by some friends and attendants, rode out into the country,
and, coming to a large lime-tree, he got off his horse, and
made his squires fasten his girths as he directed. He
then mounted again, and having had his legs tightly tied
to the girths, he seized a thick branch of the tree with
his right hand, and drove his spurs into his courser's
flanks; but in spite of all its efforts, the horse was unable
to get away. Hemricourt, therefore, sent back the animal to the king, saying that it wanted both strength and
courage, and was dull to the spur. The king then sent
him another, which he submitted to the same test, and
the struggle between man and horse was long and violent.

At length, owing to the girths and the *poitrail* breaking, the steed got away, leaving the knight and his saddle suspended from the tree.   This horse the Sire de Hemricourt kept, though an ignominious fate awaited it.   When the knight and his associates came to the place appointed for the combat, the Arragonese did not appear, and the King of Sicily, taking advantage of the circumstance, meanly required that the horses should be returned. When the messenger came to De Hemricourt, 'What,' cried he, 'has the king, your master, only lent me this carrion to defend his honour at the risk of my life—I who am no subject of his?   Is it thus he shows his gratitude?   By the eyes of God, he shall have his present back again, but in such a state that no knight shall ever mount him again with honour!'   So saying, he had the horse brought out of the stable, and, with his own hands cutting off the mane and tail, desired the groom to lead him away.[1]

'In those times of war,' writes the old author, Hamericourt,[2] 'and even ten years after the peace was made, knights and squires of honour rode great horses (*d'astriers*) or coursers (*corseirs*) of the greatest value they could procure, and they had very high tourneying saddles without foresaltiers.   They were covered with caparisons wrought in embroidery with their armorial blasons.   They were armed with breast-plates with good armour of thin iron pieces, and upon the plate they had rich wardcoats bearing their blasons.   Each had a helmet upon his

[1] Miroir des Nobles de la Hesbaye.   The Valley of the Meuse, by Dudley Costello.

[2] De Bellis Leodunsibus, cap. 41.

bacinet with a handsome crest; and several lords, knights, and others had beneath the drapery of their caparisons ringed mail for their horses.' And in a manuscript work entitled the 'Guerre des Awans et des Warons,' recording the party wars among the people of Liege at this time, the horse-shoe is described as 'large fer a cheval ot, a talons moult crochus.'

The 'great horse,' the arms and armour, and the large shoes with high calkins, are well depicted in the German knight painted by Lucas Cranach in the 15th century (fig. 157).

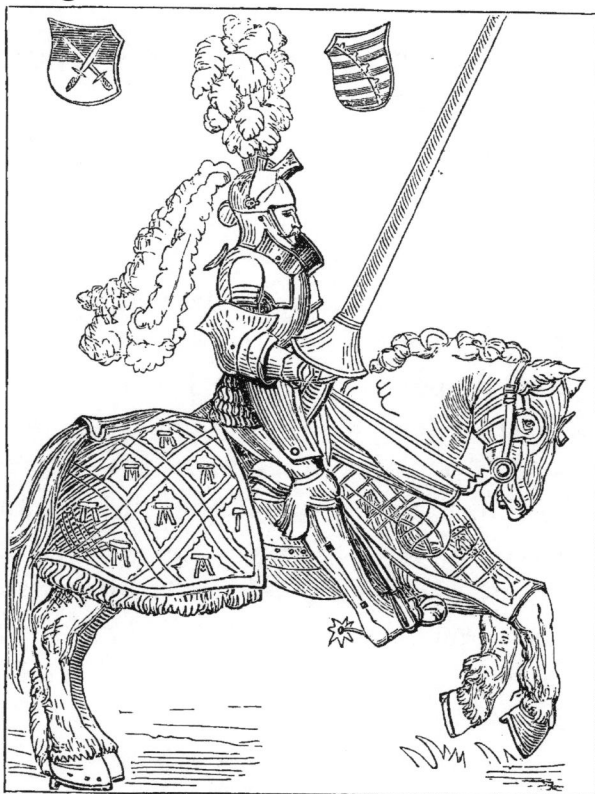

fig 157

In Scotland, it might be inferred that horses for riding purposes were generally shod, though those for draught were not ordinarily so, if we may judge from an act passed in 1487. An Act of Parliament was passed in 1481, which made the smith who pricked a horse's foot while shoeing it liable to furnish another until the cripple was cured, or if it died, to pay its value.[1] This, in many respects unjust, law was procured by the Duke of Albany and his brother, the Earl of Mar. It is difficult, if not impossible, to discover how much the unfortunate farrier was likely to lose if the animal he had accidentally lamed happened to die, as the value of horses appears to have fluctuated considerably in Scotland for three centuries. In 1283, for instance, a burgess's steed was valued at one pound; in 1329, a courier's horse was supposed to be worth five shillings; and in 1424, a colt, or horses more than three years old, thirteen shillings and four pence.

Though horses were always extremely numerous in the Scottish armies, yet they were seldom, if ever, used for agricultural purposes; ploughing being generally performed by oxen.

For a long period, much attention had been paid to breeding good horses. So early as the 13th century, we find Roger Avenel, Lord of Eskdale, possessing a stud in that valley. Patrick, Earl of Dunbar, in preparation for his departure to the Holy Land (A.D. 1247), sold to the Monks of Melrose his stud of brood mares in Lauderdale, for the considerable sum of one hundred marks sterling.

[1] *Skeen.* Parliament 1481, cap. 79.

Alexander III. had several establishments for rearing horses, to be used in hunting as well as in war.[1]

I cannot find any record of the price of shoes in Scotland at this period. It is merely mentioned that in 1488, a dozen horse-shoes, two plough-irons, and the iron mountings of two ploughs which had been stolen, were valued at twenty shillings.[2] And in the Thane of Cawdor's Western Journey in 1591, there is an entry in his journal of expenses to the effect, that at Glasgow, one of the items in the host's bill was 'giffin to the smyth for your broun geldin's schoun xiij s iiij d.[3]

The English statutes of the reign of Edward VI. (1547-52) give us an approximate idea of the size of the horses commonly in use in England and Scotland. The stallions allowed to be imported into England for breeding purposes were to be fourteen hands high, and the mares fifteen hands.

So important did Henry VIII., the father of Edward VI., consider the possession of large and good horses, that he devised a law by which it was intended that none but these should be kept in the country, fixing a standard of value for that purpose, and regulating that the lowest stallion should be fifteen hands high, and the mares thirteen hands; and before they had arrived at their full growth, no stallion at two years old, under fourteen hands and a half, was permitted to run on any forest, moor, or

[1] *C. Innes.* Sketches of Early Scotch History, p. 131. Edinburgh, 1862.

[2] *Acts of the Lords of the Council in Civil Causes,* p. 106.

[3] *C. Innes.* Sketches of Early Scotch Domestic History. Edinburgh, 1861.

common where there were mares. At Michaelmas tide, the neighbouring magistrates were ordered to 'drive' all forests and commons, and not only destroy such stallions, but all the 'unlikely tits,' whether mares, geldings, or foals, which they might deem not calculated to produce a valuable breed. He moreover ordained, that in every deerpark, in proportion to its size, a certain number of mares, at least thirteen hands high, should be kept; and that all his prelates and nobles, and 'all those whose wives wore velvet bonnets,' should keep stallions for the saddle, at least fifteen hands high.

The 'delicate stratagem' of shoeing a troop of horses with felt on particular occasions, as hinted at by Shakespeare, was tolerably well realized at least half a century before the immortal bard had made any progress in establishing his fame, and from the following incident he may have derived the idea he afterwards introduced into 'King Lear.' In Lord Herbert's 'Life of Henry VIII.,'[1] it is stated that that monarch, while in France, 'having feasted the ladies royally for divers days, departed from Tourney to Lisle (October 13, 1513), whither he was invited by the Lady Margaret, who caused there a juste to be held in an extraordinary manner; the place being a large room raised high from the ground by many steps, and paved with black square stones like marble; while the horses, to prevent sliding, were shod with felt or flocks (the Latin words are *feltro sive tomento*), after which the ladies danced all night.'

It is supposed that in the Guildhall of London, on the occasion of the marriage of Katharine of Aragon (after-

[1] *Kennet.* History of England, vol. ii. p. 17.

wards wife of Henry VIII.), and Arthur, Prince of Wales, the floor being of marble, and a tournament taking place on it, the horses were shod with felt.[1]

For the reign of Henry VIII. we have an excellent representation of shod horses in what is known as the 'tournament roll,' or descriptive illustrations of the 'Solemn Justs held at Westminster,' on the 5th February, 1510, in the 1st year of that king, in honour of Queen Katharine. Every horse in the long procession has its feet armed in the most unmistakable manner.[2] The one we select (fig. 158) exhibits this characteristic; and it will be

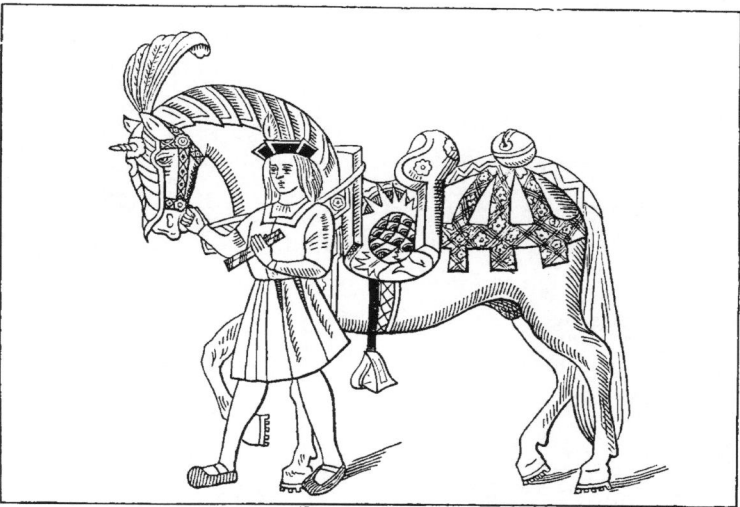

fig 158

observed that the shoes are yet very clumsy, and have the calkins and nail-heads very large, to afford a firm grasp of the ground. The nails appear to be four on each side of the shoe.

[1] Notes and Queries. 2nd Series, vol. ix. p. 394.

[2] This procession has been engraved in the Vetusta Monumenta, vol. i.

From specimens I have examined belonging to this period, it might be concluded that the weight of the shoes continued gradually to increase, while the sizes and forms occur in greater variety. Heavy armour and the tilting lance had not yet gone out of fashion, as the projecting nail-heads and calkins sufficiently indicate. Some curious specimens of shoes can be seen on the feet of the wooden horses in the armour-gallery of the Tower of London; these, I understand, belong to Henry VIII.'s reign.

It is somewhat astonishing that no toe-clips to prevent displacement of the shoes have yet appeared. The specimen found at a depth of ten feet in the Walworth sewer works in 1825, along with the bones of a horse, was probably made at this period. It has four nails on the outer branch, and apparently only three on the inner, which is much narrower towards the heel, as is often the case now-a-days. There are calkins on both branches, and the nail-head in the last inside hole projects nearly three-eighths of an inch from the surface of the shoe (fig. 159).

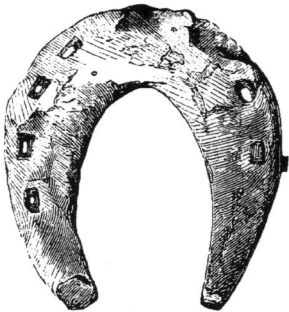

fig. 159

With the total extinction of the French language in Britain, the designation of 'Maréchal' also disappeared, or was used but very rarely. The shoer of horses was only known by that of 'farrier,' a term that had, as we have seen, been employed for centuries, and which was derived, no doubt, from the *ferreus faber* of the Latins, or the *fabbro ferrario* or *ferraro* of the Italians. In Queen Elizabeth's annual expenses—civil and military, we find that the Master of the Horse had in his gift, among many others belonging to his office, that of a Serjeant-Farrier at 1s. 1d. per diem, and three Yeomen-Farriers at 6d. And numerous instances of the newly revived name are to be discovered in writings of this and later ages. Chapman, in his translation of the ' Iliad,' has it :

> So took she chamber with her son, the God of Ferrary.

And Heywood, in the 'Troia Brittanica' (1609), writes :

> And thus resolv'd, to Lemnos she doth hie,
> Where Vulcan works in heavenly Ferrarie.

The value of shoeing yet held a high place in equestrianism and among equestrians, and much importance was attached to shoes, either as relics, or for purposes of display. We have already seen to what an extent this was carried at Okeham; it was also in vogue elsewhere, and often gave rise to strange customs which continued to a late period. For instance, in the *Preston Pilot* for 1834, it is mentioned ' that a large assembly congregated for the purpose of witnessing the renewing of the horseshoe at the Horse-shoe corner, Lancaster, when the old shoe was taken up and a new one put down, with 1834 engraved on it. Those who assembled to witness the ceremony were entertained with nut-brown ale, &c.; afterwards they had a merry chairing, and then retired. In the evening they were again entertained with a good substantial supper. This custom is supposed to have originated at the time John O'Gaunt (third son of Edward I.) came into the town upon a noble charger, which lost its shoe at this place. The shoe was taken up and fixed in the middle of the street, and has ever since been replaced with a new one every seventh year, at the expense of the towns-men who reside near the place.'

Examples of ostentatious extravagance in horse-shoes are numerous in the middle and succeeding ages. During the Roman period, we have already remarked that attempts at display in this particular direction were made by the wife of Nero and others, when golden or gilded *soleæ* were fastened on the feet of mules or horses. Gold and silver shoes and nails were fashionable, it appears, among the wealthy who were ostentatiously inclined, to so late a period as the 17th century. When Boniface, Marquis of Tuscany, one of the wealthiest princes of his time, went in 1083, to meet Beatrix, mother of the famous Matilda, marchioness of Tuscany, who married Godfrey of Lor-raine, his escort was so grandly equipped, that instead of iron, the horses had silver shoes and nails, and when any of these came off they were the property of those who picked them up.

> Qui dux cum peregret illo,
> Ornatos magnos secum tulit atque caballos,
> Sub pedibus quorum chalybem non ponere solum
> Jusserat, argentum sed ponere, sic quasi ferrum
> Esse repercussum clavum voluit quoque nullum,
> Ex hoc ut gento possent reperire quis esset.
> Cornipedes currunt, argentum dum resilit, tunc
> Colligitur passim, passim reperitur in agris,
> A populo terræ testans quod dives hic esset.[1]

Bartholomeus Scriba, in his Annales Gennenses, for the year 1230, asserts that a certain man, named Ermemolinus, gave eight thousand bizantines to Genoa, as a mark of his affection and friendship; and with this money the

---

[1] *Donizone*, Vita Mathilda, lib. i. cap. 10.

very best horse that could be procured was to be purchased, and presented from him to the community of
that town, covered with the best gold, and shod with
silver shoes (*ferri pedatus clapponis argenteis*); which
horse or destrier (charger) was bought and led through
the state of Genoa, as a remembrance of his noble act,
robed in a cloth of gold, and wearing silver shoes (*clapponis argenteis*).'[1]

Giovanni Villani, the Italian historian, who lived in the
14th century, in his writings speaks of horses adorned with
bridles of gold and shoes of fine silver: 'Havendo ornato
il suo cavallo di freno d'oro, e ferrato di fine argento.'[2]

The 'Roman de Rose,' a French romance of the 12th
century, speaks of gilt or golden shoes:

> Pour fere gens parler de foi,
> Fist tous les quatre fers dorer
> Ne vout mie dire Ferrer.

William of Tyre, for the year A.D. 1130, in describing
Boemond, a brother of Robert Guiscard, Count of Apulia,
and who was assigned the principality of Antioch after the
first Crusade, relates how 'he sent to a distinguished nobleman, through a friend of his, a white palfrey shod with
silver shoes (*argento ferratum*), and a beautiful bridle
ornamented with silver.'[3]

Johannis Bromton, describing the journey of Duke
Robert to the East, states that at Rome he placed a
valuable mantle on the statue of Constantine, putting to
shame the Romans, who refused to bestow one even in
many years. 'He rode, also, a certain mule whose shoes

[1] Muratori. Vol. vi.   [2] Lib. iv. cap. 18.
[3] Bellis Sacra Historia, p. 311. Basil, 1549.

were made of gold (*auri fecit ferrari*), and prohibited his servants from picking these up when they fell off.'[1]

In the 11th century, the first Norwegian king, Oluf Kyrre, the Quiet (1066—1087), introduced many new and extravagant customs into his country. Mr de Capell Brooke, describing them, informs us that ' the former inclination of the Norwegians to magnificence universally increased. Silken sails, *golden shoes for their horses*, cushions of down with silk hangings, silken hoods embroidered with silver, gilded helmets, etc., were almost necessary to those who sought the Court.'[2]

In the Saga of Sigurd Jorsalafar, the Pilgrim of Jerusalem, or Crusader, who reigned in Norway in 1103, it is told that he had his horse shod with golden shoes when he rode into Constantinople, on his way to the Holy Land, and so managed that one of the shoes came off in the streets, but none of his men were allowed to regard it.[3]

We have elsewhere given other examples of this silly fashion at this epoch.

Even so late as 1616, we read that James Hayes, afterwards Lord Doncaster, an English ambassador, when he made his public entry into Paris acted in a similar extravagant manner. ' Six trumpeters and two marshals, in tawny velvet liveries, completely suited, laced all over with gold (richly and closely laid), led the way : the ambassador followed, with a great train of pages and footmen in the same rich livery, encircling his horse. And some said (how truly I cannot assert) the ambassador's

---

[1] *A*bbatis Jornalensis.　Edit. Twysden, p. 911, 1652.
[2] History of Norway from the Earliest Times, by *G*. L. Baden, p. 172.
[3] *S. Sturleson.*　The Heimskringla.

horse was shod with silver shoes, lightly tackt on; and when he came to a place where persons or beauties of eminency were, his very horse prancing and curvetting in humble reverence threw his shoes away, which the greedy understanders scrambled for, and he was content to be gazed on and admired till a farrier, or rather the argentier, in one of his rich liveries, among his train of footmen, out of a tawny velvet bag took others and tackt them on, which lasted till he came to the next troup of grandees; and thus, with much ado, he reached the Louvre.' [1]

At a still later period, we find Duke Eberhard of Würtemberg causing his dead charger to be skinned and stuffed, and its hoofs shod with gold shoes, before being set up at Stuttgart. The creature had saved his master's life by swimming with him at the battle of Höchstädt, 13th August, 1704; but was accidently shot eight days afterwards, through the carelessness of one of the duke's followers.

Von Tschudi [2] mentions that during the brilliant period of the Spanish domination in Peru, like signs of wealth and foolish display were in vogue among the conquerors. Incredible sums were frequently expended on carriages and mules; and very often the tires of the caleza wheels and the shoes of the mules were of silver instead of iron. A Tartar song of the 14th century causes a Mongol khan to say, 'Bid the horses be put to my golden chariot, and let them be shod with golden shoes and silver nails.' [3]

The liberality of the knights during the hey-day of

---

[1] *Wilson's* James I. p. 94.   [2] Travels in Peru, p. 138.
[3] *Chodzko.* Popular Poetry of Persia.

chivalry often rose to as fantastic heights as in this extravagant display of James Hayes.   For instance, when Alexander III. of Scotland repaired to London, attended by a
hundred knights, at the time of the coronation of Edward
I., the whole party, as soon as they had alighted, let loose
their steeds, all most richly caparisoned, to be scrambled
for by the multitude.   This was probably new to the English chivalry, and no doubt startled them not a little: five,
however, of the English nobles immediately followed the
example set them.

In the 16th century we have a complete treatise—the
first, on shoeing, from the pen of Cæsar Fiaschi,[1] a masterly production of its kind, and in which no less than
35 chapters are devoted to this subject.   From the care
with which they are written, the sound sense that pervades
many of them, the faculty of observation, and the great
number of shoes devised to meet certain wants, we conclude that this artist was no ordinary workman, but an
enthusiast in hippology —a man of talent, and a scholar.
His masterly production forms the basis of nearly all the
treatises subsequently written on horse-shoeing.   The space
at our disposal permits but a very limited notice of its contents.   The first chapter, which serves as an introduction,
makes known that ' there are found to-day very few good

---

[1] Traité de la Manière de Bien Emboucher, Manier, et Ferrer les
Chevaux; avec les figures de Mors de Bride, Tours et Maniements et
Fers qui y sont propres.   Dédié au Roi Henri II.   Paris, 1564.   This
is the French translation of the Italian work.   There were also pub-
lished in Italy, in this century, the ' Trattato di Mascalcia' of Filippo
Sacro de Logliacozzo (Venice, 1553); and the ' Gloria del Cavallo' of
Caracciolo (1567).   In France, shortly after Fiaschi's work appeared,
Claudio Corte published ' L'Ecuyer' (Lyons, 1573).

farriers (*maréschaux*) : and yet among these there are some who more frequently think of profit and ease to themselves, than pay any regard to the wants and conveniences of the horses they shoe. So that if the horseman, because of his ignorance, is obliged to submit to the opinion of his *maréschal*, it will very often happen that he will see his horses lamed (*enclouez*) or badly shod, or otherwise inconvenienced : things due, as we witness every day, to the carelessness, ignorance, or malice of the farriers. Seeing, then, that the hoofs are the parts which support the whole of the body, and consequently bear all its weight, it is all the more necessary that the cavalier should be careful in having them well shod, and, besides, well attended to.'

Chapter II. contains advice as to the colour of the horn,—*pour cognoistre la bonté et malice d'icelle.* 'The black horn is the best.'

Chapter III. treats of the differences between the fore and hind feet, and also between the heels and toes of the feet. The heels of the fore-feet are the most sensitive, and need great care because they bear nearly the whole weight and strain. So that in shoeing horses, the nails must not come near them; and for the same reasons care must be taken not to drive the nails near the toes of the hind-feet, which are also the most sensitive parts. To do all in our power to protect them, the shoes applied must neither be too much curved nor yet too flat, but selected with care and good judgment.

Chapter IV. explains the manner in which the fore and hind feet should be armed.

Chapter V. speaks of the calkins (*crampons*), frost-nails (*clous à glace*), catches (*crestes*), points (*barbettes*) and rings (*annelets*), sometimes added to the fore-shoes. 'The calkins are useless on the fore-shoes, and they are even hurtful to the *nerfs* (tendons) of the limb, and cause the whole body to suffer pain. When we travel (*chevanche*) in mountainous or stony countries, it is far better to use a Turkish shoe, which protects the heels like a shield. The shoe to which is attached false nails [1] (*clous bastards*), not so high (in the head) as frost-nails, does not slip; the calkined shoe is apt to wound the horse when ridden; the calkin *à l'Aragonaise* is less dangerous. . . . . All other accessories, such as frost-nails, crests, barbettes, and annelets, ought not to be applied until after due deliberation, for they are often more hurtful than useful.'

Chapter VII. is devoted to the way in which the heels and the frog (*cartilage*) should be pared, and the hoof otherwise managed. 'The heel, with the cartilage or *tendron*, named in Italian the "fetton" (frog), particularly in the fore-feet, should be moderately pared or opened (*ouvert*), according to the character of the hoofs; if these are not good, care should be taken not to weaken them too much by too great opening. Besides, the cavalier should have removed from the toes of his horse's feet as much horn as may be necessary to give them a proper shape, which may easily be discovered by putting the foot to the ground.'

Chapter IX. relates to the form which the fore-shoes should have. Usually, the fore-shoe should not project beyond the toe of the hoof, except this part has been

---

[1] It would appear that nail-heads alone were rivetted into the shoes in places to prevent slipping.

broken and worn ; but it is advantageous that it should project a little beyond the foot from the quarters back, so as to preserve the horn there ; and behind the foot it should not be short, but exact and equal to the extremity of the heel, for if it surpass the heel the horse will likely forge (click or strike) with the hind feet ; and if too short, if the heels are weak and tender, the animal may suffer pain and injury. In the next chapter, the same observations are made with regard to the hind-feet. In the eleventh chapter we have the mode of adjusting the shoe to the hoof. 'The shoe should be so fitted that the foot may suffer in no way through the carelessness of the farrier—that is to say, the hot shoe should only be applied to the hoof for as long a period as may be necessary to fit it well.'

The nails are described in the following chapter. 'The nails ought to be large, moderately long, and neither flattened, hammered, or otherwise hardened. With ordinary horses eight or nine is the usual number ; and with coursers or " Frisons," ten, and sometimes more. I do not wish to deny that with some hoofs six or seven nails are sufficient, but there are few of these. When the number is odd, the majority of the nails should go to the outside of the foot, which is the least sensitive.'

Chapter XIII. speaks of the *bordure* or *pancette*, sometimes added to the shoe, and which was nothing but a very wide sole. The other chapters up to the twenty-second, are devoted to the characters of various kinds of hoofs, and how to arm them. This chapter mentions the shoes necessary for young horses which, having been reared in marshy lands, have the frogs diseased. 'Employ the half-shoe (*fer à lunette*); the heels and neighbouring parts will become hard, and the shoulders and arms will be brought better into play. Light work, but not on bad roads. Only apply these shoes for some months.'

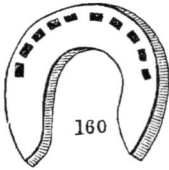

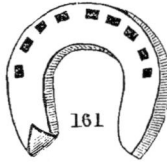

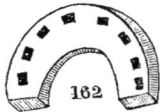

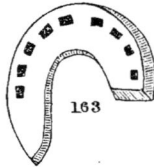

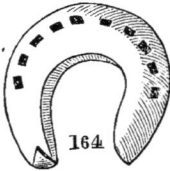

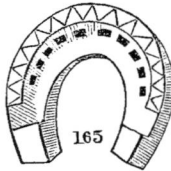

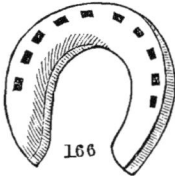

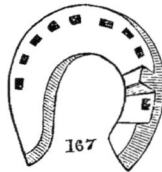

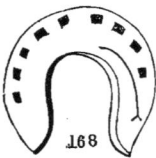

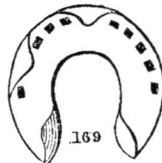

The remaining chapters are devoted to various kinds of shoes, suitable to different varieties of hoofs, or horses whose manner of going was defective; as well as the method of shoeing vicious horses. The figures of shoes he gives are 20 in number. No. 1. Fore-shoe without calkin (fig. 160). 2. Shoe with the calkin *à l'Aragonaise* on one side, and the other side thickened (fig. 161). 3. *Lunette* shoe, or 'tip' (fig. 162). 4. Three-quarter shoe (fig. 163). 5. Bevelled shoe, with the Aragonaise calkin on one branch, and the other thick at the heel (fig. 164). 6. Shoe with *sciettes*, or projecting toothed border, and thickened towards each heel, to prevent slipping (fig. 165). 7. Thick-sided shoe, thin towards the inner border, and seated like the English shoe (fig. 166).

8. Shoe with buttons, or raised catches, on the inner branch, and thickened on the heel of the same side (fig. 167). 9. A shoe which has the inside heel and quarter much thicker and narrower than usual (fig. 168). 10. A shoe with crests or points towards the ground surface on the toe and quarter, and *bar-bettes* at the heels (fig. 169). 11. A shoe with the calkins doubled over, and provided with rings (fig. 170). 12. The foot surface of a shoe with the heels turning up towards the foot (fig. 171). 13. Shoe with two calkins (fig. 172). 14. A *bar* shoe (fig. 173). 15. A jointed shoe, to suit any sized foot (fig. 174). 16. A jointed shoe without nails, and secured by the lateral border and the heel-screw (fig. 175). 17. A hind-shoe with calkins (fig. 176). 18. A shoe with one of the branches greatly thickened at the heel (fig. 177). 19. A hind-shoe with a crest or toe-piece (fig. 178). 20. A hind-shoe with the toe elongated

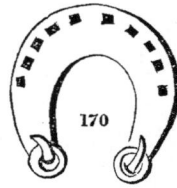

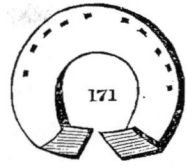

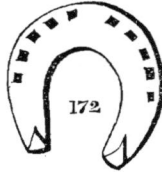

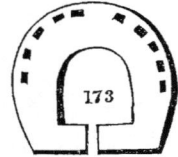

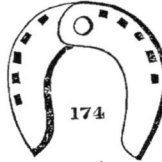

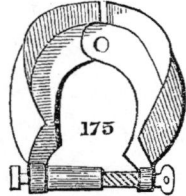

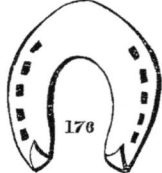

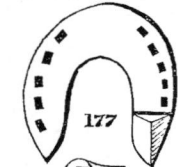

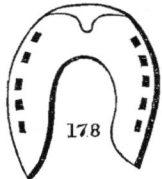

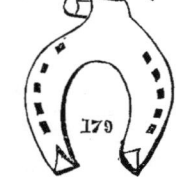

29

and curled upwards, probably for a foot the back tendons of which were contracted, and caused the horse to walk on the point of the toe (fig. 179).

In Germany, the first veterinary treatises published in which shoeing is mentioned are those by Albrecht, ' des Kaiser Friederich huffschmid ; ' [1] Hörwart von Hohenburg ;[2] and Seuter.[3]   There does not appear to be anything novel on the subject in these works, beyond what we have already epitomized from the Italian writers.

In 1598 appeared the excellent treatise of Carlo Ruini, a Senator of Bologna, on the anatomy and diseases of the horse ;[4] in which the maladies and defects of the feet were specially considered, and in a manner truly wonderful, for that time.   Indeed, his instructions for the relief or cure of many foot maladies by shoeing are repeated in modern days.   From his descriptions, we learn that the cruel and unscientific fashion of *opening the heels*, as it is termed, and paring the soles until the horn was quite thin, as well as shoeing with high calkins, was producing those effects with which we are so familiar now-a-days. His treatment of contracted heels consisted chiefly in applying lunette, or thin-heeled shoes, to allow the posterior parts of the hoofs to come in contact with the ground ; and also to employing shoes with clips at the inner angles of the heels to grasp the inflection of horn, named the ' bars,' so as to press them outwards—a mode of expansion still very common on the

---

[1] Das Kleine Rossarzneibüchlein.   Benedig, 1542.

[2] Von der Höchberümpten, Adeligen und Ritterlichen Kunst der Reyterey.   Tegernsee, 1577.

[3] Buech von der Rossarzney, etc.   Augsburg, 1588.

[4] Dell' Anatomia e dell' Infirmita dell Cavallo.   Bologna, 1598.

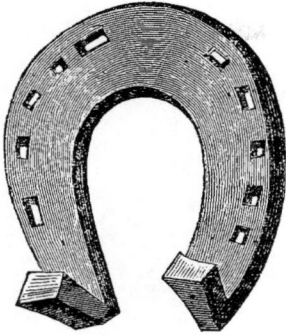

fig. 180

continent, and for which several patents have been secured during this century.

The fashion of arming the hoofs with heavy shoes and great calkins, appears to have prevailed generally for several centuries ; a specimen from the church door of Saint-Saturnin, where it had been attached by some farrier anxious to exhibit his skill, may serve to give us an idea of what was considered a proper model. It bears the date 1573 (fig. 180).[1]

[1] *Megnin.*   Op. cit. p. 62.

CHAPTER X.

FOR the remainder of this history, we will confine our
attention to England and France, alone; countries which
have vied with each other in researches into the functions
of the horse's foot, and the best mode of protecting it by
shoeing.

During the 17th century, there appears to have been
an increasing desire to enhance the services of this noble
animal, and, thanks to the influence of the Italian hippiatrists, the men who now began to study the horse in
health and disease were capable of greatly adding to the
small amount of knowledge previously possessed on the

subject of shoeing; although it is probable their efforts to improve it met with little success.

In England, the form of the shoes in ordinary use would seem to have varied to a notable degree in different parts of the country, and on one occasion this variety gave rise to a remarkable incident connected with the Civil War that broke out about the middle of the century. When Charles II. was making his escape from England in the winter of 1649, and got as far as Lynne, he put up at an inn in a village where his attempts at getting away, and his being somewhere in the locality, were well known. 'The passengers who had lodged in the inn that night, had, as soon as they were up, sent for a smith to visit their horses, it being a hard frost. The smith, when he had done what he was sent for, according to the custom of that people, examined the feet of the other two horses (the king's) to find more work. When he had observed them, he told the host of the house, "that one of those horses had travel'd far; and that he was sure that his four shooes had been made in four several counties." Which (says Lord Clarendon), whether his skill was able to discover or no, was very true. The smith going to the sermon (it was Sunday), told this story to some of his neighbours; and so it came to the ears of the preacher, when his sermon was done.'[1] This preacher was a most enthusiastic puritan, and having strongly suspected Charles to be in the neighbourhood, at once gave the alarm; the king, however, contrived to make a very narrow escape.

Whether it was in grateful recognition of the acuteness manifested by this son of Saint Eloy, or a necessity

[1] Hist. of the Rebellion, vol. iii. p. 330. Oxford, 1702.

imposed by the important development this art had assumed, certain it is, that some years after the king's return from exile to England, and the restoration of the monarchy, the Company of Farriers was incorporated (1763) by the style of 'the Master Wardens, Assistants, and Commonalty of the Company of Farriers, London.' This local corporation was, and is now, a livery company, and governed by a master, three wardens, and twenty-four assistants. In 1736, it had, besides these, thirty-nine on the livery.

The arms of the corporation are: *Ar.* three horse-shoes. *Sa.* pierced of the field. Crest. An arm embowed, issuing from clouds on the sinister side, all *proper*, holding in the hand a hammer *az.* handled, and ducally crowned *or*. Supporters. Two horses *Ar.* Motto, ' *Vi et Virtute.'*

In Scotland, the artificers had, from an early period, formed a corporation at Edinburgh, designated the Hammermen's Corporation. This was one of the chief guilds or public bodies, and included every handicraft; though at first it appears that that of the iron, or black-smith, greatly predominated. The earliest entry, which occurs in 1582, though the corporation had been embodied for some considerable time before this date, gives us to understand that among the 'essays' or specimens of skill and proficiency required to obtain admission, that of the smith was 'ane door cruick (hook) and door-band, ane spaide iron (a spade), ane schoile iron (a shovel), and *horse-shoe* and *six nails* thereto.'

Many distinguished men were presented with the freedom of this Corporation of Hammermen. An entry for

March 21st, 1657, shows that Mr Charles Smith, advocate, was admitted a blacksmith; and was pleased to produce, by way of essay, 'the portrait of an horse's leg, shoed with a silver shoe fixed with three nails, with a silver staple at the other end thereof; which was found to be a *qualified* and well-wrought essay.'[1]

If I remember aright, the crest of the corporation was an uncovered arm grasping a hammer, and the motto, ' By hammer in hand all arts do stand.'

A horse-shoe in my possession, dug up from the battle-field of Marston Moor (near York), and which belonged, without doubt, to some horse engaged in that slaughter (July 2, 1644), is of a good outline. Though extremely oxidized, we can yet see that it measured a little more than $4\frac{1}{2}$ inches in length and breadth—the width being about one inch and three-eighths, and the thickness about one quarter inch. The foot surface appears to have been concave throughout, and without any *seating* for the hoof; while the ground surface is convex to such an extent that the inner circumference is much lower than the outer. I can only trace three oblong nail-holes on each side; but whether the shoe has been grooved around these or not, it is impossible to say.

The most notable work on veterinary medicine published in England in the 16th century, was that of Thomas Blundevil.[2] This, though not the first, is yet

---

[1] Transactions of the Socy. of Antiquaries of Scotland, vol. i. p. 170.

[2] The Four Chiefest Offices belonging to Horsemanship. The Order of Curing Horse Diseases, etc. The True Arte of Paring and Shooying all maner of houes, together with the shapes and fygures of dyuers shooes, very necessarye for dyuers horses. By Thomas Blundevil, of Newton-Flotman, in Norffolke. London, 1565.

entitled to be considered the foundation, or real commencement of veterinary science in Britain. As previously explained, this science, like many others, owed its
resuscitation to Italy. After the fall of the Byzantine
empire, learning once more sought refuge in that favoured
land; and the writings of the Greek and Roman hippiatrists, transferred to this genial soil from their Eastern
nursery and repository, were not long in bringing forth
good fruit, as evidenced in the writings of Rusius, Ruini,
Fiaschi, and many others. The veterinary science of
France, England, and other countries, took its origin
from this source. And Blundevil acknowledges this in
the frequent quotations he gives from the Italian writers,
and the references he makes to their opinions. Indeed,
the technical expressions he employs are nearly all Italian,
only some few of them being French. The English language could not furnish them; and more particularly is
this observed in the section or treatise devoted to 'paring
and shooying all maner of houes.'

He mentions the various breeds of horses he was
acquainted with, and their good and bad qualities, particularly with a view to their being profitably reared in
England; these were the horses of 'Turkey and Barbary;
Sardinia and Corsica, courser of Naples, jennet of Spayne,
Hungarian, highe Almayne; Flanders horse; Frizeland
horse, and Iryshe hobbye.' In that portion of his work
which is more intimately connected with the subject now
under consideration, he writes: 'The art of shoeing con-
sisteth in these points, that is to say, in paring the hoof
well, in making the shoe of good stuff, in well fashioning
the webb thereof, a well piercing the same, in fitting the

shoe unto the horse's foot, in making nails of good stuff, and well fashioning the same, and finally in well driving of the said nails, and clenching of the same. But as neither paring nor shoeing is no absolute thing of itself, but hath respect unto the foot or hoof (for the shoe is to be fitted to the foot, and not the foot to the shoe), and that there be diverse kinds of hoofs both good and bad, requiring great diversity as well of paring as shoeing, it is meet, therefore, that we first talk of the diversity of hoofs, and then show you how they ought to be pared and shod.'

After describing the hoofs in a very quaint manner, and showing us, unwittingly, how much disease and defective form prevailed, and which arose, no doubt, from bad shoeing, paring the hoofs is next commented upon, when he talks about the 'butter.' This is the ungainly weapon or instrument long wielded with such fatal effect on horses' feet in England, and still in use on the continent. It appears to have been introduced into this country and France from Germany, the authors of the 'Origines de la langue Française' deriving it from *bozen* or *botzen*, to *push*, in Old German. In France, from an early period, it has been named *boutoir*, from whence Blundevil, who is the first to import it into our language, terms it 'butter.' Up to a recent date it was in use in England, and was known as 'butress.' Contemporaneously with its mention in the writings of the old farriers, do we find serious diseases of the feet noticed, and particularly contraction of the hoofs at the heels.

While Blundevil is advising that the heels of the fore feet should be gently pared, he recommends that '*the*

toes be pared so thin almost as the edge of a knife.'　In
paring, too, he mentions that 'the French ferrers hath a
proverb which saith, " Devant dariar, dariar devant," which
means spare the fore foot behind, and the hinder foot before, as well in paring as in piercing the shoes (i. e. making
the nail-holes).

'Make your shoe of spruse or Spanish iron, with a
broad web, fitting it to the foot, and let the sponges (heels)
be thicker and more substantial than any other part of the
shoe; yea, and also somewhat broad, so as the quarters on
both sides may *disbord*, that is to say, appear without the
hoof a straw's breadth to guard the coffin, which is the
strength of the hoof, and only beareth the shoe. . . .
And as touching the nails, make them also of the same
iron, the heads whereof would be square, and not fully so
broad beneath as above, but answerable to the piercing-
holes, so as the head of the nails may enter in and fill
the same, appearing above the shoe no more than the
breadth of the back of a knife; so shall they stand sure
without shogging, and endure longer, and to that end the
stamp that first maketh the holes, and the " preschell" that
pierceth them, and also the necks of the nails, would be
of one square fashion and bigness: that is to say, great
above and small beneath, which our common smiths do
little regard, for when they pierce a shoe, they make the
hole as wide on the inside as on the outside. . . . A good
nail should have no shouldering at all, but be made with
a plain and square neck, so as it may justly fit and fill the
piercing-hole of the shoe. . . . The shanks of the nails
should be somewhat flat, and the points sharp, without
hollowness or flaw, and stiffer towards the head above,

than beneath.   And when you drive, drive at the first
with soft strokes, and with a light hammer, until the nail
be somewhat entered. . . . The shoe standing straight
and just, drive in all the nails to the number of eight, four
on each side, so as the points of the nails may seem to
stand on the outside of the hoof, even and just one by
another, as it were in a circular line, and not out of order
like the teeth of a saw, whereof one is bent one way and
one another way.   That done, cut them off and clinch
them so as the clinches may be hidden in the hoof, which
by cutting the hoof with the point of a knife, a little beneath the appearing of the nail, you may easily do.   That
done with a rape (rasp) pare the hoof round, so as the
edge of the shoe may be seen round about.'

He always recommends free paring, and for rough and
brittle hoofs '*plenty of rasping on the outside to make them
smooth,* and the shoe put on with *nine* nails—four inside
and five out.'

For the contracted or hoof-bound foot, he recommends *paring the sole thin and opening the heels well,*
and putting on a shoe like a half moon.

Concerning shoes with calkins, he quotes Cæsar
Fiaschi as opposed to their use, and as approving of the
Turkish mode of shoeing for mountain travelling. 'Notwithstanding, some never think their horses to be well
shod, unless all the shoes be made with calkins, either
single or double.'

Of the shoes with rings, shown in Fiaschi's work, he
says they were first invented to make a horse lift his feet
high, but that they caused a horse pain on hard roads,
especially those horses which had not sound feet.   Blun-

devil calls them 'unprofitable devices,' and recommends that the shoes with sponges (from the French *éponge*, the heel portion of the shoe thickened) only be used ; if it is necessary to teach a horse to lift his feet, he should be shod heavily while at the school, and afterwards with light shoes.

'In Germany and "highe Almany," the "smythes" do make the shoes with a swelling welt round about the shoe, which being as high as the heads of the nails, or higher, saves the nails from wear.' These shoes Blunde vil praises for lasting, having used them in these coun tries on very stony ground, and he mentions that Fiaschi also lauds them ; though he advises that the *wealt* be indented, having sharp pointed teeth like a saw, and that the sponges behind be as thick as the welt ; and that the welt be of a tough hard temper, for fear of wearing too fast. 'With these kind of shoes they use in Italy to shoe such Barbary horses, jennets, and Turks, as are appointed to run for the best game at some public triumph, or any other private wager.

'Some that use to pass the mountains where smiths are not readily to be found, to shoe a horse if need be, do carry about with them certain shoes made with *vyces*, wherewith they make the shoe fast to the horse's foot without help of hammer or nails. Notwithstanding, such shoes are more for the show than for any good use or commodity. For though it save the horse's foot from stones, yet it so pincheth his hoof, as he goeth with pain, and perhaps doth his hoof more hurt than the stones would do.'

He advises the jointed shoe to be applied in such

cases, 'but this shoe must be set on with nails, and therefore it is needful that the rider learn to drive a nail if need be, whereof he must have always store about him, together with hammer, pynsons, and " butter," handsomely made, and fit for carrying; without these the horsemen of Almany never travel, neither is there any gentleman that loveth his horse but can use these instruments for that purpose as well as any smith.'

He gives various drawings of shoes, chiefly borrowed from Fiaschi, and heavy and clumsy. The 'Planche' shoe for weak heels is only a more formidable model of the modern bar shoe (fig. 181). The drawing he also gives of a nail is that of our present square-headed nail.

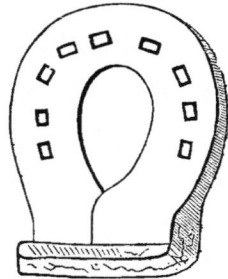

fig 181

All the shoes have the square hole and *no fullering*. This is not mentioned anywhere; so that I may be in error in assigning it so early a date in England.

Sensible as are many of Blundevil's remarks, yet we cannot avoid concluding that he was greatly in error in recommending paring and rasping, particularly to such a ruinous extent. The terrible injury inflicted on horses by this unwise and barbarous practice, in addition to very faulty shoes, has hung like a curse upon these creatures up to the present day. Blundevil has in this respect been largely followed.

Michael Baret,' in his treatise on horsemanship, published 50 years later, speaking of teaching a horse to pace

---

' An Hipponomie, or the Vineyard of Horsemanship, pp. 97, 112. London, 1618.

or amble, mentions 'tramels, heavy shoes, pasternes of lead, and shoes of advantage' being used on the hind limbs, 'to keep the hinder parts of the horse down, and to cause his hinder feete strike further forward within his fore parts.' The 'shoe of advantage' was the most dangerous; as the projections or plates at the toe struck the tendons of the fore-legs and seriously injured them. For the coursers, the day before racing, the hoofs were to be shod, 'but let them be such shooes as shall be best agreeing to the race; which if it bee a soft moore or swarth, let them be but thinne plates, or halfe shooes (like a halfe moone), but if it bee hard and gravelly, let them be whole shooes, but yet so light as is possible.'

Markham's principal work on farriery and horsemanship [1] contains little beyond what Blundevil had stated in the previous century; but in a smaller treatise [2] we have some examples given of the condition of horses' feet, and the attention they received. For 'foundering, frettizing, or any imperfection in the feet or hoofes of an horse,' he gives the following directions for the treatment of the unfortunate creature's extremities: 'First pare thin, open the heels, and take good store of blood from the toes, then tack on a shooe, somewhat hollow.' The sole was then to be filled up with all kinds of fantastic compounds. In a later edition of this treatise (1647) he omits the 'good store of blood:' 'First pare thinne, open the heels wide, and shooe large, strong, and hollow.'

The agony the poor horses must have suffered on a

[1] Masterpiece.   London, 1638.
[2] The Faithful Farrier.   London, 1639.

journey, from the outrageous treatment their feet were subjected to, as well as from the terrible basin-shaped clumsy shoes, is fully evidenced by the numerous re-cipes this admirable horseman gives for 'stoppings' to be applied while travelling. We have also directions 'how to helpe the surbating or sorenesse in the feete.' These are, as might be expected, on a par with the general manage-ment of the hapless organs. 'When you find your horse to be surbated, presently clap into each of his fore-feet two new-layd eggs, and crush them therein, then upon the toppe of them lay good store of cow-dung; thus stop him (or, rather, the horse's feet), and in foure houres he will recover.'

It is not until we arrive at the 18th century, that any-thing worthy of notice occurs relative to this subject, in England. It may be mentioned, however, that the 17th century produced the first treatise on the Anatomy of the Horse, by Snape (London, 1683), farrier to his Majesty King Charles II., a very estimable work, and one which did good service in drawing attention to the value of anatomy, particularly with regard to the horse's foot.

In France, in the 15th century, the community of *maréchaux* comprised the *maréchaux ferrants* and the *maréchaux grossiers.* The latter were only carriage-smiths, and had nothing to do with horses. The *maitrises,* or 'trade freedoms' were, however, abolished in February, 1776, and the farriers stood upon their own proper de-signation. In the following August, the trade companies were again formed, and the *maréchaux ferrants* were classed with the *éperonniers* or spur and bit makers; an improvement, as the two occupations were closely allied with the conservation and utility of the horse.[1]

In the 17th century, many publications on veterinary medicine and farriery were published, among which may be mentioned those of Francini,[2] Dumesnil,[3] Beaugrand,[4] Espinay,[5] Prome,[6] Beaumont,[7] and Delcampe.[8]

But the most distinguished treatise of the century was perhaps that of Solleysel.[9] This had an immense success, was translated into every cultivated language in Europe, and became the oracle of the veterinary surgeons and horsemen of those days. Although this hippiatrist is largely indebted to the writings of Cæsar Fiaschi; and though anatomy and physiology enter but little into his writings, yet there is a good deal of originality in the matter of shoeing, evidencing a tendency to place that art upon a scientific basis; but the high estimation in which it had been previously held was apparently on the wane. Solleysel, while attaching to its practice great importance, being persuaded that every squire, gentleman, or other person having good and fine horses 'ne doit ignorer l'ordre et la méthode qu'il faut tenir pour les bien ferrer, afin que s'il ne peut avoir un bon maréchal, il puisse ordonner de quelle manière ils doivent être ferrés

[1] *Ambert*, Esquisses Historiq. sur l'Armée Françaises, p. 68. Saumur, 1837.

[2] Hippiatrique. Paris, 1607.

[3] L'Art de la Maréchalerie. Paris, 1628.

[4] Le Maréchal Expert. Lyons, 1633.

[5] Le *Grand* Maréchalerie. Paris, 1642.

[6] Le *Grand* Maréchal Française. Paris, 1662.

[7] Le Nouveau Parfait Maréchal. Paris, 1660.

[8] Art de Monter à Cheval. Paris, 1663.

[9] Le Parfait Maréchal. Paris, 1664.

pour le bien être;' yet adds, that, in his time, kings and people of quality could shoe horses: 'On a vu, de notre temps, des rois sçavoir forger un fer; et il est peu de personnes de qualité qui ne sachent brocher des clous, pour s'en servir dans la nécessité.' And he now complains that the little progress that had been made in a knowledge of this branch of veterinary science 'has maintained it in a state of debasement which even affects the other branches;' farriery, when he wrote, was 'un métier, ou une certaine routine, que ces ouvriers apprenaient chez des maîtres dépourvus de tous principes de leur art.'

In a brief historical notice like the present, an analysis of this treatise will not be expected; and we can only give some abridged notices from the translation made by Sir William Hope, and published in London, in 1706.[1]

Speaking of a journey, he says: 'Many horses as soon as unbridled, instead of eating, lay themselves down to rest, because of the great pain they have in their feet, so that a man is apt to think them sick; but if he look to their eyes, he will see they are lively and good; and if he offer meat to them as they are lying, they will eat it very willingly; yet if he handle their feet he will find them extremely hot, which will discover to him that it is in that part they suffer. You must therefore observe if their shoes do not rest upon their soles.' And again: 'When you are arrived from a journey, immediately draw the two heel-nails of the fore-feet, and if it be a large shoe, then four. And two or three days after you may blood him in the neck, and feed him for ten or twelve

[1] The Compleat Horseman, or Perfect Farrier. London, 1706.

days with wet bran only, without giving him any oats, keeping him well littered. The reason why you are to draw the heel-nails is, because the feet swell, and if they were not thus eased, the shoes would press and straiten them too much. It is also good to stop them with cow-dung, but do not take off the shoes, nor pare the feet, because the humours are drawn down by it'

There are also frequent allusions to *foundering* (inflammation of the feet), the changes in the hoofs induced by this disease; as well as to the occurrence of treads, over-reaches, coronary abscesses, &c. With regard to the practice of shoeing at this time, there are the following directions and explanations: 'There are two methods of shoeing. The first is, to shoe for the advantage of the foot, and, according to its nature and shape, to fit such shoes to it as may make it better than it is; and if it be good, may preserve and keep it from becoming bad. The second method is, that which disguiseth the foot, and maketh it appear good when really it is not; which method, although in time it wholly ruins the foot, yet horse-coursers, who have no other design but to sell and put off their horses, do not much trouble themselves about it; for provided their horses' feet but appear good, and they get them sold, it is all they desire. I shall treat of the first only, wherein are four rules to be observed in shoeing all sorts of feet whatsoever. The first is, *Toe before,* and *quarter behind,* or as we commonly say, *before behind, behind before.* By *toe before* is meant, that you may give the nails a good hold upon the toes of the fore-feet, because there the horn is very thick, which it is not in the quarters of the fore-feet, for there the horn is thin, and you would hazard the pricking your horse. *Quarter behind* is that a horse hath the quarters of his hind feet strong, that is to say, the horn thick, and so capable of suffering a good gripe by the nails; but at the toes of the hind feet you will immediately meet with the quick, because the horn is but thin in that part; and therefore smiths should put no nails at all just in the toes of the hind feet, but only in their quarters.

'The second rule is, *Never to open a horse's heels.* People call it opening of the heels, when the smith in paring the foot, cutteth the heel low and close almost to the frush (frog), and taketh it down within a finger's breadth of the coronet, or top of the hoof, so that he separates the quarters at the heel, and by that means weakens and takes away the substance of the foot, making it to close and become narrow at the heels. Now this, which they call opening, would be more properly called closing of the heels; for the roundness and circumference of the foot being cut, by doing that which they call opening of the heels, which is to cut them wholly away, they are no longer supported by anything; so that if there be any weakness in the foot, it will of necessity make it shrink and straiten in the quarters, which will quite spoil the foot.

'The third rule is *to make use of as thin and small nails as possible;* because the nails that are thick and gross make a large hole, not only when they are driving, but also when they are riveting; for, being stiff, they split the horn and take it away with them. Neither can a tender foot be shod with such big nails without hazard of pricking, especially if there be but little horn to take hold of.

30 *

But smiths, to prevent this, pierce their shoes too near the edge, which will in time ruin the foot.

'The fourth rule is *to make the lightest shoes you can,* according to the size of your horse, because heavy shoes spoil the back-sinews and weary the horse; and if he happens to overreach, the shoes being heavy are more easily pulled off.' 'Those who think it frugality to shoe with thick and heavy shoes, and seldom, are deceived, for they lose more by it than they gain, for thereby they not only spoil the back-sinews but lose more shoes than if they had been light.'

Excessive paring with the 'butteris' seems to have been in vogue then as at a later day, for in recommending a certain method of shoeing he remarks: 'Do not pare your horses' feet almost to the quick, as some people do, who think thereby to prevent the so frequent shoeing of their horses. But if you know that your horses' hoofs are smooth and tough, you may with the more confidence pare his soles reasonably near.'

This old hippiatrist, in fact, gives a few excellent directions for the management of the horse's feet, and evidently far beyond the usual practice of his age; though mixed with many which are bad. He condemns heavy and high calkins, and admits that horses are much better without them altogether. Though the rasp was in use, he does not advise its being put to the outer surface of the wall, and only speaks of paring the frog when the heels are flat or low, and that part of the foot is likely to come in contact with the ground. For the cure of these flat feet, too, he recommends the barbarous operation of *barring* (ligaturing) the pastern veins, 'so that you may put a stop to the superfluous humour which falleth down upon the lower part of the foot, and causeth the sole to grow round and high; and also the coffin-bone, or little foot, which is the bone in the middle of the coffin, to push itself down, which, through time, maketh the foot become round at the sole.'

Flanders at that period appears to have furnished large numbers of horses, whose special characteristics were hairy legs, and wide flat-soled feet; for this author, when describing the best way to remedy this defective form of hoof by a shoe resting on the sole, instead of the customary vaulted armature, adds: 'The surest way is to rectify such bad feet in the beginning, and especially in the time when horses alter or change their horn, which is the first six months after they come from Flanders.'

His advice to keep the *sole strong* by refraining from paring it, to make the shoe fit the foot instead of the foot the shoe, and to take a short thick hold of the wall with the nails, is excellent. His remarks on pathological shoeing, too, show much judgment and experience of this important subject. The nails were to be thin and supple; large nails were destructive to the hoofs. For contracted hoofs, he recommends the employment of *fers à pantoufles*, which he says were invented by M. de la Brone, squire to Henry III. These were merely shoes with the inner border of each heel turned downwards at a more or less acute angle, so as to cause the heels of the hoof to glide forcibly outwards when the horse's weight was imposed on them. Lunette shoes were also employed by him for horses of the *manége* who had their hoofs contracted.

To the people who argued that horses were better

without shoes, Solleysel mentions that those of the German peasantry are not shod; though he asserts it would
be much to their advantage if they were, as the limbs and
feet were in nearly every case he saw more or less de
formed.

M. Bernard recently confirms this observation, by
stating that in Lorraine, Alsace, and Bavaria, he saw very
many agricultural horses unshod, and that deformities of
the hoofs were common.[1]

[1] *Journal de Méd. Vét. Militaire,* vol. iv. p. 111.

CHAPTER XI.

In the 18th century, when veterinary schools were
established in France, treatises on shoeing were abundantly multiplied. With 'L'Ecole de Cavalerie' of La
Guérinière (1733), 'La Parfaite Connaissance des Chevaux' of Saunier (1734), 'Le Nouveau Parfait Maréchal'
of Garsault (1755), and others, appears the 'Nouvelle
Pratique de Ferrer les Chevaux de Selle et de Carosse'
(Paris, 1756) of Lafosse [1] (Maréchal des Petites Ecuries

[1] This excellent essay was translated into English by Braken (who

du Roi). This veterinarian, a man of great observation, and an enlightened practitioner, may be said to have been the most advanced of that school which, for two centuries, had been endeavouring to improve the vicious courses adopted by the farriers in their treatment of horses' feet. The principal of these practices were injudicious removal of the horn, and the great weight and length of the shoes. We have seen that the Italian writer, Fiaschi, had already protested against the use of calkins, which were becoming of greater size as time advanced. An example of this, from the church-door of Saint-Saturnin, has been already given. During the reign of Louis XIV., this absurd fashion appears to have been at its height. No thought seems to have been bestowed on the injurious influence such shoeing might have on the form or quality of the hoofs, on the true or false disposition of the limbs, nor yet on the horse's natural movements. Chargers and ordinary riding-horses wore strangely-shaped masses of iron, which, for weight and clumsiness, could scarcely, one would think, be carried by a strong waggon-horse of our own times. This unreasonable and most pernicious custom, which makes us wonder how it was possible that anything like quick progression could be accomplished without serious damage to the limbs of horses and riders, is shown in the paintings of Lebrun, court-painter to the Grand Monarque, which may be seen in the galleries of the Louvre, and in which Alexander and other heroes of antiquity are represented on horses whose feet are cum-

had performed a like service for Lafosse's earlier work, ' Traité des Observations et des Découvertes sur les Chevaux '). It has been republished in the Bibliothèque Vétérinaire, Paris, 1849.

bered with tremendous 'crampons.' In the Gobelins' tapestry, manufactured under that artist's direction, these massive projections are also depicted. A shoe of this description, copied from one worn by a saddle-horse, on a piece of Gobelins at Holyrood Palace, Edinburgh, and made in 1684, will perhaps give some idea of their proportions (fig. 182).

In the reign of Louis XV., however, the large calkins were generally abolished by the farriers, though the shoes were yet as long, if not longer, than before, and towards the heels were made heavy and thick.

Against this absurd fashion Lafosse uses every argument.

fig 182

Informing us that in Prussia, the fore feet only were shod; in Germany, the fore and hind—each shoe having three calkins; in France, only calkins on the hind feet; while in England the shoes were wide, thin, and with thickened heels, so that the frogs could not reach the ground, though without calkins before or behind; he says that all strangers visiting France carried in their train a farrier to shoe their horses in their own fashion, thinking it preferable, and that French noblemen did the same. Not that the mode of shoeing of any country was preferable to another—for native and foreign horses were alike badly shod—but because it was less an affair of reasoning than fancy and habit.

'The practice of shoeing horses appears to me to be good, useful, and even necessary on paved roads; but it is

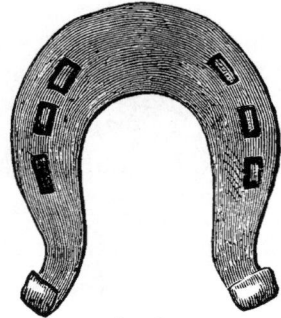

on the form and manner of applying shoes that not only depends the preservation of the feet, but also the safety of the limbs and the harmony of movement. We always find ourselves more active and nimble when we wear easy shoes; but a wide, long, and thick shoe will do for horses what clogs do for us—render them heavy, clumsy, and unsteady.

After giving a brief notice of the anatomy of the foot, the necessity for the farrier to understand this, and also the fact that the horse, in a natural condition, ought to have the whole extent of its foot placed upon the superfices of the ground it covers, he refers to the defects of the shoeing then in vogue, and as aptly as if he had lived in our own day : ' As it is not possible to employ unshod horses on paved roads or hard ground without running the risk of destroying some of the parts just mentioned, we have been compelled to shoe them ; but the actual method is so injurious that, so far from preserving their feet, it concurs to their destruction in occasioning a number of accidents, as I will demonstrate.

' 1. Long shoes, thick at the heels, never remain firmly attached to the feet in consequence of their weight, and break the clinches of the nails.

' 2. They require proportionately large nails to retain them, and these split the horn, or frequently their thick stalks press against the sensitive laminæ and sole, and cause the horse to go lame.

' 3. Horses are liable to pull off these long shoes when the hind-foot treads upon the heel of the fore-shoe, either in walking, while standing by putting the one foot upon the other, between two paving-stones in the pavement, be-

tween the bars of gates, in the draw-bridges of fortifica-
tions, or in heavy ground.

'4. They move heavily, as the weight of their shoes
fatigues them.

'5. Long shoes with massive heels raise the frogs from
the ground, and prevent the horse walking on those parts.
Then, if the horse has a humour in the frog, it becomes a
ficthrush, or *crapaud* (canker), because the humour lodges
there. In shoeing with short shoes, the horse goes on
his frog, the humour is dissipated more easily, particularly
in the fore-feet, as the animal places more weight upon
them than the hind ones.

'6. Long shoes, thick at the heels, when put upon
feet which have low heels, bruise and bend them inwards,
and lame the horse, although the heel be sprung, and
when the foot is raised we can see daylight between the
shoe and the hoof; when it is on the ground, the heel
descends to the shoes, because the hoof is flexible.

'7. Shoes long and strong at the heels, when the foot
is pared, the frog being removed a long distance from the
ground, cause many accidents—such as the rupture or
straining of the flexor tendon, and compression of the
vascular sole, a circumstance not known until I pointed it
out.

'8. Long shoes cause horses to slip and fall, because
they act like a patten on the slippery pavement, as well in
summer as in winter.

'9. Long shoes are also injurious when horses lie like
a cow, in consequence of the heels wounding the elbows.

'10. Calkins should not be used on paved roads;
they are only useful on ice or slippery ground (*terre grasse*).

'11. The calkins on the inside heels are liable to wound the coronets when the horse happens to cross his feet.

'12. A horse shod with them is soon fatigued and never goes easy.

'13. The horse which has only a calkin on the outside does not stand fair, and the calkin confines the movement of the coronary articulation, the foot being twisted to one side.

'14. If a horse has his feet pared and loses a shoe, he cannot travel without breaking and bruising the wall, and damaging the horny sole, because the horn is too thin to protect it.

'15. If the shoes are long, and the heels of the hoof pared out hollow, stones and pebbles lodge between the shoe and the sole, and make the horse lame.

'16. Flat feet become convex by hollowing the shoes to relieve the heels and the frog, because the more the shoes are arched from the sole, the more the wall of the hoofs is squeezed and rolled inwards, particularly towards the inner quarter, which is the weakest; the sole of the foot becomes convex, and the horse is nearly always unfit for service.

'17. If the wall of the hoof is thin and the shoes are arched, the quarters are so pressed upon that the horse is lame.

'18. Pared hoofs are exposed to considerable injury from wounds by nails, stones, glass, etc.

'19. The pared sole readily picks up earth or sand, which forms a kind of cement between it and the shoe, and produces lameness.

' 20. The reason why it is dangerous to pare the feet of horses, is because when the sole is pared, and the horse stands in a dry place, the horn becomes desiccated by the air which enters it, and removes its moisture and its suppleness, and often causes the animal to be lame.

' 21. A habit to be abolished is that in which the farrier, to save trouble, burns the *sole* with a hot iron, so as to pare it more easily. The result often is to heat the sensitive sole and cripple the horse.

' 22. It often happens that, to make the foot pleasant to look at, the horn of the sole is removed to the quick, and the flesh springs out from it; this granulation is called a cherry, and sometimes it makes the horse unserviceable for a considerable period.

' 23. It is the pared foot which is most affected with what is termed contracted or weak inside quarter, and which also lames the horse.

' 24. It also happens that one or both quarters contract, and sometimes even the whole hoof; then, in consequence of its smallness, all the internal parts are confined in their movements; this lames the horse, and is due to paring.

' 25. There also occurs another accident: when the quarter becomes contracted, the hoof splits in its lateral aspect; this accident is termed a sandcrack (*seima*), and the horse is lame.

' 26. The fashion of paring the hoofs, and especially the heels, within which are the bars, causes contraction, and this renders the horse lame.

' 27. It is an abuse to rasp the hoofs of horses; this alters the hoof and forms sandcracks.

'28. If a horse which has pared hoofs happens to lose his shoes and walks without them, the horn is quickly used and the feet damaged.

'29. Another defect is in the manner of making large nail-holes in the shoes, etc.

'30. The majority of farriers, in order to pare the sole well, cut it until it bleeds, and to stop the hæmorrhage, they burn the place with a hot iron, and the horse returns lame to his stable.'

We see, then, that the curse of paring and heavy shoes was causing great evils in the days of Lafosse, as much as in our own. After enumerating all the vices and defects of shoeing, as it was then practised, he proceeds to lay the foundation for a rational method; and his remarks to this end are particularly happy. In a state of nature, he observes, all the inferior parts of the foot concur to sustain the weight of the body; then we observe that the heels and the frogs—the parts said to be most exposed, are never damaged by wear; that the wall or crust is alone worn in going on hard ground, and that it is only this part which must be protected, leaving the other parts free and unfettered in their natural movements. These are the true and simple principles of good farriery he lays down, and they are as appropriate and explicit to-day as they were then. 'To prevent horses slipping on the dry glistening pavement (*pavé sec et plombé*), it is necessary to shoe them with a crescent-shaped shoe—that is, a shoe which only occupies the circumference of the toe, and whose heels gradually thin away to the middle of the quarters; so that the frog and heels of the hoof bear on the ground, and the weight be sustained behind and before, but particularly in the latter, because the weight of the body falls heaviest there. The shorter the shoe is the less the horse slips, and the frog has the same influence in preventing this that an old hat placed under our own shoes would have in protecting us from slipping on ice.

'It is necessary, nevertheless, that hoofs which have weak walls should be a little longer shod, so that the gradually thinning branches reach to the heels, though not resting upon them. For horses which have thin convex soles (*pieds combles*), these long shoes should be also used, and the toes should be more covered to prevent the sole touching the ground; at the same time, the shoe must be so fitted that it does not press upon the sole, and the heels and frog rest upon the ground; this is the only true method of preserving the foot and restoring it.' 'A horse which has its heels weak and sensitive ought to be shod as short as possible, and with thin branches (*éponges*), so that the frog comes in contact with the ground; because the heels, having nothing beneath them, are benefitted and relieved (fig. 183).

'Crescent shoes are all the more needful for a horse which has weak incurvated quarters, as they not only relieve them, but also restore them to their natural condition. Horses which have contusions at the heels (*bleimes*, corns) should also be shod in this manner, and for cracks (*seimes*, sand-

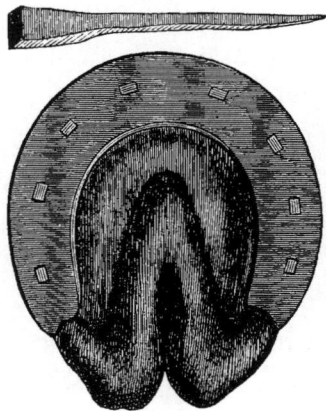

fig. 183

cracks) at the quarter it is also advantageous. *The sole or frog should never be pared;* the wall alone should be cut down, if it is too long.   When a horse cuts himself with the opposite foot the inner branch of the shoe ought to be shorter and thinner than the outer.   In order that the shoe wear a long time, I have used a nail of my invention, the head of which is in the form of a cone, and the aperture in the shoe of the same shape, and exactly filled by the nail.   However much the shoe may be worn it is always retained in its place.   This kind of nail (fig. 183) possesses three other advantages : one, that it is less liable to be broken at the neck because it exactly fits the stamped hole; the other that it is smaller, and, in consequence, not likely to press on the sensitive part of the foot; and, lastly, that it does less damage to the horn.

'By this new mode of shoeing all the defects and accidents attendant upon the old method are evaded.'

Elsewhere he speaks of another kind of shoeing, which is not without interest.   The chapter referring to this is headed : ' Half-circle shoes for the safety of the rider, for use on dry and slippery roads, either in summer or winter, in ascending mountains, or in descending them at a gallop, without slipping in any way.'   This method of shoeing was contrived as follows : ' The semi-circle (fig. 184, next page) ought to be from two to three lines in width and one and a half in thickness, so as to admit of the holes being made in them with a punch; these holes should be counter-pierced on the same side on which they are stamped, so that the nail-head be completely buried in their cavities.   Ten holes at least are required, but they should be small in proportion, as they are only needed to sustain the wall; the shoe should also be flexible. As is customary, the excess of crust should be removed, observing, however, to leave a little more than usual in order to imbed the semi-circle in it; then to apply this, a groove is made in the middle of the

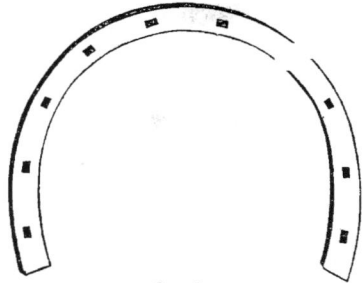

fig 184

wall of the foot to the depth of the shoe, so that it may lie therein, and the outer edge of the crust project beyond it all round, to facilitate its being worn on the road. The two ends of the shoe ought to be incrusted in the heels, as this is productive of two mutual advantages: one, that the wall should preserve the thin shoe from too rapid wear, and the other, that the shoe prevents the hoof from breaking, or too much attrition (fig. 185). This mode of shoeing is advantageous for saddle-horses; it would be also good for draught-horses, did the shoes stand wear long enough. I have seen many horses go with these shoes for three weeks; of course, the less work they did the longer the shoes would last. I may mention, however, that there is a more convenient mode

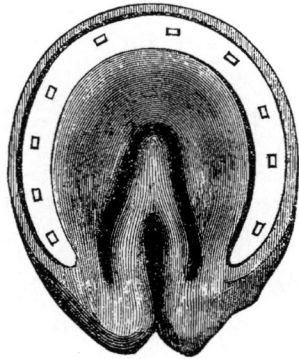

fig. 185

of shoeing draught-horses; this is with a shoe that is bedded (*enclavé*) in the whole thickness of the wall, observing to leave it projecting in its entire contour. This shoe may be termed *le croissant enclavé* (the imbedded

31

crescent) ; it should be stamped very fine (*maigre*).   It must be remarked that these two kinds of shoes are only fit for horses with strong hoofs.'

His recommendations for shoeing good hoofs to travel on all kinds of ground are as follows : 'The shoes must not be too long or project beyond the heels, but only reach the bars; neither must the hoofs, behind or before, be pared.   The wall or crust alone should be diminished in proportion as it may be too long; this should be done evenly, and neither the sole nor frog must be cut; the latter should be allowed to project, if possible, above the shoe, so that it may come into contact with the ground.   The shoe ought to be about the same strength throughout, or a little thicker and wider in the outer branch of the fore foot, and thin at the heels of the hind one.   Be careful to stamp the nail-holes on the same line, not in a zigzag manner; the holes should not be too coarse, as there is then danger of pricking the horse, or binding the hoof with the stalk of the nail.   The shoe should be stamped coarser outside than inside, because it may be necessary to leave it wider outside.   Do not bend the shoes in adjusting them, nor arch them; they ought to be nearly flat; though they might be slightly curved, so as to preserve the wall of the hoof.   They should also follow the outline of the hoof, a little more to the outside than the inside.   When fitting, the shoe should not be kept too long a time on the hoof, for fear of heating it.   With this shoeing we may travel on slippery ground or grass land, in using for each shoe two nails with long heads, which will prevent the horse from slipping.   Also during frost, on paved roads, or ice or snow, use these nails, as they prevent slipping; the roads being hard, three nails are required—two in the outer branch, and one in the inner.'

Reverting to the defective shoeing of his time, he endeavours to demonstrate, that by removing the horn of the frog and points of the heels from the ground, the animal's footing on paved roads is much less secure. 'The draught-horse first places his weight on the toe, then on the two sides of the hoof, and afterwards the heels are lowered to meet the heel of the shoe. The saddle-horse rests more lightly on the toe. The cannon (or shank bone) presses on the pastern-bone, this on the coronary, and this again on the coffin and navicular bones. From this disposition, we should note two important points which throw light on the defects of the present method, and indicate how to remedy them ; one is, that the strain of the weight is neither fixed on the toe nor heel, but between the two ; the other, that the more the frog is removed from the ground or from any point of support, the more the pressure of the coronary on the navicular bone fatigues the tendon on which it rests, in consequence of the excessive extension it experiences at each step the horse takes. The frog ought therefore to rest on the ground, as much for the facility as for the surety of the horse's movements ; as the larger the frog is, so the less do the heels meet the ground ; and the more the heels are relieved, the greater ease does the horse experience in progression. The only way to insure this is to shoe him according to the method I have indicated, as this causes him to walk on his frog, which is the natural prop or basis (*point d'appui*) for the flexor tendon.'

The whole aim of Lafosse's teaching appears to have

31 *

been wisely devoted to the importance of allowing the posterior parts of the foot to rest on the ground without the intervention of the shoe. 'It is useful and even necessary to put short shoes on all flat feet, particularly on those which have the form of an oyster-shell. Every flat foot has low heels; but nature, to remedy this defect, bestows a large frog to preserve these parts. We ought not, then, to pare the soles, much less cut them out towards the heels; neither should the hoofs be too much rasped; all these practices are so many abuses which bring about the destruction of the horses' feet. The first abuse —hollowing out the heels, is to destroy the horn which forms the bars and prevents the heels and quarters from contracting; the second abuse—rasping the foot, is to destroy the strength of the hoof, and consequently to cause its horn to become dry and the horny laminæ beneath to grow weak; from this often arises an internal inflammation, which renders the foot painful and makes the horse go lame.'

It ought to be always remembered, that the more a horse's foot is pared, so the more do we expose it to accidents; it is depriving it, in the first place, of a defence that nature has given it against the *hard* and *pointed* substances it encounters; and, in the second place, and which is of the utmost advantage for both horse and rider, in not paring the sole, and only using as much of a shoe as is necessary to protect the horn, the animal will be no longer liable to slip on bad roads in winter or summer, when they are vulgarly called *plombé*, as will be shown.

' 1. Causing a horse to walk on the frog and partly on the heel, the former is found to be rasped by the friction it experiences on the earth and paved road, and is pressed by the weight of the body into the little cavities and interstices it meets.

'2. By its flexibility, it takes the imprint and the contour, so to speak, of the ground it comes into contact with ; so that the foot rests on a greater number of parts, which, mutually assisting each other, multiply the points of support, and thereby give the animal more adherence to the surface on which he moves. We may even say that he acquires a kind of feeling in this part, through its correspondence with the fleshy sole, and from this to the tendon—a feeling that I will not compare with that we experience when we walk with naked feet, but which is yet sufficient to warn him of the counterpoise he ought to give to his body to maintain its equilibrium, and so pre-serve him from falling, twisting, or stumbling.

'The object of shoeing, by him who first resorted to it, would only be as a preservative and a defence, as much for the wall as for the sole. But he would not add the condition of paring either the one or the other, I do not say to our excess, but in any way whatever, because this would be contrary to his principle, and would destroy his work.

'This precaution (paring) can only be recommended in cases where the horn is rugged, and the shoe does not rest on it everywhere equally, thus opposing its solidity. In such a case it is right, but otherwise it is a contradiction and an absurdity. I have often questioned those amateur horsemen who were particularly careful to have their horses' feet pared, but none of them could demonstrate either its necessity or propriety. . . . The horny sole receives its nourishment from the vascular sole; its softness and pliancy are due to its thickness, and its nourishment is diminished, while it becomes harder, in direct proportion to the thinness we give it; we even see horses whose soles are pared, habitually lame. The air, when the sole is in this state of thinness, penetrates and dries it to such a degree, that if care is not taken to keep it damp when the animal is in a dry place, it contracts and presses on the vascular sole; so that, if some time after we wish to pare the sole again, it is not possible to do so, because it is so hard and dry that the boutoir will not touch it, and the horse goes lame. . . . What risk does a horse not incur who has nearly been deprived of his soles through this paring! If he encounters stones broken glass, or nails, these easily penetrate to the sensitive sole, and cripple him for a long time, if not for ever.

'When a horse loses a shoe — a circumstance frequently occurring, and if the hoof is pared, the animal cannot walk a hundred steps without going lame; because in this state the lower surface of the foot being hollowed, the horse's weight falls on the crust, and this having no support from the horny sole, is quickly broken and worn away; and if he meets hard substances on the road, he all the more speedily becomes lame. It is not so when the sole is allowed to retain its whole strength. The shoe comes off, but the sole and frog rest on the ground, assist the crust in bearing the greater part of the weight of the body, and the animal, though unshod, is able to pursue his journey safe and sound.

'It is a fact that every horse, except those which have the feet diseased and soles convex, and to which shoes are necessary to preserve the soles, may travel without shoes ; and without going for an example to the Arabs, Tartars, etc., we will find it among our own horses, which, in the country, work every day without requiring shoes ; but as soon as our wisdom and skill is brought to bear in hollowing out the foot to the quick and making a fine, equal, and symmetrical frog—doing it well and properly, as we say in France, shoes become indispensably necessary.

'I therefore ask all amateur horsemen to insure their horses as much as they can against this pretended perfection. It may be asked, what will become of the horny sole if it is never pared, and it may be feared that by its growth the foot will become overgrown. Not at all; for in proportion to its growth it dries, becomes flaky, and falls off in layers.

'The compressions so dangerous, which cause inflammation, would no more be dreaded if we left the horn of the sole, the bars, and the frog entire. By their pliability, thickness, flexibility, texture, and the situation they occupy, they appear to be solely destined by nature to serve as a defence to the vascular sole, as the frog particularly acts as a cushion to the tendo achillis—all being disposed to obviate shock on paved roads, or injury from a stone, splinter, etc.

'It is necessary to be convinced of another fact : this is, that it is rare that a horse goes at his ease, and is not promptly fatigued, if the frog does not touch the ground. As it is the only point of support, if you raise it from the ground by paring it, there arises an inordinate extension of the tendon, caused by the pushing of the coronary against the navicular bone, as has been mentioned above, and which, being repeated at every step the animal takes, fatigues it, and induces inflammation. From thence often arises the distention of the sheaths of tendons (*molettes—* vulgo, " windgalls "), engorgements and swelling of the tendons, etc., that are observed after long or rapid journeys. These accidents arise less from the length of the journey, as has been currently believed, than from the false practice of paring the sole.

' I am astonished that this method of shoeing has not been employed long ago, and I have much trouble in persuading myself that I am the inventor. I am more inclined to believe that it is only a copy of that which has been practised by the first artist who thought about shoeing horses.

' If my suspicions are correct, the oblivion into which it has fallen proves nothing against its perfection, because the good as well as the bad are alike liable to be forgotten. The multitude, more credulous than enlightened, are easily persuaded; hence the long thick shoes, those with calkins, then with thick heels, and afterwards the thin. There is every reason to believe that if the poor animals for whom all this has been done could be allowed to speak as they must think, nothing of the kind would have taken place, and they would have preferred their ancient armature, which, having only been designed to preserve the crust, had certainly none of the inconveniences of that employed now-a-days.'

Lafosse's experience of this admirable mode of protecting, while preserving, the foot, was derived from a trial of its advantages on more than 1800 horses; and his success was most astonishing, though no more than might, on reflection, be anticipated.

'These short shoes, thin at the heels, have caused the horses to walk on their frogs, which are their points of support, and those which were lame at the heels are sound again; those also whose inside quarters were contracted, bent over, and split (sandcrack), have been cured. It has been the same with horses whose quarters and heels have been contracted (*encastelé*) : these have been widened, and have assumed a proper shape. The same may be said of those whose soles were convex (*comblé*), and which went lame with long shoes. My method has also preserved those horses which had a tendency to thrush (*vulgo*, " fic ") and canker of the frog (*crapaud*).

'If the horse be shod with calkins, there is a great space between the frog and the ground; the weight of the body comes on the calkins; the frog, which is in the air, cedes to the weight; the tendon is elongated; and if the horse makes a violent and sudden movement, the rupture of that organ is almost inevitable, because the frog cannot reach the ground to support it in the very place it ought to; and if the tendon does not break, the horse is lame for a long time from the great extension of the fibres, some of which may have been ruptured   If the horse be shod without heels to his shoes (*éponges*), the frog, which carries all the weight of the horse's body, yields at each step, and returns again to its original form. The tendon is never in a state of distraction; its fibres are no longer susceptible of violent distension during a sudden movement. I will go so far as to assert, that rupture of the tendon will never occur on a flat pavement; if it does, it

will be in the space between two paving-stones. Two
things clearly follow from what I have said—that it may
happen that the tendon achillis sustains all the different
degrees of violence that can be imagined, from total rupture to the smallest abrasion of its fibres, which will cause
the horse to go lame; and it is on the frog alone that all
these different degrees depend, as has been demonstrated
more particularly in the history of fracture of the navicular bone and the anatomy of the foot.'

After enumerating all the objections urged against his
rational method of shoeing, and replying to them, he
concludes: 'My new shoeing, I repeat, has nothing to
oppose it but prejudice; anatomy, which has made
known to me the structure of the foot, has demonstrated
all its advantages, and experience has fully confirmed
them.'

I regret extremely that our limits forbid my trans-
lating at greater length from this splendid monograph;
but I hope that I have been able to some extent to show
that Lafosse's ideas on shoeing were founded on sound
anatomical and physiological principles, the result of
close observation and experience. And yet they appear
to have made but little progress in the face of the opposition offered by ignorant grooms and farriers, who were
incompetent to understand anything but the mere every-
day routine of the rapidly degenerating art; and the prejudice of those amateur horsemen who, though the last
perhaps to take upon trust statements relative to other
matters, would yet believe everything told them by these
horse attendants and shoers. The farriers of Paris, indeed,
unanimously protested against the innovation two years

after Lafosse had published his treatise, and their protest appears to have carried the mind of the crowd.[1]

Bourgelat,[2] the illustrious founder of those French veteri nary schools, which have done that country such honour and rendered her agriculture such great service, introduced another system of farriery, which has prevailed more or less in France until the present time. ' Shoeing,' says this professor, ' is a methodical action of the hand on the feet of animals, on which it is practicable and necessary. By it the foot of the horse, principally, ought to be main-tained in the condition in which it is found if its con-formation is good and regular, and its defects should be repaired by shoeing if it is found vicious and deformed. By shoeing, also, it is often possible to remedy the inevit-able consequences of disproportions between various parts of the body, or at least to modify their effects . . . . . to obviate those which result from defectiveness in the direc-tion of the limbs . . . . . to facilitate, to a certain degree, freedom and regularity in the execution of movements . . . . . and to prevent those false positions of the limbs to which certain habits appear to dispose them.' The nails were to be regularly disposed between the toe and the heel, and the shoe bent up or *adjusted* in such a way

[1] Réponse à la Nouvelle Pratique de Ferrer du Sieur Lafosse. Par les Maîtres Maréchaux de Paris. Paris, 1758.

[2] Essai Théorique et Pratique sur la Ferrure. Paris, 1771, 1804. There were also published in France about this period :—

Ronden. Observations sur des *A*rticles Concernant la Marécba-lerie. Paris, 1759.

Hérissant. Médecine des Chevaux. Paris, 1763.

Weyrother. Le Parfait Ecuyer Militaire de Campagne. Paris, 1768.

Druts. L'Anti-Maréchal. Liege, 1773.

Chalert. Ferrure des Chevaux. Paris, 1782.

that, seen in profile, it looked like a cradle, and would appear to afford anything but a solid or easy footing. The total length of the ordinary fore-shoe was to be four times the length of the toe between the two first holes and the posterior or inner border. 'The distance of the external border from the one and other branch, this measure being taken between the two last or heel-nails, should be three and a half times this length, one-half of which will give the proper width of the heels to their very extremities. With regard to the adjusture, the toe should be curved up (*en bateau*) from the second nails from the heel to twice the thickness of the shoe, reckoning from the ground to the upper edge of the shoe at this part; it is necessary also that from this situation the extremities should rise up towards the heels to one-half its real thickness, and from thence the convexity should be one and a half times its thickness' (fig. 186). This mode of shoeing was adapted to the *aplomb* and the movements of the limbs, Bourgelat thought; and his reasoning on this shows that at least he had carefully studied the mechanical problems of progression. There

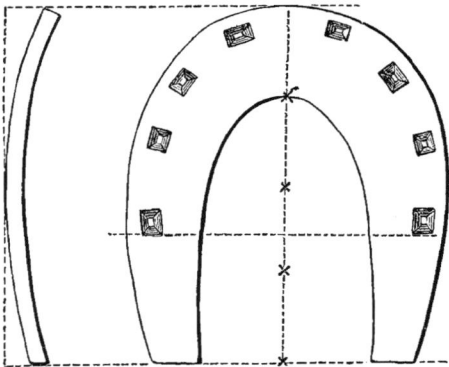

fig. 186

was nothing in the way of novelty, however, in the curvature of the shoe; we have shown in figures 56, 57, and 66, that ancient specimens found in Belgium and Germany were so adjusted, and to about the same degree. Some of Bourgelat's maxims on shoeing were very good, especially the second, in which he particularly insists on abstaining from opening up the heels. 'The second maxim in good shoeing is *never to open the horse's heels;* this is the greatest abuse, and ruins the majority of feet.' 'Opening the heels' is when the farrier, in paring the foot, cuts the heel close to the frog, carrying the opening to within a finger's breadth of the coronet, so as to separate the quarters from the heel, and by this means the foot is weakened, and made to contract. That which is called *opening a heel* is in reality contracting it, for the roundness or circumference of the hoof being cut in this ' opening,' there is nothing left to sustain the heels; therefore it inevitably happens, if there is any weakness in the foot, that it contracts. If the farriers were careful of their reputation and mindful of their duty, they would make this maxim one of the principal points in their statutes.'

Any one who has had much to do with horses, or visited a shoeing forge, will know that it is customary to adjust or *try on* the new shoe while it is in a hot state, so as to obtain for it a more solid and secure bearing on the hoof, and to fit it better. Before the 18th century, it is probable that the hoof-armature was usually adjusted in a cold state, a practice which has many disadvantages. Cæsar Fiaschi seems to corroborate this, when he says of the shoeing of his day: 'Je ne vois d'autre remède, eu égard au peu de solidité de cette ferrure, que de savoir soi-même brocher les clous ou de se faire suivre par un maréchal.' He nevertheless speaks of fitting the shoe while it was hot. At any rate, it is not until 1736 that we find the first mention of the *ferrure à chaud,* combined with burning the hoofs in order to rob them more easily of their horn. Laguerinière[1] speaks of the farriers *burning the horny sole, to make it the more easily pared,* and the dangers of this practice. 'On doit bien se donner garde de souffrir qu'on brûle les pieds aux chevaux avec un fer chaud, comme font la plupart des maréchaux, afin qu'ils soient plus aisés à parer.' Then he speaks of the clips of the shoe only being made hot to fit it to the foot of carriage horses: 'Mais, comme pour les chevaux de carrosse on est obligé de mettre un pinçon à la pince du fer, dans cette occasion on ne peut se dispenser de faire chauffer ce pinçon, afin qu'il puisse s'enfoncer dans la corne ; mais tout le reste du fer doit être froid.' And Lafosse, in 1756, as we have seen, speaks of the *sole chauffée* and the *sole brulée ;* so that in this interval the farriers had resorted to the expedient of heating all the sole, in order to make it more easily yield to the paring-knife, though it is recommended that the shoe should be fitted while in a hot state to the hoof.

In Laguerinière, we find the first mention of clips being used to aid in retaining the shoes. In all the ancient specimens I have examined, nothing of the kind is to be found ; though frequently the toe of the shoe is slightly curved upwards, perhaps to serve as a clip, and a nail is sometimes driven into the centre of the toe, as in the Hod Hill specimen, with the same object.

Lafosse[2] the younger repeats, in a great measure, the recommendations of his father, and appears to have tested the merits of his method ; so that it is scarcely necessary to

[1] Traité sur l'Ecole de Cavalerie.   Paris, 1733.
[2] Cours d'Hippiatrique.   3rd edition.   Paris, 1772.

do more than refer to his half-circle shoeing, which was intended, like that of his parent, to prevent horses from slipping on the stones ·

'*Half-circle shoeing for Carriage Horses.* As the preceding method of shoeing would not prevent the horse from slipping when he first places his foot on slippery ground, seeing that the toe comes down before the other parts, and that is entirely covered with iron, we use a half-circle shoe. This ought to be on the sides from the nail-holes more exact than the foot, and put on in such a manner that the whole of the crust projects beyond one-half of its thickness around its circumference.

'After reasonably shortening the foot with the corner of the boutoir, a groove is made within the wall adjoining the horny sole; into this channel the hot shoe is fitted. It is afterwards attached with small nails, whose heads are to be half buried in the holes, and the sharp margin of the crust is to be rasped away, to prevent chipping of the horn. With this shoeing, the horse goes on the whole of the crust, either in ascending or descending.

'*A third kind of half-circle shoeing for Saddle Horses.* The half-circle or shoe ought to be from two to three lines in width, and one and a half in thickness. It ought to have 10 holes equally distributed and counter-pierced on the same side; consequently, the nails should be very small. It is placed in the same manner as the preceding, from which it only differs in width and in having one hole more. A horse shod in this manner is lighter; his movements are more elastic, firmer on a dry slippery pavement, and are more agreeable to the rider.'

In England, a treatise on the anatomy and diseases of

the horse's foot, exhibiting some improvement in the anatomical details at least, was published by Jeremiah Bridges.[1] After enumerating the various parts of the foot and their characteristics, as they were known in his day, he proceeds to specify the best kinds of hoofs, and in doing so casually informs us, that the horses bred in Derbyshire, the mountainous parts of England and Wales, as well as in the Highlands of Scotland, have good feet; while those reared on low marshy ground, such as the fens of Lincolnshire, have commonly flat and soft feet, arising from the moist soil, which relaxes their texture.

'The best method to keep the foot sound is good shoeing; liberty, sometimes, in pasture; or proper exercise. Standing long in stables contracts the feet.' 'The usefulness of a horse's shoes is too obvious to want many words to explain; they are a guard to the foot.' Among the newer inventions yet spoken of, he enumerates the 'screw shoe.' 'The design of this shoe is to relieve and help nature, by extending the hoof and heels when drawn in or contracted, to remove the causes which obstruct a free and regular circulation, by restoring the parts affected to their proper size and position. This it performs by means of two ridges fixed on the inside of the shoe towards the back part; these pressing gradually and equally on the inside of the hoof, the contracted horny parts are mastered, and give way to the operation of the screw, which opens the heels. This may be forwarded in desperate cases, when the hoof is quite contracted, and the

[1] No Foot, No Horse; an Essay on the Anatomy of the Foot of that Noble and Useful Animal—a Horse. By J. Bridges, Farrier and Anatomist. London, 1751.

horse a cripple, by making five cuts or scissures on the outside of the hoof to the quick. In some cases, when the heels only are contracted, two are sufficient, but in many the shoe alone will answer the end. To remedy this disorder in the foot, proceeding from contracted hoofs and heels drawn in, where the complaint is slight, a shoe may be made for the horse to work in, with a feather (flange or clip) on the under side, as occasion may require, which gradually pressing on the inside of the heel, the weight of the horse as he treads forces the hoof outwards. If both heels be drawn or wired in, a feather must be made accordingly on each side.' We have here Carlo Ruini's shoe. This treatise, from the enumeration of the maladies contained in it, plainly shows what an amount of torture must have been suffered by the unfortunate horses of the last century. The fashion of excessive paring of the hoofs, heavy shoes, and faulty nailing, is strongly commented upon by Mr Bridges. The use of the 'butteris' and 'drawing knives' for removing the hoof and 'making the foot fit to the shoe, instead of the shoe to the foot,' is particularly reprobated.

In 1723, a set of new shoes cost two shillings.[1]

A century after Blundevil, and nearly contemporary with Lafosse, whom he carefully studies and to some extent copies, comes W. Osmer.[2] In several respects his work is much superior to that of Blundevil, and we have abundant evidence in it to prove that scientific shoeing, founded on a study of the anatomy and physiology of

---

[1] Notes and Queries, vol. ii. p. 186.

[2] A Treatise on the Diseases and Lameness of Horses. 3rd edition. London, 1766.

the horse's foot, was making progress. Though Osmer's observations are mainly based on the teachings of Lafosse, yet he does not blindly follow that celebrity, but having carefully tested the mode of shoeing advocated in the 'Nouvelle Pratique,' points out its defects in a very fair and reasonable manner. He is the first writer on this subject who gives us a good idea of the way in which the art was practised in England; and in doing this, he is particularly severe with those artisans whom Hogarth, in his picture of the 'Enraged Musician,' has delineated as wearing a cross-belt of bright blue decorated with golden horse-shoes, the badge of the peripatetic farrier. 'If you pretend to have your horse shod according to your own mind, it is a general saying amongst these men that they do not want to be taught; which is as much as to say, in other words, there is nothing known in their art, or ever will be, but what they already are acquainted with

If you ask one of these artists his reason for acting in this or that particular manner, or should inquire of him the use of any part assigned to some particular end, he can give no answer, nor even pretends to have any knowledge thereof, but is guided by custom alone.'

After remarking on the necessity for shoeing in some countries and not in others, and the probable simplicity of the earlier attempts to defend the hoofs, he says, 'in process of time, the fertility of invention, and the vanity of mankind, have produced variety of methods, almost all of which are productive of lameness; and I am thoroughly convinced, from observation and experience, that 19 lame horses of every 20 in this kingdom, are lame of the artist, which is owing to the form of the shoe, his ignorance of the design of nature, and maltreatment of the foot, every part of which is made for some purpose or other—though he does not happen to know it. . . . I suppose it will be universally assented to, that whatever method of shoeing approaches nearest to the law of nature, such is likely to be the most perfect method.' Agreeing perfectly with Lafosse as to the grave injury inflicted on the feet by paring the soles and frog, and opening the heels, he is careful in explaining the functions of these parts. 'The frog, together with the bars, occupying the hinder part of the foot, is designed by nature to distend and keep it open, which, when cut away, suffer the heels, the quarters, and the *coronary ring* to become contracted, whereby another lameness is produced, which shall be treated in its proper place.'

This lameness is the 'navicular disease,' supposed to be first described by Mr Turner of London some thirty years ago. Osmer distinctly mentions it: 'I have seen many instances of sudden lameness brought on horses in hunting and in racing, by a false step, which have continued lame their whole life-time; and upon examination, I have found the ligaments of the nut-bone (*os naviculare*) rendered useless for want of timely assistance and knowledge of the cause; from hence the cartilages of the same have been sometimes ossified, and the bones of the foot have been sometimes wasted, and sometimes enlarged, it being no uncommon thing to meet a horse whose feet are not fellows, the natural form of the injured foot being generally altered hereby; and nothing can contribute more to such an accident than the unequal pressure of the foot in our modern concave shoe.' Elsewhere he speaks of the

32 *

erosion of the cartilage of the navicular bone, and the symptoms indicative of this foot disease. And long before this period, contracted hoofs arising from undue paring by the *maréchal*, and lameness resulting therefrom, were, as we have seen, often mentioned. But the unknown author of the 'Grand Maréchal, Expert et Français,' published at Toulouse in 1701, not only gives us this information, but actually describes the neurotomy operation for the relief of this lameness, the *discovery* of which in 1816, by Professor Sewell, of London, has almost immortalized his name. Here is the *modus operandi :* 'Vous coucherez le cheval, ensuite lui ouvrirez la partie où l'on barre la veine, et en tirerez le nerf avec la petite corne ; après quoi vous le graisserez avec du populleum, et il guerira.'

Osmer continues his discourse on the treatment of the horse's hoof in shoeing. 'The spongy, skin-like substance (of the frog) is not to be cut away till it becomes ragged, because it is the expansion of the skin round the heel, its use being to unite more firmly the foot and its contents, and to keep the cellular part of the heel from growing rigid; it also surrounds the coronary ring, and may be observed to peel and dry away as it descends on the hoof.' This skin-like substance is the coronary frogband Bracy Clark claims the credit of being the first to notice, in 1809.

After laying it down as a rule that the crust or wall should only be removed in a degree proportionate to the growth, he goes on to say: 'In all broad fleshy feet, the crust is thin, and should therefore suffer the least possible loss. On such feet the rasp alone is generally sufficient to make the bottom plain, and produce a sound founda_tion, *without the use of the desperate buttress* (the French

boutoir, the *butter* of Blundevil). . . . The superficies of
the foot round the outside now made plain and smooth,
the shoe is to be made *quite flat*, of an equal thickness
all round the outside, and open and most narrow back--
wards, at the extremities of the heels, for the generality
of horses,—those whose frogs are diseased, either from
natural or incidental causes, require the shoe to be wider
backwards; and to prevent this flat shoe from pressing
on the sole of the horse, the outer part thereof is to be
made thickest, and the inside gradually thinner.   In such
a shoe the frog is admitted to touch the ground, the necessity of which has been already shown; add to this, the
horse stands more firmly on the ground, having the same
points of support as in a natural state.   Here now is a
plain, easy method, agreeable to common sense and reason,
conformable to the anatomical structure of the parts, and
therefore to the design of nature—a method so plain that
one would think nobody could ever swerve from it, or
commit any mistake in an art where nothing is required
but to make smooth the surface of the foot, to know
what loss of crust each kind of foot will bear with advantage to itself, and to nail thereon a piece of iron,
adapted to the natural tread of the horse; the design,
good, or use of the iron, being only to defend the crust
from breaking, *the sole wanting no defence, if never pared.*
. . . . The modern artist uses little difference in the treatment of any kind of foot; but with a strong arm and a
sharp weapon carries all before him, and will take more
from a weak-footed horse at one paring, than nature can
furnish again in some months, whereby such are rendered
lame.   If a strong-footed horse, with narrow and con-

tracted heels, be brought before him, such meets with treatment yet more severe; the bar is scooped out, the frog trimmed, and the sole drawn as thin as possible, even to the quick, under pretence of giving him ease; because, he says, he is hot-footed, or foundered. By which treatment, the horse is rendered more lame than he was before.' This causes contraction of the hoof and compression of the parts within; and, besides, a shoe was applied thin on the outer circumference and thick on the inner, which, being concave to the foot and convex to the ground, afforded but few points of support, removed the frog from pressure, and caused great mischief. I possess some specimens of this terrible instrument of last-century barbarism. It almost makes one shudder to think of the fearful agony the poor horses must have suffered, when compelled to wear and work with it.

Osmer continues: 'Let the shoe on every horse stand wider at the points of the heels than the foot itself; otherwise, as the foot grows in length, the heel of the shoe in a short time gets within the heel of the horse; which pressure often breaks the crust, produces a temporary lameness, perhaps a corn. Let every kind of foot be kept as short at the toe as possible (so as not to affect the quick), for by a long toe, the foot becomes thin and weak, the heels low, and the flexor tendons of the leg are strained; the shortness of the toe helps also to widen the narrow heels. In all thin, weak-footed horses the rasp should be laid on the toe in such a manner as to render it as thick as may be; by which means the whole foot becomes gradually thicker, higher, and stronger. In all feet whose texture is very strong, the rasp may be laid obliquely on the fore part of the foot, towards the toe, and the toe itself thinned, whereby the compression on the parts is rendered somewhat less, by diminishing the strength of the hoof or crust.

'But this rasp is to be used with discretion, lest the crust being too thin, and not able to support the weight of the horse, a sandcrack ensue; which frequently happens from too free or unskilful use of this tool, and from the natural rigid texture of the coronet. The heel of the shoe, on all strong and narrow-heeled horses, should be made strait at the extreme points; the form of the shoe in some measure helping to distend the heel of the horse. For the same reason, the shoe on no horse should be continued farther than the point of the heel. It has been already said that neither frog nor sole should ever be pared; nevertheless, it must be understood that it is impossible to pare the crust without taking away some of the adjacent sole, and it is also requisite, in order to obtain a smooth and even surface, so far as the breadth of the shoe reaches, and no farther. The frog also will become ragged, and loose pieces will occasionally separate from the body thereof, perhaps in one foot, and not in the other. When this happens, it should be cut away with a knife, to prevent the gravel lodging therein. But if it be left to the artist to do, he will be sure to take away more of it at one time than will grow again in many weeks.'

He advocates calkins, or 'corking' the shoes, in winter only, when the ground is soft and slippery; and then says of his recommendations: 'This method of treating the foot, and such a kind of shoe as has been described, I have used many years; and, to the best of my remembrance, have not had a horse lame since, except when pricked by the artist; and it is a matter of the greatest astonishment to me, how any other form of a shoe could ever come into general use　　This flat shoe is not to be made with a smooth surface, after the French manner, *but channelled round, or what is called fullered, after the English manner;*[1] by which the horse is better prevented from sliding about, and the heads of the nails are less liable to be broken off; both which inconveniences attend the shoe whose surface is smooth.'

The best mode of preventing horses from 'cutting' is next dealt with; and in treating of the value of turning horses out to grass without shoes, we learn that Osmer was perfectly cognizant of the expansive properties of the horse's foot, about which so much discussion and discovery has been made in this century, though his views are rational and perfectly correct; which is more than can be said for those of the majority of succeeding theorists. He admits the value of Lafosse's 'lunette' or 'crescent' shoes, in certain cases, chiefly in those where the hoofs are contracted: 'In such a shoe the heel of the horse rests in some measure upon the ground, receives some share of weight, and is, by means of such weight and pressure, kept open and expanded; by which expansion of the heels the compression on the interior parts of narrow-footed horses is removed, and he that was before lame is, by degrees, as the foot spreads, rendered sound—if there be no disease in the interior parts of the foot. Again, where horses have

---

[1] Osmer is the first writer I can discover in England who speaks of this 'fullering' as English. The reader will remember it as Burgundian, or rather German, and prevalent in the fifth century.

feet inclined to the other extreme, whose heels are weak and low, if the shoe be set somewhat short at the points of the heel, such will, by degrees, improve and grow higher. Yet an English farrier can never be prevailed on to believe that weak low heels will become stronger by leaving them exposed to hard objects. But it must be expected that horses with weak or diseased feet, who have been accustomed to go in long, broad shoes, will at first go very lame in shoes which are either short or narrow. And many that are lame of the shoer with various disorders in their feet, would be cured by Lafosse's shoes, *if the frog, sole, and bars were not pared out. But when those things which are designed by the Divine artist as a natural defence to the interior part, are cut away by the* superior wisdom *of our earthly artists, why then, undoubtedly, Lafosse's shoes will not do, for the horse requires some artificial defence to supply the loss of the natural one.* Now it is the weight, unequal pressure, form and action of the iron made use of to protect the foot when it is thus horribly abridged by our artists, that is productive of almost all the evils incident to horses' feet.' These words of Mr Osmer are as true and applicable at the present day as they were more than a century ago. This writer also speaks of the drawing-knife—a weapon quite as, if not more, destructive

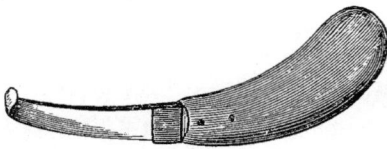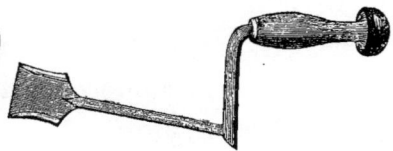

fig 187   fig 188

than the *boutoir*, both of which are here represented (figs. 187, 188).

Mr J. Clark's excellent treatise,[1] dedicated to the Earl of Pembroke, and published twenty years later, is also a protest against the destructive and cruel mode of managing horses' feet, and the vicious character of the shoes applied to them. The science of veterinary medicine was rapidly advancing; its practitioners were, many of them, men of education and observation, and the gap between the *shoer,* —the man of routine, and the man of science, was gradually widening; so that farriery, properly so called, soon lagged behind; and all the teaching of such men as Blundevil, Osmer, Clark, and others, could not move it from its degraded state. Much of this was due, however, to the pernicious influence of ignorant grooms and others, who, trusted implicitly in this matter by their employers, prejudiced them against the introduction of improvements, the aim of which they had not sufficient intelligence to understand. 'However necessary it has been found to fix iron shoes upon the hoofs of horses, it is certainly contrary to the original design of shoeing them, first to destroy their hoofs by paring, &c., and afterwards to put on the foot a broad strong shoe to protect what remains, or rather to supply the defect or want of that substance which has been taken away. Yet, however absurd this manner of treating the feet of horses may appear, it is well known that it has been carried to a very great length, and still continues to be thought absolutely necessary. The destruction of their hoofs, and many other bad consequences arising from it, are every day but too apparent.' So says Mr Clark. The Earl of Pembroke, in his work on

---

[1] Observations on the Shoeing of Horses. By J. Clark, Farrier to His Majesty for Scotland. 3rd edition. Edinburgh, 1782.

Horsemanship, published some years previously, writes:
' Physic and a *butteris*, in well-informed hands, would not
be fatal; but in the manner we are now provided with
farriers, they must be quite banished. Whoever at present lets his farrier, groom, or coachman, in consideration
of his having swept dung out of the stables for a greater
or less number of years, ever even mention anything more
than water-gruel, a clyster, or a little bleeding, and that,
too, very seldom; or pretend to talk of the nature of feet,
of the seat of lamenesses, sicknesses, or their cures, may
be certain to find himself very shortly quite on foot, and
fondly arms an absurd and inveterate enemy against his
own interest. It is incredible what tricking knaves most
stable-people are, and what daring attempts they will make
to gain an ascendant over their masters, in order to have
their own foolish projects complied with. In shoeing, for
example, I have more than once known that, for the sake
of establishing their own ridiculous and pernicious system,
when their masters have differed from it, they have, on
purpose, lamed horses, and imputed the fault to the shoes,
after having in vain tried, by every sort of invention and
lies, to discredit the use of them. How can the method
of such people be commendable, whose arguments, as well
as practice, are void of common sense? If your horse's
foot be bad and brittle, they advise you to cover it with a
very heavy shoe; the consequence of which proceeding is
evident: for how should the foot, which before could scarce
carry itself, be able afterwards to carry such an additional
weight, which is stuck on, moreover, with a multitude of
nails, the holes of which tear and weaken the hoof? The
only system all these simpletons seem to agree in, is to shoe

in general with excessive heavy and clumsy, ill-shaped shoes, and very many nails, to the total destruction of the foot. The cramps (French *crampon*, Anglice *calkin*) they annex tend to destroy the bullet (fetlock—Fr. *boulet*), and the shoes, made in the shape of a walnut-shell, prevent the horse's walking upon the firm basis which God has given him for that end, and thereby oblige him to stumble and fall. They totally pare away, also, and lay bare the inside of the animal's foot with their detestable butteris, and afterwards put on very long shoes, whereby the foot is hindered from having any pressure at all upon the heels, which pressure might still perchance, notwithstanding their dreadful cutting, keep the heels properly open, and the foot in good order.'

Mr Clark informs us that, in his day, horses in the North and West parts of Scotland, and in Wales, went always without shoes, and ' performed all manner of work without any detriment to their hoofs, which, from being accustomed to go bare, and rubbing or touching fre-quently against hard bodies, like the hands of a labouring man, they acquire a callousness and obduracy which greatly adds to their firmness.' In Prussia, too, it was only customary to shoe them on the fore-feet. ' In Ger-many they use thick, heavy, strong shoes, with three cramps or caukers, one on each heel and one on the toe of the shoe.'

In describing the anatomy of the foot, he explains that 'in the middle of the frog is a longitudinal cleft or opening, *by which the heels have a small degree of con-traction and expansion at every tread which the horse makes upon the ground;* ' and, speaking of the hoof, he remarks that the sole and frog, by being exposed to wear, acquire great firmness and tenacity, which enables them to resist external injuries. 'But no apology whatever can vindicate that pernicious practice of cutting and paring their hoofs to that excess which is but too frequently done every time a horse is shoed, and, in order to repair the injury done to the foot, fix on it a strong, broad-brimmed shoe, from the very construction of which, together with the loss of its natural defence, horses, too frequently, are rendered totally useless.' 'In preparing the foot for the shoe, the frog, the sole, and the bars or binders, are pared so much that the blood frequently appears. The shoe by its form, being thick on the inside of the rim and thin upon the outside, must of consequence be made concave or hollow on that side which is placed immediately next the foot, in order to prevent its resting on the sole. The shoes are generally of an immoderate weight and length, and every means is used to prevent the frog from resting upon the ground by making the shoe-heels thick, broad, and strong, or raising cramps or caukers on them. From this form of the shoe, and from this method of treating the hoof, the frog is raised to a considerable height above the ground, the heels are deprived of that substance which was provided by nature to keep the crust extended at a proper wideness, and the foot is fixed as it were in a mould' 'If we attend further to the convex surface of this shoe, and the convexity of the pavement upon which horses walk, it will then be evident that it is impossible for them to keep their feet from slipping, especially upon declivities of streets. It is also a common practice, especially in this place, to turn up the heels of the shoes into what is called cramps or caukers, by which means the weight of the horse is confined to a very narrow surface—the inner round edge of the shoe-rim, and the points or caukers of each heel; the consequence is, that it throws the weight of the body forward upon the toes, and is apt to make the horse slip and stumble.' The shoes in use appear to have been possessed of every bad quality, and must have inflicted fearful torture upon the unlucky animals compelled to wear them, particularly after the outrageous manner in which their hoofs were pared. 'Farriers, in general, are too desirous to excel one another in making what is termed fine neat work; and that is no other than paring the sole till it yields easily under the pressure of the thumb; and to give the frog a fine shape, it is frequently pared till the blood appears, to prevent the effusion of which the actual cautery is sometimes applied. It is to be observed, that, when the sole is so much pared, it dries and hardens in proportion as it is thinned; and the strong horny substance of the crust, overcoming the resistance from the sole, is thereby contracted. This will produce lameness, the real cause of which is overlooked or little attended to. Among the many disadvantages that attend the common shoes, one is, their being more liable to be pulled off, from their great weight, length, &c., especially in deep ground, in riding fast, or when the toe of the hinder foot strikes against the heel of the fore-shoe. To prevent this inconvenience, *sixteen or eighteen nails* are frequently made use of, which destroy and weaken the crust by their being placed too near one another; and it is not uncommon, when a shoe nailed in this manner is pulled off, that the crust on the outside of the nails breaks away with it. If this should happen a few days after the foot has been so finely pared (which is not unusual), or upon a journey, and at a distance from any place where a shoe may be immediately procured, the horse instantly becomes lame, from the thinness of the sole and weakness of the crust, and is hardly able to support the weight of his own body, much less that of his rider.'

This able writer gives two drawings of one of these terrible instruments of torture—the foot and ground surface of an ordinary shoe (figs. 189, 190).

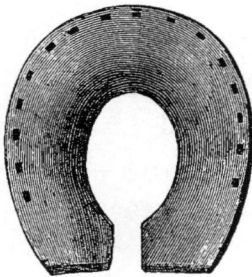 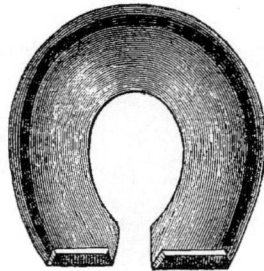

fig. 189   fig 190

The shoe recommended to be worn by Mr Clark is that described by Osmer, though he says it was employed by him many years before that veterinarian's treatise was published. 'In shoeing a horse we should in this, as in every other case, study to follow nature; and certainly that shoe which is made of such a form as to resemble as near as possible the natural tread and shape of the foot, must be preferable to any other. . . . . In order that we may imitate the natural tread of the foot, the shoe must be made flat, if the height of the sole does not forbid it; it must be of an equal thickness all around the outside of the rim (for a draught-horse about half an inch thick, and less in proportion for a saddle-horse); and on that a narrow rim or margin is to be formed, not exceeding the breadth of the crust upon which it is to rest, with the nail-holes placed exactly in the middle; and, from this narrow rim, the shoe is to be made gradually thinner towards its inner edge (figs. 191, 192). The breadth of

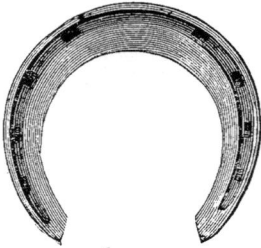 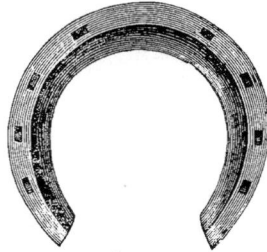

fig 191   fig. 192

the shoe is to be regulated by the size of the foot and the work to which the horse is accustomed; but, in general, it should be made rather broad at the toe, and narrow towards the extremity of each heel, in order to let the frog rest with freedom upon the ground. The shoe being thus formed and shaped like the foot, the surface of the crust is to be made smooth, and the shoe fixed on with eight, or at most ten, nails, the heads of which should be sunk into the holes, so as to be equal with the surface of the shoe. The sole, frog, and bars should never be pared.'

This, it will be at once perceived, is nothing more or less than the modern seated-shoe which Mr Clark recommends; but he appears to have met the usual amount of opposition. 'So much are farriers, grooms, etc., prejudiced in favour of the common method of shoeing and paring out the feet, that it is with difficulty they can even be prevailed upon to make a proper trial of it. They cannot be satisfied unless the frog be finely shaped, the sole pared, the bars cut out, in order to make the heels appear wide. This practice gives them a show of wideness for the time; yet that, together with the concave form of the shoe, forwards the contraction of the heels, which, when confirmed, renders the animal lame for life. In this flat form of shoe its thickest part is upon the outside of the rim, where it is most exposed to be worn; and being made gradually thinner towards its inner edge, it is therefore much lighter than the common concave shoe, yet it will last equally as long, and with more advantage to the hoof; and as the frog and heel is allowed to rest upon the ground, the foot enjoys the same points of support as in its natural state. It must therefore be much easier for the horse in his way of going, and be a means of making him surer-footed. It is likewise evident that from this shoe the hoof cannot acquire any bad form, when at the same time it receives every advantage that possibly could be expected from shoeing. In this respect it may very properly be said that we make the shoe to the foot, and not the foot to the shoe, as is but too much the case in the concave shoes, where the foot very much resembles that of a cat's fixed in a walnut-shell.' 'I would observe, upon the whole, that the less substance we take away from the natural defence of the foot, except on particular occasions which may require it, the less artificial defence will be necessary: the flatter we make the shoe we give the horse the more points of support, and imitate the natural tread of the foot; therefore the nearer we follow these simple rules, the nearer we approach to perfection in this art.'

33

To Osmer and Clark, therefore, belongs the merit of having introduced this great innovation in the shape of the shoe, and persistently pointed out the injury caused by excessive paring and unscientific shoeing. To Mr Clark is most certainly due the credit of having unmistakably asserted that the foot of the horse expands and contracts in a lateral direction during progression. In nearly every treatise published on the horse's foot, or on shoeing, particularly on the continent, during the last 20 years, this notion has been erroneously ascribed to Bracy Clark, who is always referred to as its originator.

CHAPTER XII.

ESTABLISHMENT OF THE LONDON VETERINARY SCHOOL. M. ST
BEL. MOORCROFT. THE QUALITIES OF A GOOD SHOE. COLEMAN.
ERRORS IN PHYSIOLOGY. CONCLUSIONS OF COLEMAN AS TO
SHOEING. IMPRACTICABLE SHOEING. BRACY CLARK. EXAGGER-
ATED NOTIONS AND RE-DISCOVERIES. FUTILE EXPERIMENTS.
VARIOUS WRITERS. MR GOODWIN'S METHOD. ITS RECOMMEND-
ATIONS AND APPROPRIATENESS. ITS COMPOSITE CHARACTER.
PREPARATION OF THE HOOF AND APPLICATION OF THE SHOE.
ERRORS IN THIS METHOD. THE BAR AND JOINTED SHOE.
DISCOURAGEMENT OF VETERINARY SCIENCE IN BRITAIN. THE
UNILATERAL SHOE. YOUATT AND HIS TEACHING. MILES
METHOD OF SHOEING. ITS FALLACIOUSNESS. HOT-FITTING.
HALLEN AND FITZWYGRAM'S METHOD. ITS DISADVANTAGES.
MAVOR'S PATENT SHOE.

TOWARDS the termination of the 18th century, a
veterinary school, which might be termed private, was
commenced in London, and its first teacher, M. St Bel,
published a small treatise on shoeing. This, however,
appears to be nothing more than a commendation of
Bourgelat's method. The shoe advised to be worn,
nevertheless, was concave on the ground surface, to correspond to, or resemble, the concavity of the sole, and plane
towards the hoof, something like the hunting-shoe of the
present time. It was constantly used when the College
was first established. More important was the little work

by William Moorcroft,[1] assistant professor, and afterwards
the daring explorer of Central Asia.   After describing,
like some of his later predecessors, the anatomy of the
foot and the principles which ought to prevail in its defence, and pointing out that in proportion as a greater
quantity of crust is brought to bear flat on the shoe the
firmer the horse must stand; and the less pressure that
takes place between the sole and the shoe, the less chance
will there be of his being lamed, he speaks of various
shoes.   As those intended for the fore-feet have always,
and rightly, been looked upon as the most important,
considering that they have to bear the principal portion
of the weight, and that the fore-feet are by far the most
frequently lamed, the defences for this region will only
be noticed here.   Moorcroft describes the narrow shoe,
or plate—a flat shoe, the exact breadth of the crust,
and of a moderate thickness: this was only serviceable
for racing-horses and hunters.   'A flat shoe, of the exact
breadth of the crust, and of a moderate thickness, would
defend this part sufficiently as long as it lasted; but as it
would wear out in a few days, or even in a few hours, when
the friction happened to be violent, and as very frequent
shoeing is expensive, as well as hurtful to the hoof itself,
this kind of shoe is only fit for racing, or hunting on soft
ground.'[2]   Then the shoe with a flat upper surface, and
broader than the crust, is figured.   This he thinks objectionable, as it would press on a portion of the sole
and cause lameness; so that, to avoid such a mishap,
the sole is required to be pared or hollowed out, which

[1] Cursory Account of the Various Methods of Shoeing Horses.
London, 1800.   [2] Op. cit., p. 6.

Moorcroft thought very injurious. Next, the shoe in common use is noticed. This is the same as that so strongly commented upon by Osmer and Clark, with its upper surface sloping downwards from the outer to the inner edge. Its defects are indicated in a similar manner, and it is shown that a shoe ought to possess the following qualities: it ought to be so strong as to wear a reasonable time; it ought to give to the crust all the support it can receive; it ought not to alter the natural shape of the foot; and it ought not to press at all on the sole, or to injure any of the natural functions of the foot. The shoe best calculated to answer these purposes was that so strongly recommended by Osmer and Clark, and which Mr Moorcroft designated the 'seated shoe;' all the experiments he had instituted for a number of years led him to this conclusion. His directions as to paring the sole and frog are similar to those of Mr Clark; though the nature and functions of the latter appear to have been imperfectly understood by him, as he complains of the frog becoming hard and losing its spongy texture when allowed to remain unpared and in contact with the ground. 'Eight nails for each shoe are found to be enough for saddle and light draught horses; but for such as are employed in heavy draught, ten are required. A smaller number does not hold the shoe sufficiently fast; and a greater number, by acting like so many wedges, weaken the hoof, and rather dispose the crust to break off than give additional security. . . . . It may be laid down as a general rule, that the last nail should not be nearer to the heel than from two inches to an inch and a half.'

This new method of shoeing, so long advocated by Osmer and Clark, had gained but trifling success up to the time when Moorcroft wrote his treatise. That gentleman, full of enthusiasm in the new-born profession, and sanguine as to the benefits to be derived from the seated-shoe, had the aid of machinery invoked to make this kind of armature more rapidly and less expensively than it could be manufactured by hand; and this, together with his deservedly high reputation as a veterinarian, brought it into general use, and so firmly established it in public opinion, that it is still the common shoe. It has also made some progress on the continent, where it is known as the 'English Shoe.'

In the opinion of Mr Moorcroft, this particular kind of defence was better adapted for ordinary wear than the semi-lunar or 'tip' shoe of Lafosse, or even the thin-heeled shoe; though he was a strong advocate for frog and heel pressure on the ground.

About this period Professor Coleman, successor to M. St Bel, published his elaborate work[1] on the horse's foot and shoeing, which was dedicated to His Majesty George III. An analysis of this voluminous monograph cannot be attempted here; suffice it to say that, amid much error as to the physiology of the foot, and consequent incorrect deductions in the application of this to shoeing, there is yet much truth. Every allowance must be made in criticizing many of Coleman's notions with regard to shoeing. Though a most promising surgeon

[1] Observations on the Structure, Economy, and Diseases of the Foot of the Horse, and On the Principles and Practice of Shoeing. London, 1798, 1802.

before joining the Veterinary College, his opportunities for studying comparative pathology, and especially the subject now under consideration, must have been rare. Medical men, it must be remembered, unless they study these matters as carefully as they have done those connected with their own profession, are apt to commit very grave mistakes, their special knowledge being, at times, more liable to mislead than to guide them.

Coleman repeats the statement as to the evil influences of paring and bad shoeing; and, owing to his exaggerated notions of the elasticity and expansive properties of the foot, adopted almost entirely Lafosse's ideas as to the manner in which it ought to be shod. These were, as we have noticed, frog and heel pressure. The conclusions at which he arrived were these:—

'1. That the natural form of the fore-feet of horses, before any art has been employed, approaches to a circle.

'2. The internal cavity of the hoof, when circular, is completely filled by the sensible parts of the foot.

'3. The hoof is composed of horny insensible fibres, that take the names of crust, sole, bars, and frog.

'4. The crust is united with the last bone of the foot by a number of laminated, elastic substances.

'5. The uses of the laminæ are, to support the weight of the animal, and, from their elasticity, to prevent concussion.

'6. The horny sole is externally concave, internally convex, and united by its edge with the inferior part of the crust.

'7. The uses of the horny sole are *to act as a spring,*

by descending at the heels;[1] to preserve the sensible sole from pressure, and (with its concavity) to form a convexity towards the earth.

'8. The external bars are nothing more than a continuation of the crust, forming angles at the heels.

'9. The internal bars are a continuation of the laminæ of the crust, attached to the horny sole at the heels, within the hoof; and that these insensible laminæ are intimately united with sensible laminated bars, connected with the sensible sole.

'10. The use of the external bars is to preserve the heels expanded; and the use of the internal horny bars, to prevent separation and dislocation of the horny sole from the sensible sole.

'11. The external frog is convex, and of an insensible, horny, elastic nature.

'12. The internal sensible frog is of the same form, very highly elastic, and united with two elastic cartilages.

'13. *The frogs are not made to protect the tendon.*

'14. The use of the frog is to prevent the horse from slipping, by its convexity embracing the ground; and from the elasticity of the sensible and horny frogs, they act as a spring to the animal, and keep expanded the heels.

'15. The common practice of shoeing is, to cut the frog and totally remove the bars.

'16. The removal of the bars and frog deprives these organs of their natural function.

'17. The shoe commonly employed is thicker at the heel than the toe.

---

[1] The italics are my own, and are merely intended to indicate in what respects Coleman probably or assuredly erred.

'18. This shoe is convex externally, concave internally, and four nails placed in each quarter of the crust.

'19. The shoes, being nailed at the heels, confine the quarters of the crust, and produce contraction.

'20. The frog, being raised from the ground by a thick-heeled shoe, becomes soft, and very susceptible of injury.

'21. The shoe being thick at the heel only preserves the frog from pressure in the stable and on smooth surfaces, while sharp and projecting stones are perpetually liable to strike the frog at every step.

'22. The frog being soft becomes inflamed whenever it meets with pressure from hard bodies.

'23. The concavity of the shoe within, tends to prevent the expansion of the quarters, and to bruise the heels of the sole.

'24. The convexity without makes the horse very liable to slip.

'25. Contracted hoofs, corns, and frequently thrushes and canker, are to be attributed to this practice.

'26. The intention of shoeing is to preserve the hoof sound, and of the same form and structure as nature made it; and as the common practice is altering its form, and producing disease, there can be no doubt but that the common practice of shoeing is imperfect, and requires alteration and improvement.

'27. It is very practicable to preserve the hoof circular and free from corns, contraction, thrushes, and canker.

'28. To accomplish this very desirable object, it is necessary, in all cases, first to endeavour *to remove a por-*

tion of the sole between the whole length of the bars and crust.

' 29. *The sole should be made concave at the toe, with a drawing-knife, in all cases where the horn is sufficiently thick to admit of such removal.*

' 30. The internal surface of the shoe may be flat whenever the whole of the sole is concave, and will admit of a picker between a flat shoe and the sole.

' 31. *When the interior portion of the sole is thin, or flat, or convex, and cannot be made concave, the shoe at this part should be made concave.*

' 32. As the crust, in flat feet, is always thin, *the shoe at the toe should have a very small seat, only equal to the nails.*

' 33. As the sole at the quarters, even in flat or convex hoofs, *will very generally admit of removal,* the quarters and heels of the shoes will be flat.

' 34. That while the quarters and heels of the shoe, on the upper surface, are flat, the concavity of the shoe at the toe has no kind of influence in contracting the heels.

' 35. The external surface of the shoe should be regularly concave, to correspond to the form of the sole and crust, before the horse is shod.

' 36. This external concavity of the shoe is well cal culated to embrace the ground, and to prevent the horse from slipping.

' 37. The relative thickness of the shoe, at the toe and heel, should be particularly attended to.

' 38. The wear of the shoe, at the toe of the fore-feet, is generally three times greater than the consumption of iron at the heels.

' 39. The heels of the shoe should be about one-third the substance of the toe.

' 40· This form of shoe is preferred to a high heel, as it allows the frog to perform its function, by embracing the ground, and acting as a spring.

' 41. The weight of the shoe being diminished at the heel, the labour of the muscles that bend and extend the leg is diminished.

' 42· Where no part of the crust can be removed from the toe, and the horse has been in the habit of wearing high shoes, the heels should be made only one-tenth of an inch, every time of shoeing, thinner than the shoes removed.

' 43· If the frog be callous and sound, and the toe admits of being shortened, the iron may be diminished at the heels, in the same proportion as the toe is shortened.

' 44. The muscles and tendons will be exerted beyond their tone if the heels of the shoes are not gradually thinned as the horn grows, or as the toe of the crust can be removed.

' 45. Young horses, with perfect feet, should not have thin-heeled shoes at first, unless the crust at the toe can be removed in the same degree as the iron at the toe exceeds the heels.

' 46· Where half an inch of horn can be taken from the toe of the crust, a shoe thin at the heel may be at once applied without any injury to the muscles and tendons.

' 47. Where the heels exceed two inches in depth, and the frogs are equally prominent, and the ground dry, a short shoe, thin at the heels, may be applied.

'48. The heels of this shoe should not reach the seat of corn, between the bars and crust.

'49. That in warm climates, and in this country in summer, the wear of the horn exposed to the ground will not be greater than the growth from the coronet.

'50. Where the heels are more than two inches high, and the ground wet, it is better to lower the heels by the butteris than to wear them down by friction with the ground.

'51. It is not safe to employ the short shoe on wet ground, except in blood horses with very thick crusts, and then only with great attention to the consumption of horn.

'52. The long thin-heeled shoe should rest on the solid junction of the bars with the crust.

'53. The nails should be carried all round the toe of the crust.

'54. They should be kept as far as possible from the heels, and particularly in the inside quarter.

'55. Where the crust is thin, the nail-holes of the new shoe should not be made opposite, but between the old nail-holes of the crust.

'56. The nail-hole should be made with a punch of a wedge-like form, so as to admit the whole head of the nail into the shoe.

'57. The head of the nail should be conical, to correspond with the nail-hole.

'58. The shoe and nails of a common-sized coach-horse may weigh about eighteen ounces.

'59. The shoe and nails of a saddle-horse may weigh twelve ounces.

'60. The shoe should remain on the hoof about twenty-eight days; but if it wears out before this period, the next shoe should be made thicker.

'61. Horses employed in hunting, in frost, and in the shafts of carriages, require an artificial stop on the hind-foot, and in some situations on the fore-feet.

'62. Whenever this shoe is employed, it should be turned up on the outside heel, and the horn of the same heel should be lowered.

'63. The horn on the inside heel should be preserved, and the heel of the shoe more or less thick, in proportion to the horn removed on the outside heel.

'64. This shoe, when applied, is generally as high on the inside as on the outside heel.

'65. A bar-shoe is very beneficial where the frog is hard and sound, and where the heels have been much removed to bring the frog in contact with pressure.

'66. The upper part of the bar should rest on the frog, and the part opposite the ground turned up in order to act as a stop.

'67. When this shoe is applied the frog receives pressure, the heels will be expanded, and the muscles and tendons not more stretched than before the heels were lowered.

'68. This shoe may be applied for sandcracks, but no part of it should be supported by the crust opposite the crack.

'69. Where, from bad shoeing, the bars are removed and corns are produced, a bar-shoe may be employed to prevent pressure opposite to the seat of corn.

'70. *Where the sole is too thin at the heels to admit of*

any removal with a drawing-knife, the bar-shoe may be applied with advantage.

'71. In this case the heels of the shoe should be raised from the heels of the crust, and the bar rest on the frog.

'72. The hoof being cut and the shoe applied, as directed, will preserve the hoof in its circular form.'

Keeping the sole from pressure, and allowing the frog to bear the greater portion of the horse's weight, was the prevailing idea with Professor Coleman. The foot was distorted and mutilated to attain this object, and the most curious contrivances devised to confine the bearing solely to the toe of the foot and the frog. With regard to these principles of shoeing he was particularly dogmatic. 'There are only *two principles* to govern the practice of shoeing, which *for all horses in all ages and in all countries must be invariably followed* . . . . . and which are of much greater moment than the shape of the shoe itself. So long as nails and iron are employed to protect the hoof, the crust is the part that should receive the nails and the pressure of the shoe; *and the sole of every horse employed for every purpose is a part that should not be in contact with the shoe.* All other rules for the practice of shoeing are subordinate and conditional.' Artificial frogs were invented and patented to make due pressure on that part of the foot, and everything was done to cause the expansion of the heels; and yet the sole was recklessly scooped away, *while to fasten on a half-shoe, eight nails* were employed (fig. 193). Though the method of shoeing with 'tips' and thin-heeled shoes had been recommended by Lafosse and others, these authorities are never once mentioned by

Coleman ; and at present, with those who have had better
opportunities of making them-
selves acquainted with the construction and functions of the
foot, it is recognized as a fact,
that sole-pressure is almost
as necessary to a healthy condition of the hoofs as frog-
pressure. Coleman was a stout
opponent of the seated-shoe,
and offered the strongest arguments he could frame to
make it unpopular. It may be observed, however, that he
afterwards returned to the thick-heeled shoe, but added
to it clips at the inner angles of the heels, intended to
grasp and pull the bars outwards. This antiquated invention was also patented,[1] and was subsequently re-invented
by many anti-contractionists. It had no success with
Coleman.

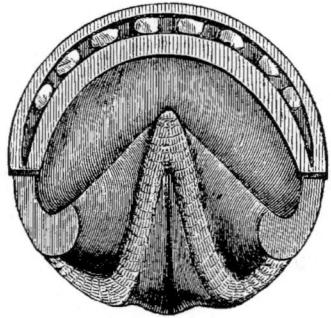

fig 193

[1] This was the same kind of shoe as that proposed by Carlo Ruini, of
Bologna, in 1598, for the same condition of the hoofs. After dilating the
heels and strengthening the feet by allowing the horse to roam at large
in a meadow, or unsoling the hoofs, that writer adds : ' Se gli mettera un
ferro debole sottile, e stretto di verga ; il quale sia tanto largo nelle cal-
cagna, che il corno, o guscio del piede vi posi sopra ; e habbi nella parte
di dentro due oruchie eguali, ma d'ogni lato acconcie talmente, che
pigliano nella parte di dentro del corno, e guscio del piede, senza poza
potere in modo alcuno offendere, e danneggiare il vivo, e l'osso del
piede. Dipoi essendo per buon spatio di tempo stato à molle il piede
nell' acqua calda, e mollificato, si pigliera con le tenaglie il ferro nel
calcagno e tirandolo per forza verso fuori, s'allargherà à bastanza in-
sieme con li quarti e con le calgagno del piede.'—*Anatomia et Infirmita
del Cavallo,* p. 653. The same description of shoe, and one opening
with a screw, is noticed by J. Bridges.

One of his pupils, Bracy Clark,[1] to some extent adopted his views, though in other respects he far out stripped him in exaggerating certain functions of the foot, and devising means to aid those functions. With out the slightest compunction, apparently, he claims the merit of having discovered the elastic properties of the foot, and re-discovers various parts. His weakness, or rather his mania, with regard to the horse's foot was lateral expansion, and descent of the sole in progression. This exaggerated idea so influenced his notions of shoeing, that he spent several years endeavouring to prove that shoes were unnecessary, and when at last forced to employ this defence, he invented several to be attached to the hoof without nails. The unyielding iron rim riveted to the lower margin of the foot by rigid nails was to him the only source of disease; the shoe in common use, the unskilful nailing, the destructive paring, were but little to blame; *the prevention of that heel movement which resembled the waving of an osier branch in the wind when a horse galloped, and which contributed so much to the rapidity of movement, was the sole cause.* The nailless shoe, however, was too complicated, and to remain secure on the hoof had to be as immovably fixed as the nailed one; so a jointed shoe was *invented*, identical in every respect with that of Cæsar Fiaschi, and so often spoken of by writers subsequent to that maréchal. This shoe was useless, and could no more facilitate the lateral expansion and contraction, even had it existed to the degree Bracy Clark imagined, than the ordinary one. With the joint

[1] A Series of Original Experiments on the Foot of the Living Horse. London, 1809. 2nd Edit., 1829.

only at the toe, where there was no motion, and the branches nailed as usual to the sides and heels, where this excessive play was supposed to be going on, it might have been foreseen that no good could result. The thin-heeled shoe, the bar shoe, and indeed every shoe, proved unsatisfactory to him, and the chief value of his experiments and labours rests on the demonstration of the changes brought about in hoofs by a vicious system of paring and shoeing them, which the highly-developed expansion theory caused Bracy Clark entirely to overlook. This author was of opinion that the sole and frog should not come into contact with the ground.

It is scarcely necessary to say that the false doctrine of lateral expansion and sole descent propounded by Bracy Clark and Professor Coleman, has had a most serious and pernicious influence on farriery, not only in this country, but on the continent ; and has largely tended to the production and perpetuation of foot diseases that are torturing to the animal, and baffling to the veterinary surgeon.

The theories published by Bracy Clark, with regard to the elasticity of the foot, were certainly ingenious, but not to any degree original ; though they were rashly speculative, and must have been based on the most slender instalment of proper experience and observation.

This century has been very prolific in treatises on farriery, inventions, and modifications of horse-shoes and horse-shoeing. In England, among other writers, at its commencement, were White, Blaine, and Peall. These veterinarians appear to have been more or less in favour of Coleman's thin-heeled shoe, and sanctioned the well paring-out method of preparing the hoof.

34

The best work produced at this period was undoubtedly that of Mr Goodwin, veterinary surgeon to
King George IV.[1]   It is written in a fair and scientific
spirit, and gives an excellent resumé of the merits and
demerits of the various systems of shoeing then in vogue.
With regard to the different kinds of shoes in use, he dis
covers faults in the seated, jointed, thin-heeled, and com
mon shoe, which forbade his recommending them for
general purposes.   The French mode of shoeing, which
was Bourgelat's, came nearest to his standard of superiority, yet he had two objections to this system in
general: 'the convex form of the shoe on the ground
side, and the concave form on the foot side.   I object to
the first, because the horse is by no means so safe or
secure on his feet, more particularly when going over
stones.'   The second objection was that offered by the
older writers to the common English bowl, or quoit-shaped,
shoe.   His new system appears to have been similar to
that recommended by Professor St Bel, so far as the
ground surface of the shoe was concerned.   'In the shoe
I have adopted, I have reversed the form on each side
(speaking of the French pattern), *making it concave on
the ground surface, and convex on the foot surface,* with an
inclination from the inner to the outer rim (figs. 194,
195).   To effect this form on each side, it is necessary
that the shoe should be sloped or bevelled on the ground
side, from the outward to the inward part all round the
shoe, except about an inch and a half at the heels.   To
accomplish this inclination on the foot side, it is necessary
to thicken the inner part at the heels, as far as the flat sur-

[1] A New System of Shoeing Horses.   London, 1820.

face extends.' This inclination was to be moderate at first,

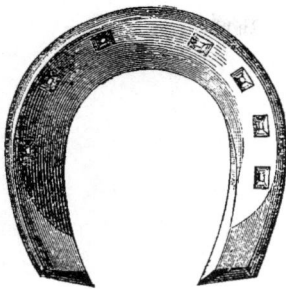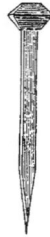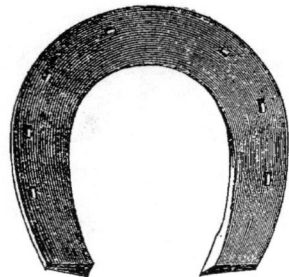

fig 194   fig. 195

though lameness from an extreme degree had not been
observed. The shoe was only adapted for hoofs with strong
concave soles; yet with all other kinds of feet, if it was
clear of the sole, the inclination was a matter of no moment. The curve at the toe, and the manner of punching
the nail-holes, resembled the French shoe. This pattern
lasted in wear as long as the ordinary armature. It will be
seen that this is simply a modification, or rather a combination, of Solleysel's *fer à pantoufle*, Bourgelat's curved or
adjusted shoe, and the concave-surfaced shoe of St Bel.
'The concave ground surface renders the animal more
secure on his legs, as he has a greater purchase on the
ground, and by this form the weight is thrown on the
crust, or wall, which prevents any unnecessary strain on
the nails and clinches.' He refers to the resemblance
between this and Solleysel's shoe, points out that his is
formed with the same intention to prevent contraction
and other permanent diseases of the feet, 'because it appeared evident to me, that when the weight of the animal
comes on a shoe of this form, it must have a tendency to
expand instead of to contract the hoof, and I have found
from much experience, that the obstacles opposed to this

34 *

form existed only in theory, as there are none in practice. It is necessary, however, to remark, that the degree of inclination must be regulated by the previous state of the foot, and its propensity to contraction. . . . When it is recollected that the horny sole, if not diseased, is concave, it will in course admit of a convex surface being applied to it; and when the superfluous parts of the horny sole produced since the last shoeing are removed, and the crust at the quarters is preserved firm and good, there is scarcely an instance where this mode of shoeing cannot be put into practice, and sufficient room be left also to pass a picker between the shoe and the sole to the nails.'

The preparation of the foot, previous to shoeing, consisted in the removal of all the superfluous growth: 'When hoofs are protected by shoes, the consumption of horn by wear and tear is nearly prevented; but as the growth of the hoof is constantly going on, it is evident that all the superfluous parts will require to be removed at every period of shoeing, otherwise it would run into a state of exuberance similar to the human nails if they were not cut. The first part to be reduced is the toe, which should be removed with a knife or rasp on the sole side of the foot, keeping in view the necessary curve: the next parts are the heels, which should, if they descend below the frog, be rasped to bring them on a level with it: having attended to these two points, it will be seen how much it is necessary to remove from the quarters, leaving them full and strong, but in a straight line from the heels to the curve, which allows the foot, when in action, a flat part to land on, and describes a space equal to the landing part of the foot when shod with a parallel shoe. This direction differs a little from the French 'adjusting balance,' inasmuch as they direct four points of adjustment at the toe, and two at the heels, which leaves the quarters rounded, and renders the foot not so secure on the ground. The sole next must have attention; the *superfluous parts* of which that have appeared since the last shoeing should be removed; this will leave it concave, and the crust or wall below the sole. Mr Moorcroft observes, that paring the soles has a tendency to bring on 'pumiced' feet, but I have not observed any such effect; on the contrary, if the sole is allowed to grow too thick, *it loses its elastic property, and the sensible sole suffers in proportion to the degree of thickness and want of elasticity.'* The frog, if *too large* or ragged, was also to be sliced away, and when the shoe was put on, a portion of the crust was to be removed at the heels and quarters. Horses with long pasterns were to have these shoes thicker at the heels, with a view to give support, and to counteract too great a flexure in that part.

By this method of shoeing, in Mr Goodwin's experience, the proportion of lame horses had been considerably reduced, and defects and deformities removed. The curve or curb at the toe was no disadvantage to draught-horses going up-hill; the ordinary shoe, when in wear for a few days, lost its sharp edge, and was then far more likely to slip than one with the broad surface of the curved toe. 'Those persons who may be averse to the adjusting curve of the French shoe will find that the next best shape is a perfect plane on the foot side, and the same on the ground side, of the width of the nail-holes all round (which should be of the French form), and the remaining part of the web or width of the shoe should be sloped or bevelled from the inside of the nail-heads all round the shoe to the inner rim, with the exception of from one to one inch and a half of flat bearing on the heels, and the shoe should be of an equal thickness from toe to heel.' The bar or circular shoe, when properly constructed, Mr Goodwin considered of the greatest use ' in affording a greater surface of defence than any other shoe, which enables us to determine the weight of the animal more generally on the foot by equalizing the pressure on more bearing points than a plain shoe.' Screw shoes are noticed, as well as their effects on contracted feet. Their use had been recently revived by Mr Jekyl, whose pattern, with a joint at the toe and a screw at the heels, was objectionable. Sir B. Bloomfield had suggested a shoe with two joints— one on each side of the toe : the toe-piece had two nail-holes in it, and each branch, furnished with a bar-clip, had three nails ; screws acted on the inner side of the branches towards the heel.

Very judicious remarks are made as to nailing shoes to the hoofs, and those on the management of the horse's feet are commendable; but it may be noticed that his curved-toe shoe was supposed to correspond to the natural form of the *os pedis,* or coffin-bone, and in one of his drawings to illustrate this principle he figures what is certainly a diseased or abnormal specimen of that bone. Perhaps on this diseased specimen he founded his imitation of the French shoe.

The French method was, in his opinion, far superior to the English one, and in lauding its merits he forgot to notice its defects, which at least equal those of the latter.

Mr Youatt,[1] in his in many respects deservedly popular treatise on the horse, refers to shoeing; and as his opinions must have had much influence on the practice of the art in Britain, if we can form any criterion by the large sale of the work, it will be well to give them a brief notice. In the anatomy of the foot, he dwells upon its expansive properties—especially at the quarters, though he does not mention having tested this in any way. Speaking of the bars, or inflections of the wall, he writes: 'The arch which they form on either side, between the frog and the quarters, is admirably contrived, both to admit of, and to limit to its proper extent, the expansion of the foot.' 'When the foot is placed on the ground, and the weight of the animal is thrown on the little leaves (laminæ), *we can imagine* these arches shortening and widening, in order to admit of the expansion of the quarters; and we can see the bow returning to its natural curve, and powerfully assisting the foot in regaining its usual form.' He protests against removing these bars, and the evil results which follow their destruction. 'Too many smiths cut them perfectly away. They imagine that that gives a more open appearance to the heels of the horse,—a seeming width which may impose on the unwary. Horses shod for the purpose of sale have usually the bars removed with this view, and the smiths in the neighbourhood of the metropolis and large towns, shoeing for dealers, too often habitually pursue, with regard to all their customers, the injurious practice of removing the bars. The horny frog, deprived of its guard, will speedily contract, and become elevated and thrushy; and the whole of the heel,

[1] The Horse, London, 1846.

deprived of the power of resilience or re-action, which the curve between the bar and the crust affords, will speedily fall in.'

Then the functions of the frog are enumerated, and their description is strangely compounded of truth and error. ' The foot is seldom put flush and flat upon the ground, but in a direction downwards, yet somewhat forwards ; then the frog evidently gives safety to the tread of the animal, for it, in a manner, ploughs itself into the ground, and prevents the horse from slipping. This is of considerable consequence, when we remember some of the paces of the horse, in which his heels evidently come first to the ground, and in which the danger from slipping would be very great. . . . The frog being placed at and filling the hinder part of the foot, discharges a part of the duty sustained by the crust ; for it supports the weight of the animal. It assists, likewise, and that to a material degree, in the expansion of the foot. . . . It is also composed of a substance peculiarly flexible and elastic. What can be so well adapted for the expansion of the foot, when a portion of the weight of the body is thrown on it ? How easily will these irregular surfaces yield and spread out, and how readily return again to their natural state ! In this view, therefore, the horny frog is a powerful agent in opening the foot ; and the diminution of the substance of the frog, and its elevation above the ground, are both the cause and the consequence of contraction : the cause, as being able no longer powerfully to act in expanding the heels ; and the consequence, as obeying a law of nature, by which that which no longer discharges its natural function is gradually removed. It is, however, the cover and defence of the internal and sensible frog. . . . We have said enough to show the absurdity of the common practice of unsparingly cutting it away. To discharge, in any degree, some of the offices which we have assigned to it, and fully to discharge even one of them, it must come in *occasional* contact with the ground. In the unshod horse it is constantly so; *but the additional support given by the shoes, and more especially the hard roads over which the horse is now compelled to travel,* render this complete exposure of the frog to the ground not only unnecessary, *but injurious.* Being of so much softer consistence than the rest of the foot, *it would be speedily worn away :* occasional pressure, however, or contact with the ground, it must have. The rough and detached parts should be cut off at each shoeing, and *the substance of the frog itself,* so as to bring it just above or within the level of the shoe. It will then, *in the descent of the sole,* when the weight of the horse is thrown upon it in the putting down of the foot, descend likewise, and pressing upon the ground, do its duty; while it will be defended from the wear, and bruise, and injury which it would receive if it came upon the ground with the first and full shock of the weight. A few smiths carry the notion of *frog pressure* to an absurd extent, and *leave the frog beyond the level of the sole,*—a practice which is dangerous in the horse of slow draught, and destructive to the hackney or hunter.'

We can see that Mr Youatt differs widely from Lafosse in his opinion of the functions, utility, and management of the frog; and he evidently writes from very superficial observation or hearsay evidence.

His ideas as to the function of the sole are also stamped

by inexperience, and the incorrect views of Coleman appear to have tainted his teaching, as they damaged his practice. The reason that the horse's sole was hollow, was because it descended or yielded with the weight of the animal. 'Then if the sole be naturally hollow, *and hollow because it must descend,* the smith must not interfere with this important action. When the foot will bear it, *he must pare out sufficient of the horn to preserve the proper concavity, a small portion at the toe and near the crust,* and cutting deeper towards the centre; and he must put on a shoe, *which shall not prevent the descent of the sole;* which not only shall not press upon it, *but shall leave sufficient room between it and the sole to admit of this descent.* If the sole is pressed upon by the coffin-bone, by the lengthening of the elastic leaves, and the shoe will not permit its descent, the sensible part between the coffin-bone and the horn will necessarily be bruised, and inflammation and lameness will ensue. It is from this cause that, if a stone insinuates itself between the shoe and the sole, it produces so much lameness.'

The principles of shoeing enunciated by Mr Youatt were entirely founded on the supposed elastic properties of certain parts of the foot—expansion at the quarters, flattening of the frog laterally, and descent of the sole. Grave errors certainly, resulting from imperfect study or mal-appreciation of the anatomy and physiology of the foot; and which were simply destruction to that organ, when these principles were applied to it.

The defence recommended was the 'seated' shoe of Osmer and Moorcroft, which was a vast improvement on that still in use, it appears. 'The ground surface of the common shoe used in the country is somewhat convex, and the inward rim of the shoe comes first on the ground: the consequence of this is, that the weight, instead of being borne fairly on the crust, is supported by the nails and the clenches.' 'Shoeing,' he says, 'has entailed on the animal some evils. It has limited or destroyed the *beautiful expansibility of the lower part of the foot;* it has led to contraction, although that contraction has not always been accompanied by lameness; in the most careful fixing of the best shoe, and in the careless manu-facture and setting on of the bad one, much injury has often been done to the horse.' The web or cover of the seated shoe was to be sufficiently wide to guard the sole from bruises, and as wide at the heel as the frog would permit, in order to cover the seat of corn. The shoe was to be fastened on with *nine nails*—five on the outside, and four on the inner side; though for small hoofs seven might suffice. The inside part of the foot surface of the shoe was to be levelled off, or made concave, so that it might not press upon the sole. 'Notwithstanding our iron fetter, the sole does, although to a very inconsider-able extent, descend when the foot of the horse is put on the ground. It is unable to bear constant or even occa-sional pressure, and if it came in contact with the shoe, the sensible sole, between the horny sole and the coffin-bone, would be bruised, and lameness would ensue. Many of our horses, from too early and undue work, have the natural concave sole flattened, and the disposition to de-scend and the degree of descent are thereby increased.' 'The web of the shoe is likewise of that thickness, that when the foot is properly pared, the prominent part of the frog shall lie just within and above its ground surface, so that in the descent of the sole the frog shall come sufficiently on the ground to enable it to act as a wedge, and to expand the quarters, while it is defended from the wear and injury it would receive if it came to the ground with the first and full shock of the weight.'

With respect to paring the hoof, Youatt commits the most dangerous blunders to be found in his work. Admitting that no specific rules could be laid down, he adds: ' This, however, we can say with confidence, that more injury has been done by the neglect of paring than by carrying it to too great an extent. The act of paring is a work of much more labour than the proprietor of the horse often imagines; the smith, except he be overlooked, will give himself as little trouble about it as he can; and that which, in the unshod foot, would be worn away by contact with the ground, is suffered to accumulate month after month, *until the elasticity of the sole is destroyed, and it can no longer descend,* and the functions of the foot are impeded, and foundation is laid for corn, and contraction, and navicular disease, and inflammation.

That portion of horn should be left on the sole, which will defend the internal parts from being bruised, and yet suffer the external sole to descend. How is this to be measured? The strong pressure of the thumb of the smith will be the best guide. The buttress, that most destructive of all instruments, being banished from the respectable forge, the smith sets to work with his drawing-knife, and he removes the growth of horn, *until the sole will yield, although in the slightest possible degree, to the very strong pressure of his thumb. The proper thick-*

ness of horn will then remain. If the foot has been previously neglected, and the horn is become very hard, the
owner must not object if the smith resorts to some means
to soften it a little; *and if he takes one of his flat irons,
and having heated it, draws it over the sole, and keeps it a
little while in contact with it.* When the sole is thick,
this rude and apparently barbarous method can do no
harm, but it should never be permitted with the sole that
is regularly pared out.

'The quantity of horn to be removed in order to leave
the proper degree of thickness will vary with different feet.
From the strong foot a great deal must be taken. From
the concave foot the horn may be removed until the sole
will yield to a moderate pressure. From the flat foot little
need be pared; while the pumiced foot will spare nothing
but the ragged parts. The paring being nearly completed, the knife and the rasp of the smith must be a little
watched, or he will *reduce the crust to a level with the sole,
and thus endanger the bruising of the sole by its pressure
on the edge of the seating.* The crust should be reduced
to a perfect level all round, but left a little higher than
the sole.' The horn between the crust and the bar
must be carefully pared out, in order to remedy or to give
the animal temporary relief from corns, and the frog was
to be diminished to a proper degree. More depended
upon the paring out of the foot, according to Mr Youatt,
than on the construction of the shoe; that few shoes, except they press upon the sole, or are made outrageously
bad, will lame the horse; but that he may be very easily
lamed from ignorant and improper paring of the feet.

Nothing could be more erroneous than this author's

views with regard to the elasticity of the foot, and nothing could be more destructive to that organ than the adoption of the rules he lays down for its management. To carry them out was simply to produce the diseases he attributes to other causes ; and it is difficult to understand how Mr Youatt, who was in many respects an intelligent veterinarian, should so far commit himself to the emission of opinions which a little investigation would have shown to be without the slightest foundation. His directions, appearing as they did in a work of a popular character, and which was to be found on nearly every horse-owner's book-shelf, must have done an incalculable amount of injury, and which could scarcely be compensated for by the correctness of other details he gives on the matter of shoeing.

For more than fifty years, and even up to the present day, the elasticity, or *lateral-expansion* and *sole-descent* mania, may be said to have proved the curse of horse flesh, and the *bête noire* of farriery. The hoof was mu tilated in every possible manner to favour this all but undemonstrable idea ; and the purblind individuals who resorted to these practices evidently could not see the damage they were inflicting, and which became all the more serious the more exaggerated their expansion theory was developed. Nearly all the ills the horse's foot was liable to, it was believed, were due to the restraint the un-yielding shoe imposed upon the lower border of the hoof, as well as the constriction caused by the nails. To remedy these every imaginable device was tried ; but nearly all of them were as unreasonable as they were unfruitful. Such had been the wonderful productions of Coleman and Bracy Clark: frog-pressure shoes, shoes with one or more joints, shoes in segments attached to a leather sole, shoes entirely of leather, shoes without nails to fasten on the foot like a sandal, and shoes in halves, as if for the cloven foot of an ox. In fact, the ingenuity of man appears to have been racked to accommodate this alternate opening and closing of the heels, and the ascent and descent of the sole; all the while the lower face of the hoof was robbed of its protection, and consequently made to undergo these very changes attributed to the iron plate and nails. The amount of torture inflicted by these well meaning, but mistaken men has been immense—the loss inestimable.

One of the many modes of promoting expansion proposed and practised many years ago, was that of Mr Turner, and which was designated 'unilateral,' because of the nails being limited to the outside and toe of the shoe, leaving the inside to expand and contract *ad libitum.* It was but the revival of a method practised centuries ago in certain cases, in this country and in France, where it was known as the *ferrure à la Turque.* For a time this new fashion had a tolerable run, but somehow it soon began to decline, as the maladies it was intended to prevent were as prevalent as ever, the sole and frog-paring being still in a flourishing condition.

It would serve no useful purpose to enumerate all the books that have been written in England in this century on the subject of farriery, or to describe all the different shoes and different methods invented, reinvented, and borrowed without acknowledgment. Machine-made shoes of various patterns have been largely tried, and have invariably failed after a short time. No general form of shoe will suit every horse—no general arrangement of the nail-holes will suffice for every foot; and these quickly and cheaply-made articles, in addition to the many defects which machine-made shoes will always have, possess one which is perhaps the most serious of all—the softness of the iron. This is so great, that the horse must either carry a most clumsy and injurious mass of material of the consistency of lead, or be shod far more frequently than the soundness of his feet will permit. Malleable cast-iron shoes, capable of sustaining a low temperature in order to alter them to suit different feet, have also been patented and tried with no better success than the machine-made shoes. Unlike them, however, they proved too hard; and if they escaped the dangers of a temperature which could scarcely be designated a red-heat, or of a few gentle taps of the hammer, and were nailed to the hoof without flying about in a number of pieces, they either smashed when brought into contact with the pavement, or proved so slippery that many horses were injured by falls with them.

Before concluding our history of the art of shoeing in England, it will, perhaps, be instructive to refer to two works, one of which has had a large sale and has passed through many editions, having been translated into one or two foreign languages; the other being the more valuable of the two, though apparently not so well known.

The first of these, by Mr Miles,[1] is what might be

---

[1] The Horse's Foot, and How to Keep it Sound. Eighth edition. London, 1856. *Also,* A Plain Treatise on Horse-shoeing. 3rd edition. 1860.

termed a re-introduction of Mr Turner's ' unilateral' shoe, modified by Bourgelat's and Goodwin's bent-up or curved toe. The method of shoeing and the shoe itself is founded entirely, like that of Mr Youatt's, on the theory of the lateral expansion of the foot and the descent of the sole.

The horny crust, according to Mr Miles, is ' elastic throughout its whole extent, and yielding to the weight of the horse, allows the horny sole to descend, whereby much inconvenient concussion to the internal parts of the foot is avoided ; but if a large portion of the circumference of the foot be fettered by iron and nails, it is obvious that that portion at least cannot expand as before ; and the beautiful and efficient apparatus for effecting this neces sary elasticity being no longer allowed to act by reason of these restraints, becomes altered in structure ; and the con tinued operation of the same causes in the end circum scribes the elasticity to those parts alone where no nails have been driven ; giving rise to a train of consequences destructive to the soundness of the foot, and fatal to the usefulness of the horse.' Serious anatomical and physio-logical mistakes occur in this section of this work, and nothing is said as to the function of the frog. The sole is made to ascend and descend as the weight was applied to or removed from it. ' This descending property of the sole calls for our especial consideration in directing the form of the shoe ; for if the shoe be so formed that the horny sole rests upon it, it cannot descend lower, and the sensible sole above, becoming squeezed between the edges of the coffin-bone and the horn, causes inflamma-tion, and perhaps abscess. The effect of this squeezing of the sensible sole is most commonly witnessed at the

angle of the inner heel, where the descending heel of the
coffin-bone, forcibly pressing the vascular sole upon the
horny sole, ruptures a small blood-vessel, and produces
what is called a corn.' It is, however, in his remarks
on paring of the horse's foot that his erroneous views of
its physiology are shown, and his directions for the performance of that operation are marked by a singular
absence of reasoning, unless it be that which was founded
on the descending properties of the sole.

As this work has, perhaps, passed through as many
editions as Mr Youatt's, and as it treats entirely of shoeing,
claiming for itself the teaching of ' how to keep the foot
sound,' we have every inducement to inquire into his practice ; influencing, as it must have done, the art of farriery in
this country to a very considerable extent. We shall then
be able to pronounce how far the usual abuses had been
mitigated and the art improved ; though it will be apparent
that his principles are those laid down by Youatt. 'The
operation of paring out the foot is a matter requiring both
skill and judgment, and is, moreover, a work of some
labour when properly performed. It will be found that
the operator errs much oftener by removing *too little* than
too much; at least it is so with parts that ought to
be removed, which are sometimes almost as hard and
unyielding as a flint-stone, and in their most favourable state require considerable exertion to cut through.
The frog, on the other hand, offers so little resistance
to the knife, and presents such an even, smooth, clean-
looking surface when cut through, that it requires more
philosophy than falls to the share of most smiths to
resist the temptation to slice it away, despite a know-

ledge that it would be far wiser to leave it alone. It would be impossible to frame any rule applicable to the paring out of all horses' feet, or indeed to the feet of the same horse at all times. For instance, it is manifestly unwise to pare the sole as thin in a hot dry season, when the roads are broken up and strewed with loose stones, as in a moderately wet one, when they are well bound and even; for, in the former case, the sole is in perpetual danger of being bruised by violent contact with the loose stones, and consequently needs a thick layer of horn for its protection; while the latter case offers the most favourable surface that most of our horses ever have to travel upon, and *should be taken advantage of for a thorough paring out of the sole,* in order that the internal parts of the foot may derive the full benefit arising from an elastic and descending sole, a state of things very essential to the due performance of their separate functions. Again, horses with upright feet and high heels grow horn very abundantly, especially towards the toe, and are always benefited by having the toe shortened, the heels lowered, and the sole well pared out; while horses with flat feet and low heels grow horn sparingly. . . . . In the first case the thickness of the sole prevents the due descent of the coffin-bone when the horse's weight is thrown upon the foot, and it requires in consequence to be pared down thinner and rendered more yielding; while in the latter case it is already so thin and unresisting, that it can with difficulty support the coffin-bone in its proper place, and offers at best but a feeble resistance to its downward tendency.'

Here we have this writer recommending that sound

beautiful feet should be reduced to the same morbid
state as those which had been ruined—though he did not
suspect so—by paring, and could 'barely support the
coffin-bone in its proper place, and offers at best but a
feeble resistance to its downward tendency.' 'Perfect feet,
or indeed tolerably well-formed feet, with a fair growth of
horn, should have the toe shortened, the heels lowered, *and
the sole well pared out ; that is, all the dead horn removed,
and, if need be, some of the living too, until it will yield in
some small degree to hard pressure from the thumb. The
corners, formed by the junction of the crust and bars, should
be well pared out, particularly on the* inside, for this is the
common seat of corn; *and any accumulation of horn in
this situation must increase the risk of bruising the sensible
sole between the inner point or heel of the coffin-bone and
the horny sole.'* A most extraordinary statement, certainly.
We are told that horn protected the feet at one season of
the year, but was not needed at another. We are now
informed that an accumulation of horn at the corners of
the heels would bruise them, and that therefore these
corners must be well denuded of their protection.

Beside this damaging treatment of the foot, the bars
were to be removed to a level with the sole. The single
feature in this portion of his subject that redeemed it from
the ordinary barbarous treatment of the farrier, was his
earnest desire that the frog might remain untouched; and
this is the only good that commends itself in his work,
unless it be the diminution of the number of nails required
to attach the shoe.

We have seen that he deprives the sole of its natural
protection in the most unreasonable manner, merely be-

cause he imagined that it descended towards the shoe to a serious degree. The weight of the shoe was of little importance. 'The inconvenience to a horse of an ounce or so of increased weight in each shoe is not worth a moment's consideration, compared with the discomfort to him of travelling upon a hard road with a bent shoe on his foot, straining the nails, *and making unequal and painful pressure;* the other evil arising out of light shoes is a deficiency of width in the web, *which robs the foot of much valuable protection, and leaves the sole and frog exposed to numberless injuries, that a wider web would effectually prevent.'* For his own horses, he took 'special care that the same width of web is continued throughout the whole shoe back to the heels, *giving increased covering and protection to the sole of the foot.'* He points out readily enough, the great danger there is in a horse injuring his foot and dropping suddenly lame on putting it upon a stone, and speaks of it as unphilosophical in not covering nearly the whole of that surface with a very wide-webbed shoe.

After this mutilation of the sole, it is asserted that the situation of the nails determines the form of the foot. The shoe was the ordinary seated one of Osmer and Moorcroft, bent up at the toe in the form of a worn shoe, or on Goodwin's principle; it was to be of the same thickness from one extremity to the other, and to have a good flat even space all round for the crust to bear upon, 'for it must be remembered the crust sustains the whole weight of the horse.' The ground surface was to be fullered for the reception of the nails, which were to be as few as possible—five or six: three or four on the outside, and two or three on the inside; the latter near the toe, according to Mr Turner's method.

Indeed, for many years this gentleman's own horses were only shod with *three* nails in each fore-shoe (of which alone I am now speaking). This was certainly a great improvement on the absurd fashion of studding the shoes all round with nails; and so long as the armature could be retained with safety, there was no reason why more than three, four, or five should be used. If Mr Miles could retain a heavy shoe with a wide cover, unsupported by the sole, which we have seen was removed altogether from it by paring, in addition to the bevelling of the iron, surely a light shoe resting on an unpared sole, in addition to the crust, would be still easier retained! The great secret of this retention of the shoe in Mr Miles's application of the one-sided nailing, lay in the excellent and careful method he adopted of fitting it accurately to the foot. The iron had a perfectly level and solid bearing on the crust, and this was accomplished without much trouble. Another curious circumstance to be remarked in his teaching is, that though he believed in the expansion of the heels to a very exaggerated degree, the shoe when fitted was to follow as closely as possible, and not project in the slightest degree beyond, the crust in this region. Consequently, it must have happened, that when the foot was put on the ground, and the asserted expansion took place, the hoof must have hung over the shoe to the amount of that dilatation, without receiving any support from it!

It was always a favourite theme with people who did not understand much about shoeing, or the nature of the horse's foot, to dwell upon the injury done to the hoof by fitting a hot shoe to it, in order to adapt the armature more accurately to the surface on which it was afterwards to be nailed; and some of these people would nevertheless injure the hoof in a very serious manner in other respects, to suit their own particular crotchets, which were probably as meaningless as they were injurious. For a great number of years, this declamation had been stoutly maintained by sundry individuals, some of whom perhaps had good reason to do so, seeing the injurious manner in which the feet were pared, and the likelihood that a careless workman would reach the sensitive parts through the thin pellicle of horn remaining with his hot shoe; but these accidents must have been very rare, and were no doubt least to be dreaded of any incidental to shoeing as it was usually practised. Mr Miles notices this fear of hot fitting: 'The danger apprehended from the shoe being applied to the foot so hot as to burn the crust and cause it to smoke, is utterly groundless. I would not have it made to burn itself into its place upon the foot without the assistance of rasp or drawing-knife, but I would have it tried to the foot sufficiently hot to scorch every part that bears unevenly upon it, because the advantage of detecting such projecting portions is very great, and this mode of accomplishing it is positively harmless; indeed it is the only one by which the even bearing necessary to a perfect fitting of the shoe can be insured.'

Some amusing stories are told of nervous old gentlemen, who were not only not satisfied with having their horses shod in their stables, but actually had the shoes immersed for a certain period in the coldest water procurable, in order to dispel the latent heat. So it had become

somewhat fashionable to shoe horses in stables, and Mr
Miles says of it : ' The practice of shoeing horses in
the stable, away from the forge, where there is no possibility of correcting any defect in the fitting of the shoe, is
so utterly opposed to reason and common sense, that I
should only have adverted to it as a custom of by-gone
days, exploded with the use of the buttress and the notion
of chest founder, if I had not actually witnessed its per-
petration within the last year, and that, too, in the stables
of gentlemen by no means addicted, upon other matters,
to yield their judgment a ready captive to other men's
prejudices.   Now if either of these gentlemen had hap
pened to ask the smith what he was doing, the answer
would, in all probability, have awakened him to a sudden
conviction that he was giving his countenance to a most
unphilosophical proceeding ; for the smith would have
told him that he was *fitting a shoe to the horse's foot*, which
the gentleman would at once perceive to be *impossible*, inasmuch as he had no means at hand whereby to effect the
smallest change in the form of the shoe, however much it
might require it; and the truth would instantly force
itself upon him, that the man was fitting the *foot* to the
shoe, and not, as he supposed, the *shoe* to the *foot*.   To
fit the shoe to the foot without the aid of anvil and forge
is impossible ; and any one acquainted with the exactness
and precision necessary to a perfect fitting would not
hesitate to declare the attempt to be as absurd as it is
mischievous.'   Some excellent examples are given of the
injury and inconvenience likely to arise from this stupid
fashion.

In this accuracy of fitting the shoe by burning it to

the hoof, lay the secret of dispensing with so many nails; and this was a veritable progress in the art of farriery, for which Mr Miles deserves every credit. His great error lay, as we have seen, in cutting away the sole, through a false idea that it descended, and in applying heavy, clumsy shoes. The improvement could not make amends for the mistakes.

The hind-shoes had no calkins, properly so called, but only long thick projections from the ground surface— a mere elongated form of calkin. They were not side-clipped at the toe for hunting; rather a mistake, as a hind-shoe secured in this way is much safer for horse and rider than one with a single clip at the middle of the toe. They had usually two or three nails more than the fore-shoe.

Through a defective knowledge of the anatomy of the hind-foot, the shoe was nailed on in the same manner as in the fore one—the inside nails being all clustered together near the toe on the unilateral system, to allow the hoof to expand. This was undoubtedly a mistake, as every farrier knows that the hind-hoof differs from the fore one in being thickest towards the heels of the crust, and thinnest anteriorly, and that the least injurious and most secure nailing is always found at the former part. This mistake may have caused the failure of his method of shoeing in Algeria.[1]

The composite method of shoeing devised, or rather made somewhat popular, by Mr Miles, was chiefly, as may be perceived, founded on the fantastic lateral-expansion

[1] *Merche.* Mémoire sur les Principaux Systèmes de Ferrure. Paris, 1862.

theory of Bracy Clark, whose ideas of the functions of the horse's foot became at last so exaggerated, that he could not devise any mode of shoeing that would not inflict injury on that organ. The treatise we have just noticed cannot, therefore, be said to afford us any signs of improvement in the art of shoeing, except in the matter of reducing the number of nails; and is chiefly composed of materials derived from various sources, some of them not very reliable.

It is a pleasure in turning to the next work, written by Colonel Fitzwygram,[1] to find a more rational and common-sense method of managing the foot and shoeing it. This treatise, founded as it is on the long experience and enlightened observation of Army Veterinary Surgeon Hallen, is perhaps the best on shoeing which this century has produced. It reminds one very much of Lafosse's master-piece, and indeed it only repeats the truths that able veterinarian first promulgated with regard to the propriety and method of maintaining the horse's foot in a sound condition. The leading principle is the entire conservation of sole and frog, which are not to be foolishly tampered with, and the maintenance of the wall or crust in all its integrity. The shoe recommended is that proposed by Mr Goodwin, with the single exception, perhaps, that instead of the upper surface following the concavity of the sole, it was to be flat. The ground surface, with the bent-up toe, was the same. This treatise, which, so far as the management of the foot is concerned, is calculated to do much good, is yet somewhat marred by an error that, though apparently unimportant, yet in reality is not so.

[1] Notes on Shoeing Horses. 2nd edition, 1863.

Speaking of the admirable arrangement of the crust-fibres for sustaining the weight by their almost perpendicular direction, he adds : 'In the sole, on the other hand, all these conditions favourable for sustaining weight are wanting. The fibres are much less substantial than those of the crust, they are not so closely connected together, and, lastly, *they are placed in layers in a horizontal position. The sole, therefore, from its construction, is unable to sustain weight or pressure.* . . . . Whilst the structure of the crust is in fibres, standing with their ends on the ground, the structure of the sole consists of fibres placed in layers horizontally. The difference in power of sustaining weight, which arises from this difference in the position of the fibres, will be easily seen. Anything standing perpendicularly will sustain a much greater weight without yielding, than it will if placed horizontally. . . Whilst, then, from its construction it is evident that the insensitive sole is not intended to bear weight, it is also most important, on account of its position, that no undue weight should be put upon it. . . . The fibres of the insensitive sole may be compared to layers of fibres of hay, placed horizontally. These will necessarily crush in under a comparatively light weight, for neither by their position nor by substance are they calculated to sustain weight or pressure.'

This is quite a mistake ; and is founded on a misconception of the anatomical structure of this part, which was first promulgated by Girard. The horn-fibres of the sole are secreted, and grow in exactly the same direction as those of the crust, and are capable of sustaining a considerable share of the animal's weight, as well as contact with the ground. This is a fact worthy of bearing in mind ; as with a mode of shoeing I have adopted, as well as in the French method of Lafosse, and a modification of it which will be noticed presently, the sole does support more or less of the strain and wear, and not only with impunity, but to the advantage of foot and limb. The horse's sole, in common with that of every quadruped, was destined by nature to sustain more or less weight and wear, and if it is not cruelly deprived of what nature has wisely given it for that purpose, it will do so perfectly.

Colonel Fitzwygram's method of shoeing does not appear to have gained much ground. The difficulties in rounding or curving-up the toe of the shoe to a proper degree, and the objection of farriers and grooms to allow the foot to remain in a healthy unmutilated state, will, it is to be feared, operate, more or less, against its adoption.

The treatise, however, should be in the hands of every horseman, not only because of the excellent advice it contains relative to the preservation and defence of the foot, but also for the clear and philosophical discussion of the various predisposing causes of disease in that organ. Miles's method of nailing, and Colonel Fitzwygram's directions for maintaining the sole and frog intact, mark, perhaps, the greatest improvements in shoeing in England during this century.

In 1862, Mr Mavor, a veterinary surgeon in London, patented a form of shoe and method of shoeing intended to serve several useful and important purposes. The shoe was made of iron rolled by machinery into a particular shape; so that when formed it appeared as a narrow, though somewhat thick rim of metal, slightly concave towards the ground, the lower margin being thin; while the foot-surface was flat, and the holes were made in the middle line of the shoe. According to Mr Mavor, the advantages of his mode of shoeing were cheapness, lightness, and simplicity of manufacture. As a proof that it was superior to every other mode, this inventor asserted that it did not in any way injure the horse's foot, but, on the contrary, allowed its natural freedom of action; promoted the growth of horn; prevented disease and concussion to the limbs; gave the horse a firm foot-hold on the most slippery pavement; was particularly adapted to strengthen flat, weak feet; and enabled the horse to travel over loose gravel without injury to, or the collection of dirt and stones in, his feet. The hind-shoes were of such a form that, though light, they were more durable than the old flat shoes; and it was impossible for the horse to cut his legs, over-reach, or click with them.

In preparing the shoe, little hammering was required; the nail-holes were punched in the centre, and inclining inwards; the iron being only the width of the crust of the foot, there was no danger of these apertures proving too coarse for nailing. In applying the shoe, the crust and bars were to be lowered and levelled from the ground-surface only, as rasping the outside of the crust and cutting away the sides of the frog weakened the foot and destroyed its naturally circular form. The sole was not to be cut, and care was to be taken to fit the shoe accurately to the outer line of the hoof, so that it might rest only upon the crust, and not upon the sole.

This method of shoeing was carried on for a short time, and fell into disuse, chiefly, perhaps, through the prejudice of the grooms and farriers in London.

CHAPTER XIII.

IN France, where veterinary science has flourished, and has been productive of most beneficial results, many excellent works on farriery have appeared during the century. Chief among them may be mentioned those of Girard,[1] Gohier,[2] Jauze,[3] Bouley,[4] Rey,[5] Merche,[6] Meg-

[1] Traité du Pied. Paris, 1813.
[2] Tableau Synoptique. Lyons, 1820.
[3] Cours de Maréchalerie Vétérinaire. Paris, 1827.
Traité de l'Organisation du Pied du Cheval. Paris, 1851. Also the article ' Ferrure,' in the Nouveau Dictionnaire Pratique, etc., Vété-rinaires. Paris, 1858.
[5] Traité de Maréchalerie Vétérinaire. Lyons, 1852.
[6] Mémoire sur les Principaux Systèmes de Ferrure. Paris, 1862.

nin,[1] and Goyau;[2] and for Belgium those of Defays.[3]
With an intimate knowledge of the structure and organization of the horse's foot, the majority of these writers
attempt to establish the practice of shoeing on a really
scientific basis ; and to make it not only subservient to
the defence of healthy organs, but also to remedy their
diseases and defects. In all these works we can trace a
gradual admission of, or approach to, the opinions held
by Lafosse with respect to the preservation of the horse's
hoof, by abstaining from mutilating it.

I regret I cannot give anything like a just idea of
these writings in the limits I have allowed myself; but as
they are comparatively recent, they are easily accessible to
the inquirer who is anxious to learn more of the subject
than I have attempted to sketch.

The curved or 'rocking' shoe of Bourgelat, so objectionable because the horse's foot shod with it had no level
or firm base to support the weight of the limb and body,
was in general use in France up to a late period; and
though Gohier had diminished the excessive toe and heel
curvature, we find Jauze still recommending it, and, more
or less modified, it has continued in use to the present day.

[1] Ferrure du Cheval. Paris, 1865. La Maréchalerie Française.
Paris, 1867. The French Government has always manifested the greatest anxiety to advance veterinary science, as it has now for many years
found the national interest to be deeply concerned in its progress. The
subject of farriery has, therefore, not been neglected ; and we observe
that the Minister for War has marked his appreciation of the value of
this, and the clever little monograph by M. Merche, by bestowing on
each of the authors a gold medal.

[2] Ferrure du Cheval, Paris, 1869.

[3] Les Ferrures Pathologiques. Brussels, 1866. Mém. sur l'En-
castelure. Notice sur une Nouvelle Ferrure à Glace, etc.

In M. Bouley's writings we find excellent principles laid down with regard to shoeing, though he recommends a certain amount of paring of the sole. M. Goyau's little treatise is, perhaps, the best practical work on shoe ing that has appeared in France; while M. Megnin's is remarkable for the great research and ability displayed in investigating the history of French farriery.

In 1840, M. Riquet, a veterinary surgeon of some repute, introduced what he termed a 'podometrical' method of shoeing.[1] We have already casually intimated that, from the time when the improvement of fitting shoes hot to the hoofs was introduced, a few amateurs and professional men fancied that injury was done to the horse's foot. In rare cases this was the case, no doubt; for the custom of paring the sole almost to the quick was so prevalent, that we cannot wonder if a careless workman did now and again retain the hot shoe long enough against the lower margin of the crust, to permit the bor- der of the sensitive sole to suffer from the high tem- perature in its vicinity. These accidents, however, appear to have been remarkably unfrequent, if we may judge from their being so seldom alluded to.

The idea prevailed to some extent, nevertheless, that hot fitting was hurtful, and it was to guard against its effects that the foot-measure shoeing was introduced. The instrument contrived to note the dimensions of the foot was ingenious, though defective, and the system altogether was so well conceived that it attained a large amount of popu larity in a short time. The size, though not the shape, of

[1] De la Ferrure Podométrique. Tours, 1840.

the horse's feet being accurately ascertained by means of the podometer, this was entered in a register, so that the shoes could be made in the forge, and the animal shod with them without being required to leave his stable.

The idea appeared to be excellent, and was at first willingly, if not gladly, received by the veterinary profession in France, where it was extensively tested. M. Riquet had so highly exaggerated the risks and injurious effects of applying the hot shoe to the hoof, and so vaunted the advantages to be derived from his podometric *ferrure à froid,* that a large number of cavalry officers became temporary converts, and indeed unreasonable enthusiasts. Even the French Minister of War did not escape the contagion, and on the 30th August, 1845, issued an order that ' in all mounted corps the cold method of fitting was to be immediately substituted for the hot.' This was no proof in favour of the invention, but rather a testimony to the plausible statements and peculiar tact of M. Riquet.

Of course the matter was soon tested; though it was some time before it was finally decided. ' At the Cavalry School of Saumur,' writes M. Barthélemy,[1] ' experiments have been made from the 22nd September, 1841, to the 5th October, 1844. During these three years all the near-side horses of the school have been shod by the cold, and the off-side ones by the hot method. In that space of time, out of 22,579 shoes which had been fitted in a cold state, 386 were lost, detached, or broken, and only 123 out of the same number fitted while hot; that is, in the first case, 1 shoe in 58 was detached, while

---

[1] Bulletin de la Soc. Vétérinaire, 1846.

in the second there was only 1 in 183. This enormous difference would have been still greater, if the hot fitting had been practised in the ordinary manner. But the School was then labouring under an impression of dangers which I might almost term chimerical, from burning the sole, and which the theory of podometric shoeing had developed. So that an order was given to the farriers to apply the hot shoe lightly, and immediately remove all that portion of the horn which had been in contact with it; this was almost a return to cold fitting. The order was punctually executed, under the uninterrupted superintendence of the acting brigadier.'

This evidence is in perfect harmony with that furnished at a later period by Colonel Ambert[1] of the Saumur School, who was at first a zealous partisan of Riquet's system. 'Out of 650 horses, the effective strength of a regiment, during every month from 55 to 60 lost their shoes in marching or manœuvering, since the employment of cold fitting; or, in other terms, the regiment has not marched for an hour without losing a shoe. With the system of hot-fitting, the same regiment lost only one shoe in a journey of eight stages.' After an extensive experience, this observer arrives at the following conclusions·

' 1. The hot fitting is not attended by any danger or inconvenience when properly practised (that is, on hoofs the soles of which are pared).

' 2. The solidity of hot shoeing (or fitting) being greater than that of cold, the workman having more

---

[1] De la Ferrure des Chevaux.   Journal de Méd. Vét., p. 246. 1851.

facility for the former than the latter, and also owing to its requiring less time, we are of opinion that in the army, as everywhere else, the preference must be given to the *ferrure à chaud.*'

Lafosse, Bourgelat, Chabert, Gohier, Rainard, Reynal, Delafond, Renault, Bouley, and Rey—in fact, all the most distinguished veterinary professors or practitioners who have studied the subject—have unhesitatingly given the preference to the mode of fitting the shoe while hot.

The Central Society of Veterinary Medicine of France, composed certainly of men most competent to judge, after discussing this question in 1846, came to the following conclusions, which were accepted unanimously by the profession :—

' 1. The *ferrure à chaud* is undoubtedly superior to the *ferrure à froid,* executed in the manner recommended and practised at this time, in that it always allows the workman to make the shoe to fit the foot—a fundamental rule in good farriery, and an immense advantage that the *ferrure à froid* does not offer.

' 2. The cold shoeing, as now practised, at the same time that it is generally more difficult and requires a longer time, is for this reason more expensive, while it is generally less solid and less durable.

' 3. Nevertheless, skilfully practised by an able workman, cold shoeing may be resorted to without much danger, and even with benefit, in some exceptional cases.

' 4. The inconveniences attributed to the hot shoeing are also applicable to the cold method, excepting always burning the sole.

'5. That this very rare accident never produces the bad effects attributed to it.

'6. Consequently there does not now exist any plausible or valid reason for substituting cold for hot shoeing.

'7. Lastly, the advantages attributed to podometric shoeing, especially that which allows the preparation of the shoes without the horses being present, and applying them away from the forge, are not sufficiently demonstrated; and in any case, if they were, they could not compensate for the inconveniences inherent in this procedure.' [1]

And one of the highest authorities on shoeing, Professor Rey,[2] of Lyons, thus sums up the advantages and disadvantages of both methods :—

'*Advantages of cold-shoeing.*—Cold shoeing does not expose the horse to the danger of having his feet burned. It may be executed either in the stable or in the middle of the highway. It evades the necessity of taking the horse to the forge to be shod, and where the flame of the fire might frighten it. This is an argument of little value, as, with scarcely an exception, horses are not afraid of the forge. Cold shoeing is preferable for weak, flat, or foundered feet, with thin soles. This is, in our opinion, the only real advantage.

'*Inconveniences of cold shoeing.*—The greatest defect in cold shoeing consists in its want of solidity. When we fit a shoe cold the horn is hard and resists every blow of the hammer, while. by the action of heat, it is a little

---

[1] Recueil de Médecine Vétérinaire, p. 476.   1846.
[2] Traité de Maréchalerie, p. 196.

softened, and permits a more exact adaptation. It is less solid, particularly in wet weather. When the atmospheric temperature, however, is less inconstant, its durability is greater. This phenomenon is not observed with hot shoeing (Reynal). The authors who wrote at the period when cold shoeing only was known, notice its want of solidity. Cæsar Fiaschi thus expresses himself in the middle of the 16th century: 'Je ne vois d'autre remède, eu égard au peu de solidité de cette ferrure, que de savoir soi-même brocher les clous ou de se faire suivre par un maréchal.'

'In campaigns, cold shoeing offers less resistance to the deteriorating action of humidity, mud, and bad roads. The veterinary surgeons who accompanied the expedition to Rome, in 1849, have described the inconvenience of cold shoeing in time of war, in connection with its de fective solidity, and the difficulty in adopting it. . . . This system of shoeing always necessitates making the foot to fit the shoe. It is difficult of application in cases where regiments are on the march, if the farriers are obliged to seek for the horses in their billets. It takes a longer time, and is not so easy. Its duration is less among town's-horses which run on paved roads, as they wear out their shoes in less than from 15 to 20 days.

'After this shoeing the horn is more brittle, and shoes are more frequently lost. Lastly, cold shoeing is less economical.

'*Advantages of hot shoeing.* In *hot shoeing*, the shoe is more readily adapted to the foot.

'The shoes which have been fitted hot to the hoofs are applied more equally. The shoeing is more solid, because the nails are not broken by the displacement of the shoe; there is a better adaptation of the clip at the toe, and a more intimate adhesion is obtained between the iron and the surface of the horn.

'Hot shoeing endows the hoof with more resistance; the horn, heated by the iron, is less hygrometrical, and less permeable by fluids.

'M. Reynal thinks that the caloric that impregnates the horn favourably disposes it for the reception of the shoe; that it destroys the absorbent, spongy, hygrometrical properties of the horn, and renders it insensible to external influences. . . . With some show of reason, the effects produced on horn by the hot iron have been compared to those of fire on pieces of wood whose extremities are superficially carbonized before being buried in the ground. Every one knows that this operation contributes to the preservation of the wood by preserving it from the action of humidity.'

Professor Renault put the two methods to the test of what was looked upon by competent authorities as a convincing experiment. He took two feet from a dead horse, one of which had been shod in the ordinary manner by fitting the iron plate to it while hot, and the other by the cold plan, according to the prescribed rules. These feet were immersed for twelve days in the water and mud of a pond, and afterwards washed and exposed for eight days to the action of heat. At the end of that period, the foot that had been fitted with the cold shoe, the hoof of which was previously swollen under the influence of humidity, had lost a great part of its primitive volume by the action of the heat. The shoe projected slightly all round the foot, although it had been closely fitted to the inside quarter, according to rule. It was not so firm on the hoof; the rivets were not so solid, or so well incrusted in the wall. With the other foot, shod on the hot method, nothing like this was observed; after, as before the experiment, the solidity of the shoeing was excellent. It was this test that led M. Reynal to believe that the caloric which impregnates the horn disposes it favourably for the reception of the shoe; that it destroys its absorbent, spongy, hygrometrical properties, and renders it insensible to external influences.[1]

With regard to the risk of injury from burning the sensitive parts enclosed within the hoof, the opponents of hot fitting, the majority of whom really knew little, if anything, of the matter practically, and either forgot or were unaware of the fact that horn is a slow conductor of heat, might have been converted by the experiments of Professor Delafond. He showed in a most conclusive manner, that a very long-continued application of the hot shoe was required to affect the vascular parts of the foot. Applying a small thermometer to the inner surface of the sole, and bringing a hot shoe in contact with the ground aspect of the foot, he found it required *three minutes* burning to produce any effect on the thermometer. Reynal also experimented to test this fact, and the result was, that the thermometer inside the hoof did not mark any change until after the sole had been roasted by a hot iron for a period three times longer than that needed for a farrier to fit his shoe. And M. Barthélemy has watched

[1] *Vatel.* Rapport sur la Ferrure à Froid. Soc. Centrale Vétérinaire, 1846.

workmen who were unconscious of his presence, in order
to note the exact number of seconds during which they
held the hot shoe to the foot.   These observations proved,
that in shoeing 100 hoofs, the hot shoe was kept in contact with the horn on an average of from 46 to 47 seconds;
that the maximum of this application was 80 seconds, and
the minimum 29 seconds.   He never knew of a horse being injured in this manner.

It may be useful to know Delafond's conclusions as to
the relative influence of various degrees of temperature
on the foot:—

' 1. The shoe warmed to a dark red heat, the carbonized portion of the sole not having been removed by the
buttress, transmits more caloric to the living tissues within
a given time than the shoe heated to a bright red (*rouge
cerise*).

' 2. The thickness of the sole being the same, the
shoe heated to a dark red causes a deeper and more severe
burn than the bright red one.

' 3. These experiments confirm what was stated in
1758 by Lafosse, that it is not the shoe heated to bright
red that most frequently causes burns of the vascular sole,
but rather that which is scarcely red or black heated.' [1]

Latterly, the few advocates of cold fitting blamed the
hot method for causing dryness of the horn and contraction of the hoof; but they either kept out of sight, or
were not cognisant of the fact, that these conditions had
been complained of when nothing but cold fitting was
known.

In a few years the cold fitting method in France had

[1] *O. Delafond.*   Recueil de Méd. Vétérinaire, p. 951.   1845.

completely failed, and was a mere tradition, only advocated by some eccentric individual, whose fancies were unassailable by facts.

Even M. Riquet, who had retired from the army, and had become veterinary surgeon to a large Omnibus Company in Paris, no longer recommended it; and the army horses were shod on the infinitely superior principle of hot fitting.

Professor Bouley remarks, that it is impossible to do iustice to a horse's feet, when shoeing them in a stable, away from the forge, by this cold adjustment of the shoes. There are so many variations in size, form, and general configuration, which no workman can remember when making the shoes; and if these are not rigorously adapted to the disposition of the foot, then is that organ likely to suffer.

Alluding to the experiments that had been instituted to ascertain the relative value of the two methods, he says: 'From whence arises so great a difference in the results, which is completely to the disadvantage of the cold fitting? It is because the hot shoe, in fusing the horn with which it comes in contact, imprints itself, it may be said, like a seal into sealing wax, and in this way the foot and shoe are in the same relation to each other as surfaces that exactly coincide; while no matter how expert the workman may be in using his tools to level the horn in a cold state, he can never do this so completely as may be done by making an impression with the heated shoe, and consequently establishing between the plantar margin of the hoof and the shoe an exact coaptation. It may be added, that when the horn has been softened by the action of caloric, the nails enter it with more facility, the clips and inequalities are more easily incrusted, and when it recovers its habitual consistency after cooling, the union between it and the metallic parts which are in juxtaposition, and which penetrate its substance, become all the more intimate because of the slight contraction that follows the dilatation produced by the caloric. In these conditions, the horn contracts on the shanks of the nails, ensheathing them still more firmly. Nothing like this occurs in cold fitting. The shoe so fixed is held to the hoof by the clenches alone, and, as often happens, the coaptation between these two not being very intimate, the branches of the shoe spring under the foot at each step, the clenches are easily broken by this movement, and the shoe is detached.'

Professor Goyau is entirely in favour of the shoes being fitted while in a hot state.

It is impossible to notice all the new shoes introduced in France. As in England, many of them were scarcely submitted to trial before they failed; others underwent a longer ordeal, and gradually subsided into forgetfulness, while the best-devised never attained to any degree of popularity. In 1820, M. Sanfarouche introduced a shoe which had its brief day. Believing in the expansion of the foot to the same extent as did Bracy Clark, this device was merely an English fullered shoe, or, as sometimes occurred, one stamped in the French fashion. It was of the same thickness throughout, was bevelled and seated like the ordinary shoe in use in this country, and wider at the heels than elsewhere, in order to facilitate the expansion of the hoof. It was also narrow, to prevent slipping. A short time after this shoe had fallen into disuse, another inventor introduced a 'hipposandal' system of shoeing; a large establishment was opened for the manufacture of this article, and Paris was duly placarded with the marvellous results to be derived from the application of this humane invention to the feet of horses. It had but a very brief existence, and was quickly forgotten. Then another shoe was proposed to prevent slipping. This was almost identical with the winter shoe in use in Canada, in having its ground-surface quite concave, and the animal resting on nothing but a sharp margin, which could not fail to give excellent foothold so long as it lasted. Unfortunately this was only for a brief period, as the shoe was made of iron. Had it been manufactured of steel, as the Canadian shoe is, it would, in all likelihood, have proved too slippery for the pavement.

The prevention of slipping has determined, more or less, the form of nearly all the shoes and methods of shoeing proposed in recent times. Indeed, it appears to have been, next to the preservation of the wall of the hoof, the chief *desideratum* from the very earliest period. We have observed that the primitive shoes had calkins to grasp the earth, and, in addition, well-lodged nail-heads, that stood high above the level of the shoe, and while keeping the animal's foot on a plane parallel with the ground, endowed it with the grasping powers of a double row of catches such as no modern shoeing has furnished. A farrier of Tours some years ago endeavoured to imitate this very primitive mode, and made nails with an iron shank and a large steel head. These, their inventor said, possessed two advantages: 1. They preserved the shoe from wear, as the heads of the nails sustained the effects of contact with the ground, and were, in this way, economical. 2. They secured the animal wearing them a safe footing on the pavement, either in summer or winter.

No doubt, the early inhabitants of Gaul and Britain have testified to these advantages two thousand years ago.

M. Perrier, believing that the ordinary expansion theory was a fallacy, and that the supposed movement took place at the anterior part of the foot, introduced a method of shoeing which was intended to promote the toe and quarter resiliency. The hoof was pared as thin as possible at these parts, while the heels were permitted to grow strong. The shoe was very narrow in front, but wide and thick towards the ends of the branches. The method of shoeing appeared to be, in many respects, almost exactly the reverse of that in every-day use. Its trial appears to have been very brief and unsatisfac tory.

Still more recently, M. Watrin attempted to modify the ordinary method of shoeing, though in a very unreasonable manner. His object appears to have been merely directed to prevent contraction of the heels; and we can scarcely doubt that the means by which he sought to attain that end were those most likely to induce this deformity. The sole was well pared, the frog and bars mutilated, the external quarter of the fore-foot was reduced to a lower level than the inner, though in the hind-foot it was the reverse. The shoe was that generally in use in France, only at the inner corner of each heel it had a clip that bent down and grasped the inner aspect of the bar. This shoe and method of shoeing could not possibly succeed, destructive as it was to the foot in general, but particularly to the inflections of the crust.   It was merely Ruini's shoe.

Veterinary Surgeon Naudin proposed a very narrow, light shoe, with a level bearing on the ground; for it must be remembered that the ordinary French shoe is 'adjusted,' or curved up at the toe, like that proposed by Goodwin, Miles, and Fitzwygram.   It did not vary to any notable degree from other shoes of this type; and the most important feature in the method of applying it was its being attached to the foot by from four to six nails.   The sole of the foot was left intact.

Yet later, M. Benjamin introduced a shoe which may be said to be the same as that proposed by Sanfarouche; though it was a great step in advance of what had yet been offered during this century in France.   The entire sole and frog were left in their natural condition, and the crust only was diminished to its natural proportions.   M. Benjamin justly claimed for this light, narrow shoe, and unmutilated sole and frog, great advantages over other systems, and the discussions among the French veterinary surgeons, which followed the introduction of his plan, shows that there was a singular unanimity as to the necessity for maintaining this most important region of the hoof in its full strength and solidity.

Nor has France been without its machine-made shoes of iron and steel, contrived to prevent slipping, while resisting wear.   M. Peschelle, some years ago, introduced a shoe with circular projections or double calkins on its ground surface, which was made by machinery.   This shoe not answering its purpose, the same inventor had laminated bars forged with a deep groove, or grooves, running along the middle of one of their faces, and from these bars shoes were made. The foot surface being flat, and the ground side deeply cut by the groove, afforded a tolerably secure grip of the pavement.

I have not been able to learn whether these were ever much employed, or whether they are now in use. From what I have heard, it would appear that, like all the machine-made shoes in this country, their utility was limited, and they scarcely attained notoriety before they became partially or totally obsolete.

Professor Tabourin, of Lyons, introduced *fers à pinçon circulaire,* which were made by machinery. The result of this experiment in hoof-armature has not been made public, I believe.

To a wonderful extent, it has been otherwise with a shoe and method of shoeing which, perhaps, more than any other in this century, has attracted public attention. In 1865, M. Charlier, a veterinary surgeon in Paris, brought to notice a patented method of shoeing which he designated 'périplantaire.' It proved to be the greatest innovation on the established routine of the age, so far as the farrier's art is concerned. And yet, after all, like the 'ferrure Benjamin,' the 'ferrure Charlier' in France is but a page of old Lafosse's treatise, which the oftener we read, the more we wonder at the existence of the grossest ab surdities in shoeing, and at the presence of painful and de structive diseases that ruin the horse and prove sad sources of bewilderment to his owner.

The 'ferrure Charlier' is a gentle *modification* of the 'fer incruste enclave' or 'croissant' of Lafosse, and the narrow shoe of Moorcroft, Mavor, and others. It consists, or rather consisted, in the insertion or imbedding of a narrow, but comparatively thick, band of iron or mild steel, around the front of the foot, in a recess cut out for it in the crust or wall of the hoof, and is very simple to look at and to consider. Only remove so much comparative soft and brittle horn, and substitute a hard, tough rim of iron or steel, almost as light (if we look at the ordinary shoes) as the material you remove, and you have insured the *soliped* against the effects of travelling, and almost restored his foot to its pristine condition.

Such is the Charlier method of shoeing; and if it has been modified in one or two essential features since its introduction, in others it has withstood the test of time, and testified in the most unequivocal manner to the correctness of the teaching afforded by the great author of modern and humane farriery. The idea of this method of shoeing, M. Charlier says, was suggested by the fashion of arming the extremity of a walking-stick by a ferrule, which everybody knows is a most efficient protection to the mass of wood it encloses.

On the 10th August, 1865, he makes the following communication to the Société Impériale et Centrale de Médecine Vétérinaire: 'Many among you have already heard of a new system of shoeing that I have imagined to prevent horses from slipping, at the same time affording them a natural bearing on the ground, and opposing contraction of the heels, and preventing several diseases caused by the shoeing now in use. Have I solved this difficult problem? I hope so; for the theory of abler authors founded on the anatomy and physiology of the foot is completely in favour of my procedure, and numerous experiments made in every condition have afforded me the following results. . . . This shoeing consists in the methodical application of a small bar of iron or steel, bent on the flat, thicker and wider at the toe and sides of the toe than at the quarters and heels, especially in its outer branch; it is about the width of the crust at its upper face, is perforated by from four to six nail-holes, rarely more, and is fitted into a groove or recess made at the inferior border of the wall, by means of small English nails with very thin shanks, driven in the usual way. Simple in conception, as it is in execution, this shoeing has many advantages, and its consequences are immense. I will endeavour to prove this to you. First, let us re-member what our learned colleague, Professor Bouley, has said in his admirable works on shoeing : " The art of the farrier ought to be to preserve to the hoof the integrity of its form, essentially allied to that of its functions; and this result can only be obtained in leaving to the bars, the buttresses (*arcs-boutants*—the angle formed by the bar and crust), and the frog and sole all their power of re-sistance ; in protecting them without interfering with their action, their contact with the ground, their suppleness, or their natural flexibility."

'No mode of shoeing as practised to-day can com-pletely respond to these various demands. To apply to the sole of the foot a metallic plate, more or less wide, but al ways inflexible, restrains it, elevates the frog, prevents its participating in weight-bearing, and, do as we may, hinders its natural functions, destroys more or less rapidly its supple-ness, the elasticity of the horny box, and, in a word, injures the vitality, the nutrition, and the good conformation of the foot.

'The frog which is thrown out of its functions, says Coleman, becomes diseased. It is the same with the external border of the sole and the bars when hindered from contact with the ground and deprived of their normal functions. When a horse has its shoes taken off, it is easy to see that all these organs suffer, that they have not their amplitude, their form, or their natural consistency. Most frequently they are hard, contracted, atrophied, dried up, or rotten. In the country, where it is possible to allow horses to go without shoes, and in foals which have not yet been shod, with the exception of the crust being worn, we see nothing abnormal; the frogs are large, the heels solid, the horn of the sole supple though resisting, and all, in a word, tends to show that vitality is there as in other parts of the body, and that the foot receives the nutritive fluids necessary to it.

'Having been struck for a long time with this difference, and the troublesome consequences which result therefrom, I sought in vain, like so many others, to modify the actual shoe, until one day I said to myself: Since the unshod horse travels perfectly well on unpaved or non-macadamized roads, and as it is always the crust which commences to break and become worn, owing to the hardness of the stony streets, is it not possible to protect this wall without touching the other parts? and would this not solve the problem?

'It was natural, therefore, that I should reflect that on the handles of several instruments, on the ends of certain articles, a ferrule of iron or copper was put to prevent them from splitting.

37

'Full of hope that the sole and the other parts would offer sufficient resistance to the hardness of our pavements and stony roads, I tried, and little by little, after many attempts, I at last imagined the shoe I now have the honour to lay before you.

'This shoe, thicker than it is wide, is very light compared with the ordinary shoe, weighing more than a third less; it is forged without trouble even by one man, and is turned, fitted, and attached as easily as the other. I am inclined to believe, then, that I have reached the end I proposed to myself, and which was to make horses travel unshod, or, since that was not possible with our paved and macadamized roads, at least with a simple rim of iron which allows all parts of the plantar surface, especially the frog and buttresses, to participate in sustaining the weight and adhering solidly to the ground.

'It is a long time since the great practitioner Lafosse had recognized the necessity of allowing the frog to play its part; we have not forgotten the famous lunette shoe which has been so much lauded, and the only inconveniences of which were that it allowed the horn of the heels to be split and prevented wearing of the toe, thus giving the limb a false position and interfering with free movement.

'My shoe has not these defects; for while accomplishing the same object, it protects the heels, wears regularly along its circumference, like the foot itself in favour able conditions.

'It is a solid artificial border, replacing the inferior margin of the wall, which is not strong enough to resist our hard roads. It is no more than this.

'The horse thus shod, after the early days succeeding its first application, when it sometimes goes less freely than usual, and appears more sensitive to the asperities of the ground, moves evenly, and with lightness, grace, suppleness, and liveliness, and is more easily managed ; all his paces, in a word, indicate that he finds himself more at liberty than with the sub-plantar shoeing.

'When at rest, we observe that he has nearly always his four feet resting on the ground, while other horses have usually a foot resting—no doubt to relieve alternately the dull pain or fatigue they experience in the hoof; neither is this so hot or feverish after journeys.

'Like the Lafosse shoe, although much more efficiently, it prevents slipping. During the frost of the first days in January and February, I have been able to travel with confidence without frost nails or calkins, when the horses of others could not move unless their feet were armed with these appliances so destructive to feet and limbs. I one day travelled along boldly with a mare whose limbs were used-up, but which was shod on my system, alongside a troop of cavalry, the soldiers being forced to dismount and lead their horses by the bridle. In snowy weather, every horse had its feet balled and walked with difficulty, while mine experienced nothing of the kind, and this result has since been observed with farm horses working on heavy clay land, where, during damp weather, they previously had their feet laden with masses of soil several inches thick, from which they could only with difficulty be freed.

'It must be an immense advantage in Paris to be able to prevent horses from slipping, not only during the

37 *

frosts of winter, but when the roads are greasy or leaded (plombé), on the granite pavement, where so many horses fall, or on the rolled asphalte, which. although a calamity at present, may become a great boon, in saving horses and carriages, be easier kept clean, diminish the noise, dust, etc., if my shoeing is adopted.

'What falls, sprains, and accidents of every description will be avoided in preventing horses from slipping! Perfectly firm on all kinds of pavement, they will be more light in hand, more easy to drive, will be less fatigued, and tire their riders less, will travel more quickly, and we will not so often see those premature failures of the limbs for which the curative art can do so little, and which cause such heavy losses to the owners of horses.

'My shoeing is also opposed to the development of corns (bleimes) and contusions, caused either by the ordinary shoes or the interposition between them and the sole of stones, pebbles, or other hard bodies, since the branches of my shoe do not bear on the corners of the sole, and no foreign body can fix itself there, or bruise the living structures.

But that which more particularly makes my method of shoeing superior to all the other known methods is, I repeat, the fact of the foot being allowed its liberty of action, all its vertical and lateral elasticity, however trifling this may be at the lower part of the hoof. or whatever may be the combinations it determines there; in this respect it evidently opposes wasting of the hoof and contraction of the heels, that destructive affection which ruins a considerable number of valuable horses.

'At first sight, this precious result of my shoeing may

not appear manifest, for already several of my *confrères* have thought that the foot must be constrained by the little bar of iron that constitutes the shoe. To convince them that this is not so, it is sufficient to take the branches of the shoe in both hands, and to separate or push them together, when it will be found that they yield to pressure. In operating in the same manner by the pressure of the thumbs against the branches of the sole, the hands being joined around the hoof, I have also re-marked and demonstrated to others the elasticity of the shoe, which follows the movements, dilatation, and con-traction of the heels: the animal's weight, in coming upon the foot in every part, produces on it, as on the wall itself, the effect of a wedge driven into a piece of wood. All that can be said against my shoe is its too great elasticity when it is worn thin. In striking on the pavement it may spread out from the heels, inconvenience the animal, or break. I remedy this trifling inconvenience by making the last hole as far back as possible.

'For saddle horses, for those of light draught, and for all those *chevaux de luxe,* or of agriculture, which do not work very severely, this shoeing will certainly prove a great benefit.

'It only remains to be seen if it will sufficiently resist the repeated and excessively fatiguing journeys performed by the horses in public conveyances, and especially those omnibus horses which travel on the bad pavement of Paris.

'For the first case, placed as I am, I am already in a position to be able to solve the question. Numerous experiments are being made with the horses of the Compagnie Impériale des Voitures de Paris, and it has already been proved that for the fore-feet, the duration of the shoe leaves nothing to be desired, and it is at least equal to that of the ordinary shoe. For the hind-feet only, because of the hard work imposed upon these horses, more resistance is required; and I hope to obtain this result when the hoofs become stronger, and allow me to employ shoes which are thicker at the toe, and also adding a kind of clips, for those which twist their feet. At present this is not possible; the feet have been too long narrowed at the toe, rasped, chiselled, deteriorated, in a word *chinoisés;* and it is necessary that I wait until nature, with the help of the simple protection she requires, repair the damage which has been done. It is not usually until the third or fourth shoeing, when the wall begins to grow thicker, and the horn of the sole stronger and more solid, that we may venture to put on strong shoes and imbed them well.'

As this mode of shoeing has attracted much attention, and as it presents several features which, if they are not particularly novel, are yet interesting, closely connected as they are with the functions and preservation of the horse's foot, the principles followed in its application will be noticed somewhat in detail, particularly as they are sufficiently simple to be readily understood.

The instruments required differ but little from those now in use, though they may be much lighter and more convenient. The *boutoir* employed by the French *maréchal* to pare the foot has, in this instance, its borders raised at right angles to a certain height, and is provided with a guide or regulator in the middle of its lower face, so as to give to each side of the blade a width proportioned to the thickness of the wall of the foot intended to be shod in this manner. M. Charlier insists that this instrument should only be employed to make the groove or trench for the reception of the shoe, the sole, frog, and bars not being allowed to be pared, but only relieved of the dead horn which is detached or projects in the region of the heels; and he wisely suggests that this *boutoir* might be replaced by a flat double or single *rainette*, provided with a guide. He gives a figure of an instrument of this kind, which resembles the English farrier's drawing-knife, the only difference being the presence of a stud fixed into its under surface near the curve or point, to prevent cutting too deeply into the margin of the sole. This contrivance, however, according to my experience, is imperfect, owing to the stud being a fixture, and not allowing any latitude to be observed in channelling into a large, small, thin, or strong hoof. My farrier-serjeant has devised a much safer and more convenient instrument in the form of a knife somewhat like the ordinary drawing-knife, but about one-half its length, with only about an inch of cutting edge at its extremity, the end of which, instead of turning over in a curve, stands up at nearly a right angle to the blade for about half an inch. The guide is a plate of iron about three inches long, narrower than the blade of the knife, with a slot or slit passing through the greater part of its length, and attached to the lower face of the instrument by two small screws—one of these a finger-screw, which stand in this slit, and are fixed into two holes in the knife. This arrangement, as will be readily under-stood, permits the cutting edge to be regulated from the extremity of the blade to the extent of an inch backwards, just as necessity may require when preparing the hoof. The guiding power in this respect is considerably enhanced by a portion of the anterior extremity of the plate being bent downwards at a right angle to the knife, and to about the same extent as the end of the blade is turned upwards; this shoulder rests against the face of the wall of the hoof, and very materially aids the shoer in performing the most difficult and hazardous part of the operation—the cutting so close to the sensitive and vascular structures of the foot without injuring them.[1]

Charlier's directions for forging the shoes are these · 'The most convenient-sized iron is that in bar $\frac{3}{4} \times \frac{5}{8}$ inch for large shoes, and $\frac{5}{8} \times \frac{3}{8}$ for small ones; or even square iron, more or less thick, according to the strength required. From such bars the shoes can be forged with an ordinary hammer: the iron is cut off in lengths proportioned to the size of the shoe; one side is made at a heat, but without stamping the holes; the second side is formed at the second heat, the *turning* of the shoe to its proper shape being effected by principally striking its upper border around the toe on the beak of the anvil, so as to give it the natural inclination of the foot. A shoe thus turned is narrower on its upper or foot surface than its lower or ground one.

'The nail-holes are made in each branch or side, and are two or three, rarely four, in number; one at the side of the toe, another at the quarter or middle of the branch, and a third at the heel, all placed at regular intervals. In my trials of this system I have usually had only three nails

---

[1] Mr Brennand, Instrument-maker, 217, High Holborn, London, now makes this knife from my model.

on the outer side and two on the inner, and always found
that number quite sufficient, even in the largest shoes.
With small ones I have only employed two nails on each
side. To stamp these, the shoe must be frequently heated,
as from the thinness of the metal it quickly cools; the
holes so made are smaller than those of ordinary shoes, are
oblong from before to behind, and rounded at the angles so
as not to weaken the iron; they are formed by an untempered cast-steel punch provided with a very tapering and
almost square extremity, the sharp corners being removed,
and the point terminating like a grain of barley. An
assistant holds the shoe in a pair of tongs on the anvil,
and it is pierced from fine to coarse by light blows, the
punch being withdrawn quickly, and straightened if bent,
moistened to keep it cool, and dipped in grease to make
it cut more promptly.

'To counter-pierce the shoe, it is necessary to have a
thinner punch than that for stamping, and a little care is
necessary to prevent the shoe being broken.

'It is of importance that the best iron be used,
notwithstanding its high price; the expense is compensated for by only half the weight being required. It
must not be brittle. Two old shoes furnish sufficient
material to make a new one; hind-shoes are to be preferred.'

The most delicate and difficult stage in the operation
is, of course, attaching the metal to the hoof. Charlier's
directions are as follows:

'1. The horse ought to have been shod a long time,
in order that the sole may have acquired that so-called
excess of thickness that is usually cut away by the farrier.

The old shoes must be carefully removed, in order that the crust of the hoof be not broken.   Only two shoes to be taken off at once,-and these diagonal ones—near hind and off fore, and *vice versâ;* all the old nails and fragments of these, if present, to be extracted.

'2. With an ordinary rasp cut away the angle of the lower border of the wall around the whole circumference of the foot, so as to straighten it and form a bevel or slope, which greatly facilitates the employment of the grooving-knife.

'3. On this bevelled edge form the groove to receive the shoe, but do not cut it so deep or so wide as the thickness of the sole and width of the wall, the limit of the latter being the zone or white-line that marks the separation of these two portions, just within the track of the old nails (fig. 196).

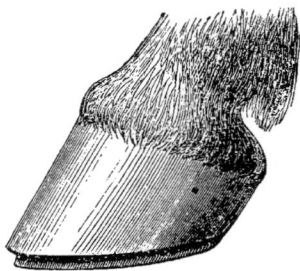

fig. 196

'4. Mould the hot shoe on the beak of the anvil by gentle blows, so as to give it, either from memory or by measurement on an old shoe, the shape of the foot, heating and reheating it until it is perfectly adapted, border to border, to the wall.   If the horse wears its shoes quickly, the outer branch may be left thicker than the inner one.

'5. Make the shoe hot, and fit it into the groove by holding it there, *but without pushing it towards the sole,* taking great care not to leave it so long as to burn, or even heat, the living tissues which are very near this cavity.   A few seconds are sufficient for this operation.

' 6. A solid and equable bearing for the shoe having been obtained, with a small drawing-knife gently remove the superficial layer of horn that has been in contact with the hot shoe, making in this way a little canal (*cannelure*) at the angle of the groove around the sole, but without touching the latter. The intention of this is to leave a space which will allow a little play at the corresponding angle of the shoe.

' 7. Take the shoe and shorten the branches if they are too long, for they should not pass beyond the heels of the foot; round them in a sloping manner from side to side, and with a half-round file take away the inner angle of the upper face of the shoe, so as to form a slight bevel which, corresponding as it does to the canal at the bottom of the groove in the hoof, prevents the sensitive parts being compressed when the weight is thrown upon the foot.

' 8. Attach the shoe with nails in the ordinary manner. The nails should be small and of the ordinary English shape, but the heads a little flatter and longer; they ought to be strong at the neck and thin in the shank.'

'On good feet these different manœuvres, which have taken so long to describe, are easy of execution; and it is only necessary that the intelligent farrier should bring to his task a little willing attention in order to practise them.

' In delicate feet with low heels, thin soles, and narrow walls, such as we so commonly have to deal with when paring and rasping has been allowed for some time, the farrier must take the greatest precautions not to injure the quick. He will not be able to imbed his shoes so deeply as can be otherwise done. In a strong foot this incrustation may be safely carried so far, that the ground-surface of the shoe and the sole are on the same level, and share in supporting the weight and strain imposed upon them. With feet damaged by previous maltreatment, this cannot be done until the horn has been sufficiently regenerated; and in the mean time the shoe may be allowed to project a little above the sole, and particularly towards the heels; though it does not last so long, does not hold so fast, and the frog, not coming entirely on the ground, is longer in regaining its healthy conformation. In these cases, lighter shoes might be used, though they must be replaced more frequently; but in this the hoof does not suffer, the nails being so small and few in number, and no paring or rasping being allowed. With feet of this description it sometimes happens that after the first application of the shoes, the horse does not travel well for three or four days, or sometimes even longer; he is afraid to touch the ground. Rest, or gentle exercise on soft soil, will suffice to give him assurance and free action; and as a longer time elapses, every inconvenience disappears; the sole and crust which are never mutilated become thick and natural, and then stronger shoes may be applied, and imbedded deeper.'

M. Charlier remarks, that it is not rare to see parts of the sole exfoliate in flakes during the first months of his method of shoeing; this, he says, is the dead horn which is being removed to give place to a good secretion as elastic as it is resisting, and in this case it may be useful to aid nature, by carefully excising these flakes, which, if allowed to project, would produce the effects of a foreign body. In this, I think, he is mistaken, as in my experiments with this system of shoeing, if it may be so named, I have always found every particle of horn useful, and never could discover that it caused any inconvenience.

At first this important modification of the ordinary mode of arming the hoof gave rise to very animated discussions. It was argued that it possessed very little novelty, and that it was but a slight improvement, or otherwise, on Lafosse's imbedded shoe. There is certainly not much difference if one compares a section of the two methods. Lafosse's we see in figure 197, and Charlier's in figure 198. The shoe of the first-named veterinarian

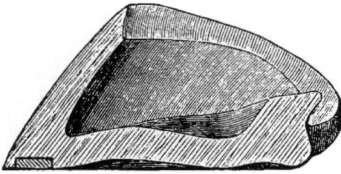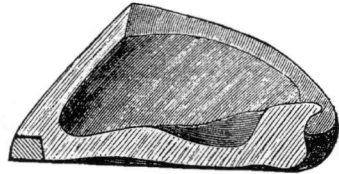

fig. 197   fig. 198

was lighter and narrower, and lay in a space between the sole and crust; whereas Charlier's shoe rested on the crust alone, and was thicker, a trifle wider, and much heavier.

Then grave doubts were entertained as to the amount of injury likely to be inflicted by a rim of iron placed so near the sensitive and vascular parts of the foot. To imbed the thick shoe, so that a portion of the sole might reach the ground, required the removal of so large a piece of the crust, that the union between it and the sole was seriously threatened; the shoe being thicker than the latter, it will be easily seen that to incrust it thoroughly a most extensive chasm had to be made around the margin of the sole, whose attachment with the crust was therefore greatly weakened. This objection appears to have forced itself so strongly on M. Charlier, that only partial incrustation was resorted to in 1866; the shoe being made a trifle wider and thicker, and the groove for its reception much shallower, and certainly not exceeding the thickness of the sole. It appears clips were also added, to prevent the shoe driving back against the sensitive part of the foot. So great an alteration had been made, that instead of 'preplantar,' Professor Bouley designated it 'presolar' shoeing. Its use on the hind-feet was nearly, if not quite, discontinued, as these organs are of little importance, so far as shoeing and disease are concerned, when compared with those in front; and the wear was so severe at the toes, the thinnest part of the hind-feet, that the encircling bands could not be made strong enough to last for a reasonable period, neither could they be imbedded deep enough with safety.

Veterinary Surgeon Signol, who devoted much time and attention to the new shoes and their application when experiments began to be made with them, reports that those used on the omnibus horses of Paris weighed on the average 850 grammes (30 ounces); they were from 18 to 20 millimètres thick (7 to 8-10ths of an inch), and were incrusted in the wall of the hoof to a depth of 15 millimètres (6-10ths of an inch); they had toe-clips. On the fore-feet, these shoes lasted 30, and on the hind-feet 28 days. More than 500 feet were shod within the space of six months; and the advantages noted during that period (1866) were: 1. Economy in material to the extent of at least 250 to 300 grammes each shoe, and even more, as some of the ordinary shoes weighed as much as 2 kilogrammes (4·409 pounds). 2. In consequence of the comparatively trifling weight of their shoes, the horses acquired a lightness of movement they did not exhibit previously. 3. They gained an extraordinary *solidity* on the pavement, and did not slip. 4. Many horses which always had corns and sandcracks, and could not be used without bar-shoes, spontaneously recovered from their infirmities after the application of this shoe. 5. Those frogs which were before shrunken and *étranglé*, became considerably developed, a fact which proves that this shoe is perfectly adapted to the physiological movements of the foot.

It will be seen that these horses were excessively over-weighted with the ordinary shoe.

Professor Bouley, perhaps the highest veterinary authority in France, and a gentleman of great scientific attainments, laid much stress on the particular advantages to be derived from this large diminution in weight. He had given the system of shoeing his careful attention, particularly after the modifications it had undergone, and appears to have been much impressed with its favourable results, notwithstanding its having deviated from the rigorous application of the fundamental principle of rational farriery he had laid down: that at each renewal of the shoes, the foot be brought, by the aid of instru-ments, to the length and form which it would have had if the animal had not been shod, and the horn had been worn in a natural manner. He believed the disadvantages of the ' ferrure Charlier' were more than counterbalanced by its advantages. He noted that, in general, the feet of all the horses so shod acquired a tendency to become enlarged and regain their primitive form, a circumstance which might be explained on reflecting that the sole, bars, and frog, having recovered all their thickness, afterwards oppose an insurmountable obstacle to that movement of contraction on itself, which the hoof tends fatally to assume when the sole and frog are thinned, and the bars are destroyed by the *boutoir*.

For it could not be denied that, with ordinary shoeing, the paring of the hoofs brought about this result, as it was a common practice to test by pressure of the thumbs the proper degree of thinness of the soles.

M. Bouley thought the shoes could be forged and put on as readily as in the old system, and he sums up his report, in 1866, as follows: The preplantar shoeing had been modified by diminishing the depth of the groove, which was not cut so near the living parts of the foot; that this modification, necessitated by experience, prevented pain being inflicted, though it had the disadvantage of making the foot longer than it ought to be, according to the principles of physiological shoeing; that this inconvenience was increased by the necessity there was for giving the shoe a greater thickness—2 centimètres (about 9-10ths of an inch), that its narrowness might be compensated for so as to resist wear for a given time; that this inconvenience, which could not be overlooked, was yet counterbalanced: *a.* By the lightening of the shoe, which diminished fatigue. *b.* By the greater surety of the horse's footing, a more solid bearing on the ground, greater liberty of movement, and as a result, a more efficacious employment of its strength. *c.* By the preservation of the integrity of its feet, or the gradual disappearance of deformities or diseases affecting them.

This authority concludes, that whether the preplantar system of shoeing succeed, or, like so many other systems, fail, its inventor had none the less done good service, in showing what was vicious in the present mode of French shoeing, and how easy it was to benefit horses by making their shoes lighter; already, the opponents of the new method were beginning to see the advantage of reducing the metallic surface, and that this narrowing of the shoes was entirely due to the example given by M. Charlier.

Professor Bouley was, perhaps, not aware of what had been done in England, in this respect; and that in this century M. Charlier's modification had been largely anticipated. Goodwin and Fitzwygram had demonstrated the necessity for leaving the soles unpared, and had conclusively shown that these parts would, to a certain extent, sustain pressure from the shoe. Coleman, Gloag, and others, had shown that the frogs could only be maintained in a healthy condition by performing their natural functions; Turner, Miles, and Fitzwygram had proved that shoes could be retained by a comparatively small number of nails; and Moorcroft and Mavor, that narrow shoes were advantageous in preventing slipping.

Another good result of this method of shoeing in France, was to enlighten the veterinary profession and the farriers of that country, with regard to the pernicious cradle-like shape they gave to their clumsy shoes, in what they termed the *ajusture*. This unseemly, and apparently unreasonable, fashion had been maintained and strenuously defended since the days of Bourgelat; and its effects must have been very prejudicial, especially when improperly applied. The plane-surfaced preplantar shoe

38

found as many advocates in this respect as the English shoe, equally plane, had, perhaps, previously found opponents in France.

Despite the opposition offered to M. Charlier's innovation, it made progress on the continent, and attracted much attention; though it has scarcely been noticed in England. The inventor, if such a designation may be applied, was liberally rewarded by the French Government, and his method of shoeing obtained for him marked honours at the Paris Exhibition of 1867. It has received the highest measure of praise from the principal veterinary teachers of France, among whom were MM. Bouley and Gourdon; in Italy, Professors Bassi and Demarchi, of the Turin veterinary school, have commended it; and in Spain, Professor Bellido, chief of the veterinary school of Cordova, has acknowledged its merits.[1]

The somewhat marvellous effects that result from allowing the sole and the posterior parts of the foot to maintain their integrity, and to assume their natural functions, appear to have astonished even those who were accustomed to study the physiology of that organ; though for that matter the same happy results had been constantly, though never generally, recognized, and in this country, at least, it was not at all uncommon to employ horses with these parts unmutilated, and wearing only thin half or whole shoes.

Fiaschi, no doubt, had noted the same beneficial

[1] For the original papers of M. Charlier, and the numerous letters and discussions resulting from this system, see the 'Bulletin de la Société Impériale et Central de Méd. Vétérinaire,' for 1865, 1866, and 1867. For reports of the experiments in Italy, see the journal 'Il Medico Vétérinario,' for 1867.

effects follow the use of his lunette shoes, and Lafosse was as well acquainted with the benefits to be derived from his method of shoeing as Charlier; while Osmer and Clark were earnest in their protestations against the fashion of removing the heels of the foot from the ground.

Experiments are still being conducted on an extensive scale on the continent, but particularly in France, in order to test how far the 'ferrure périplantaire' may be substituted for the ordinary method. My own trials, though they certainly have been on a limited scale, have proved very satisfactory. Draught and saddle horses have been shod, and in every case with advantage. The shoes employed weighed nearly one-half less than those previously worn, and have been retained firmly in their bed by from four to six small nails for each shoe. Two cases of foot-lameness accompanied by very deformed hoofs and extraordinarily contracted heels, have immensely improved by using a shoe a little shorter than the ordinary rim—only reaching to the quarters, and, being light and narrow, incrusted on a level with the sole. An Arab horse with small feet, and whose frogs had been greatly injured by the native shoes he had been compelled to wear, has been shod for several months with a strip of iron weighing, for each foot, $3\frac{1}{4}$ ounces, and with wonderful benefit. The peculiar tendency of the Eastern horses' feet to become contracted when shod on the ordinary European principles, appears to have been successfully evaded, and the frogs so diseased and wasted previously, are regaining their normal size and firmness. The horses shod with these imbedded rims of iron have travelled with perfect freedom and safety on the hilly roads, often thickly covered by layers of sharp flints, in

38.*

the vicinity of Chatham; though the soles and frogs of their hoofs were unprotected, save by the natural thickness of horn, which appears to be more abundantly secreted the more it is exposed to attrition.

When considering the best mode of protecting and preserving the foot by shoeing, we will again have occasion to refer to this system.

Since the foregoing sheets were sent to press, we learn that another 'new' method of shoeing has been 'invented,' and this time, we are told, in America—that quarter of the globe where horses were unknown until more than a quarter of a century after Fiaschi's work had been published at Spire, and where the European settlers have carried their ideas of the utility of this creature to as extreme a degree as the dwellers in the old country. This new invention, it would appear, has been for some time before the American public; though the majority of horsemen in this country were ignorant of its startling merits until the 10th of December, 1868, when a leading journal brought it into prominent notice by devoting a portion of its space to a description, that certainly reads far more like an imitation of some of the choice American advertisers than a sensible notice by a modest writer who understood his subject.

It has been our somewhat wearisome task to examine and describe several of the numerous patents sought and obtained for particular modes of shoeing, or special kinds of shoes, but which, in reality, had no right or claim to be so protected, presenting as they did no novel features, and having been in use—some of them, many centuries before.

This invention is only another illustration, afforded this time by our Transatlantic cousins, of the wonderful originality pertaining to everything new with regard to hoofs and their armature. It will be seen that the 'idea' of the shoe is, if we refer to Fiaschi, at least three centuries old, or, if we look to our primitive models, perhaps as many thousands of years ; while the method of applying it—or rather the art of leaving the frog and sole in their integrity—is an old story, repeated by almost every writer who had made the horse's hoof his study.

This will be at once apparent if we transcribe what the writer in the London newspaper has written, in order to attract attention to the new method. ' In 1860, Mr Goodenough invented and patented the shoe we are now about to describe, and has succeeded, we think, in securing all necessary protection to the hoof, and in removing, or reducing to a *minimum*, the bad effects of earlier methods. The principle laid down by Mr Goodenough is that the shoe should resemble, and preserve, as far as possible, the natural shape of the hoof, of which it is a continuation. The unshod horse has the under surface of his foot on a generally level plane, the frog and the whole margin of the hoof in contact with the ground, and the under surface of the sole, between the frog and the margin, somewhat raised by its own concavity. The Goodenough shoe is made precisely to follow the outline of the hoof for which it is intended, and to reach exactly to the bars, never projecting at all beyond the heel. Its upper surface is generally plane and true (fig. 199, see next page) ; its under surface is generally concave from the outer to the inner margin, the outer margin having, however, a narrow, flat bearing upon the ground, and this bearing is interrupted

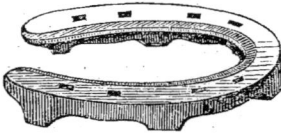

fig. 199

by portions of the margin being cut away, so as to leave a central toe-calk, and two smaller calks on either side. The elevation of these calks is inconsiderable, and their general level is the same, so that they may be compared to a series of short claws on the under surface of the shoe (fig. 200). In the notches, or spaces between

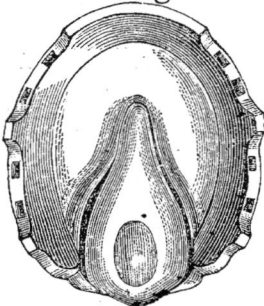

fig 200

the calks, the nail-holes are bored and counter-sunk, so that the nail-heads are completely buried in the shoe. For frost, shoes are made in which the calks have no flat bearing, but are brought up to a feather-edge. The inner margin of the shoe is thin, so that its outline passes insensibly into that of the sole, and presents no projections by which stones or snow can be retained.' A reference to our notice of Cæsar Fiaschi's work, and the drawings of shoes which he gives, as well as the mention Blundevil makes of foreign shoes, will be sufficient evidence to prove that these ground-surface projections were in use in the 16th century, while the shoe on which they were formed differs but little, if at all, in principle from the one now under discussion.

A reference also to Mr Goodwin's method of shoeing, which was in use before 1821—to Mr Mavor's and Colonel Fitzwygram's shoes,—will likewise demonstrate that there is nothing novel in the American shoe, so far as either the ground or foot surface is concerned. Several shoes have been introduced with projections on the ground surface, and one employed by Mr Broad, Veterinary Surgeon, Bath, more than ten years ago, may be said to be identical with this; while in almost every town and city, except London, toe-pieces and calks are regularly worn by draught-horses.

The preparation of the foot and application of the shoe are described as follows: 'A shoe which precisely fits the outline of the hoof is selected from the stock. If a proper fit cannot be found, any slight alteration is made by a few blows on the cold iron; or, if heating be necessary, the shoe is made cold again before it is applied, and care is taken that it remain perfectly level and true. The farrier then prepares the hoof by cutting or rasping away the surface of that portion of the crust on which the iron will rest, leaving the centre of the sole and the frog and bars untouched. Having given what he judges to be a true level to this marginal seating for the shoe, the shoe is applied cold, and the hoof is rasped again and again until horn and iron come into perfect contact in every part. As a guide to the use of the rasp, the surface of the shoe is ruddled, so that any portion of horn not touched by it remain uncoloured. The adjustment being correct, the shoe is nailed on in the ordinary way, and the process is complete. Mr Goodenough claims for his system the negative merit that the shoe, being applied cold, *does not injure and weaken the horn by burning*, as in the common method. He claims the positive merits that "it prevents slipping, *over-reaching*, and *interfering*, *cutting*, or *picking up stones*, balling snow or mud, contracted feet, corns, sandcracks, thrush, *springing of the knees,* and *shrinking of the shoulders.   It also prevents the nails striking the ground while the foot is sensitive from shoeing.*" ' We may conscientiously doubt the correctness of some of these statements, others are palpable absurdities, while others again are so obscure as to puzzle us.   In the first place, ' cold-shoeing,' as it has been termed, was, so far as I can ascertain, the only method employed in this country and on the continent before the 16th century; so that if our researches into the antiquity of shoeing prove anything, they prove that a patent was scarcely needed to make a monopoly of this method in the middle of the 19th century.   We have also shown that, in the opinion of the highest veterinary authorities, it is impossible to shoe a horse so well in this way as by fitting the hot shoes to the hoofs. This is known to every one who has had any experience of horses or horse-shoeing; and the injury supposed to be caused by the judicious employment of this means of adjusting the shoe is purely imaginary, and the result of inexperience.   The horn has no vitality, being inorganic.

This subject has often been discussed, but not, as we have seen recently, as it has been definitely decided that there was no foundation for the blame attached to hot-shoeing—as it may, though inappropriately, be termed.   As horse-owners may, however, be misled by the statement that fitting the shoe to the hoof while warm injures and weakens the horn, it may be as well to assert that the very opposite is the result, and that the method recommended by Mr Goodenough is really the one that injures and weakens the horn.   We have already given some proofs of this. In Britain (except in the army), and on the continent, cold-shoeing is a mere historical *souvenir*.

The writer of the above article, whose knowledge of horse-shoes appears to have been almost, if not quite, as limited as his experience among horses, adds, in speaking of the manufacture of these shoes by machinery : 'Gentlemen will then be able to keep a stock of shoes for their horses at their own stables, and to have them put on there by the farrier, who will need no forge. The work of the farrier will, indeed, be so much simplified that in large stables it will probably be desirable to have a *groom* instructed (1), and to make the removal of the shoes a portion of the ordinary routine of the establishment.'

It can scarcely be surprising that one who is so readily captivated and can write so confidently in praise of this long-exploded system, should recommend cold-shoeing, and these shoes with *calks at toes and heels*, for the hunting-field. 'Another advantage of the system is one that will be greatly felt in the hunting-field. The hoof, having its natural form and surface preserved, draws out of clay or mud without the suction by which so many ordinary shoes are loosened, and so much extra labour is entailed upon the horse. It has been calculated that this suction may be nearly 1 lb. per lift to each foot, in addition to the weight of the shoe; and its total amount at the end of a day's work would be such as to seem scarcely credible.' Is it not a fact that horses have been for years, and are now, shod with hunting-shoes; that these shoes have been, and are, concave on the ground and flat on the foot surface, —even more so than Mr Goodenough's patent; and that so far as their form is concerned, they are less likely to be influenced by clay or mud, and to do far less damage to the horse than this newly-invented one? Few men, I think, would be found who would ride a horse to hounds unless it had been previously shod for that purpose; and all who have ridden hard know that these shoes must be of a certain pattern, and be particularly firmly attached to the feet. The ordinary, light hunting-shoe is incomparably superior to the new invention in every respect; indeed, from the presence of toe-calks, the defective position and form of the nail-holes, and its clumsiness, this shoe is a very perilous and unsuitable one for the hunting-field, or even for ordinary road purposes, while the resuscitated method of cold-fitting makes it still less secure.

It will be observed from the figures given of this patented shoe, that the projections which stud its lower surface, and which have been more eloquently than correctly compared to ostrich claws, make it a most dangerous article; as in over-reaching, a horse must inflict serious wounds on itself, and in all probability come down with its rider, if it be a riding-horse, as their front edge is quite sharp; while horses that, through defective formation or temporary physical causes, are liable to strike their legs with the opposite feet, must inevitably produce grave wounds or contusions with a shoe of this kind. Being machine-made, the iron is not of such good quality as that of ordinary shoes, and to compensate for this, and insure wear for a reasonable time, thicker and heavier defences have to be worn. The nail-holes (eight in each shoe) are most defective in form and position, and being grouped in twos, must weaken the hoof by having the nails so closely jammed to each other, and if any elasticity or lateral expansion exists at the lower margin of the forefoot (as the patentee asserts), it must be apparent that it would no longer be permitted when this shoe is nailed on. The projecting calks at the toes must greatly tend to induce stumbling, particularly with saddle-horses, while they would cause dreadful wounds in kicking. So far the shoe is a defective one; and when the calks are worn off, which happens in a brief period if horses are employed on paved roads, it is but little different from the ordinary shoe. Being bevelled or concave on the foot as well as the ground surface, it as readily allows stones and mud to insinuate themselves between itself and the sole, while from the method of applying it, it is just as likely to produce corns, sandcracks, and the other maladies mentioned, as to prevent or cure them.

In December, 1868, the mode of attaching it to the foot looked most unscientific, if not cruel and barbarous. A visit to the place where some omnibus-horses were being experimented upon, a few days after the newspaper article we have quoted from was published, proved a great disappointment. One of the merits of this system was said to rest upon the wonderful discovery that the horse's frog was intended naturally to come into contact with the ground; and as the full benefit of this novel announcement was, it appeared, to be immediately bestowed on the unfortunate horses, the problem as how this could be done with a shoe very much thicker than that in ordinary wear, and provided with additional projections from its ground face, was being readily solved. The knife and rasp were as actively employed as ever; thin crusts and thin soles were being unmercifully trenched upon to imbed the clumsy mass of iron as deeply as need be to bring the sometimes shrunken frogs on a level with the lower face of the shoe. The middle of the sole was certainly not pared, but that portion which nature intended should be thickest and strongest, was reduced to a thin pellicle on which the rigid iron was laid. *A small hand-saw was employed to open up the heels.* The shoes were being fitted cold (though I am informed they have been fitted while at a *dark red heat*), and consequently, in every respect, the foot was made to fit the shoe, and the sole and crust had to suffer the penalty of the frog reaching the ground. The foot, altogether, was treated as if it were only a block of wood, to be cut and carved into a particular model, and without any regard whatever to its anatomy, functions, or sensibility. It was, certainly, no improvement on the commonest method of shoeing in England.

The most absurd statements were, of course, circulated with regard to the merits of this method. In quoting from the newspaper article, we have noticed some of these pretentious claims, for which there was not the slightest foundation in fact. It was advertised as the 'humane horse-shoe ;' and these advertisements asserted that it was 'the only horse-shoe which obeys the laws of nature in its construction, and is shaped as nearly in conformity with the natural foot as scientific knowledge and skilful labour can produce !' No pains were spared to make a good speculation of the wonderful *new invention ;* every public announcement of its merits seemed to be written by the same hand that had penned the first tribute of admiration, and recommended this sharp-studded weapon for the hunting-field. It is scarcely necessary to say that none of these articles gave evidence of the most trifling acquaintance with the subject of horse-shoeing, and many of them appeared to be influenced solely by the special exigencies of an embryo horse-shoe company, destined to invest money and make fortunes out of one of the most pretentious *inventions* perhaps ever introduced to the notice of the British public. No horseman, nor yet any competent man of science whose opinion is worth having, has yet ventured, so far as I am aware, to commend it in this country; and all the proper experiments hitherto made with it have, I believe, turned out unsatisfactory, or complete failures. As might have been anticipated, it has proved a most injurious method of shoeing; the percentage of crippled horses has been very great, and far beyond that attending the ordinary improper mode of shoeing; the number of shoes cast and lost has been far above the usual average, and horses have cut, stumbled, tumbled, and limped from corns, to my certain knowledge, quite as much, if not more, than with the worst application of the old system. This appears to be acknowledged so far, as the 'only humane method' now tolerates hot fitting apparently to any extent, and also sanctions the employment of calkins at the extremities of the heels, with other modifications, which leave one in doubt how much of the American invention will remain after a few months' longer trial in England. Where it has now and again succeeded in gaining a testimonial, has no doubt been largely due either to these modifications, or to circumstances in which any other ordinary shoe would have been equally successful.

It will be seen by referring to our history of shoeing, that the only claim to scientific farriery which can be admitted in this *new* system—allowing the frog to reach the ground—is no novelty, and is achieved by the mutilation of the best portions of the sole and crust.

A very much less pretentious, though promising to be a far more useful, invention, is the quite recent one of Mr Gray of Sheffield, the patentee and manufacturer of grooved steel and steel-faced bars, to be made into horse-shoes. Shoes made from these rolled bars have the ground surface cut into a series of ridges and teeth of various forms (figs. 201, 202, 203), adapted to secure a

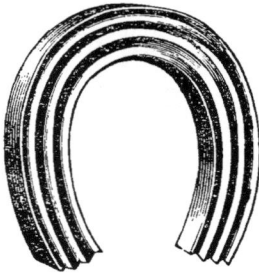

fig. 201

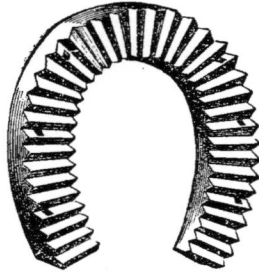

fig. 202

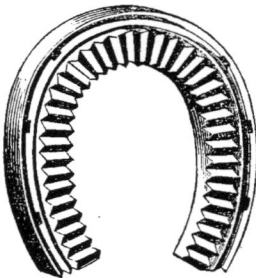

fig. 203

firm foothold, and prevent horses from slipping or falling on the pavement of large towns. Owing to their being manufactured either entirely or partially of steel—in the latter case the steel is on the ground surface—they can be tempered so as to preserve their denticulated surface in an efficient condition for some time; a rather important feature to be noted. According to Mr Gray, ' shoes made from this material will not require sharpening in winter, and will be found of universal advantage on the road or in the field; they are one-third lighter, will last longer, and look much better than any other shoes.'

The combination of steel and iron appears to be that best adapted for horse-shoes that require to be tempered, as they are less liable to fracture, and should be less expensive—indeed the patentee asserts that shoes can be made at a very little more expense than the ordinary ones, over which they are said to possess such advantages. I regret I have not had sufficient time to submit this invention to the test of experiment, but from what I have seen of it, I am in hopes that it may prove useful in the triple view of lightness, durability, and increased surety of footing, more particularly in winter. The fitted shoe looks very neat, and, as may be seen, the ground face can be ridged or serrated in any fashion. The foot surface is nearly, if not quite, plane.

These shoes can be turned, fitted, and put on by any ordinary farrier, and the holes may be made wherever they are required.

CHAPTER XIV.

IMPORTANCE OF SHOEING TO CIVILIZATION. THE GREEKS AND RO-
MANS. INCONVENIENCES ATTENDING THE EMPLOYMENT OF UN-
SHOD ANIMALS. ROADS AND CITIES. MANUAL LABOUR. INTRO-
DUCTION OF SHOEING, AND ITS EFFECTS. VARIETIES OF BREEDS
OF HORSES. CHANGES IN THE ART OF WAR. INCREASE IN
CAVALRY. ARMOUR. RIDING DOUBLE. HEAVY EQUIPMENT. IN-
CREASING IMPORTANCE OF SHOEING. EXAMPLES. NAPOLEON'S
RETREAT FROM MOSCOW. DANISH RETREAT FROM SCHLESWIG.
FARRIERS' STRIKE IN PARIS.

THUS far, then, have we endeavoured to trace the
history of horse-shoes and horse-shoeing. We have seen
that there is not sufficient evidence to testify that the Greeks
and some other ancient races whom we may designate
' horse-loving,' employed an iron defence nailed to the feet
of their solipeds ; that, though the Romans of a comparatively later age must have, to some extent, been aware
of, and perhaps practised, this art, yet their writers do not
mention it ; and, from the testimonies before us, we might
almost be inclined to conclude that the Romans only
resorted to it in those countries which they had invaded
or conquered, and where they already found it in use ;
that shoeing with iron plates and nails was known to
some, at any rate, of the Celtic and Germanic tribes
settled in the West probably long before our era ; and

that from these people the art, more or less modified, and perhaps improved, has descended to our own days, a thousand-fold more necessary to us than it was to them. It is quite possible, and even extremely probable, that for a long period shoeing was but rarely resorted to by the people who were aware of its utility; and if, as is surmised, the art was kept a secret by the Druid priests, this may account for the Romans being unacquainted with its application for some time after their having been in contact with the so-styled barbarous nations of Gaul, Germany, and Britain. Before this device was adopted, horses must have been almost exclusively employed to carry riders, who were nearly always warriors; or to drag those light tiny chariots said to be the invention of Erichthonius, the Athenian, or their modifications—the *currus arcuate,* the *lectica,* the *carpentum,* and the *carrucæ,* which, drawn by one or more horses, were seldom used except in the Grecian or Roman games. In the heroic ages, indeed, they appear to have been almost solely employed for the speedy conveyance of warriors on the march or into action, that they might be vigorous for the fight, and attack where most suitable. When these war-chariots appear with three horses, one of that number was often a spare steed to replace either of the other two that might be disabled from wounds, or perhaps have its feet worn to the quick. For long journeys, mules were preferred either for riding or draught purposes, because of the natural thickness and resistance of their hoofs; so that it may not have been a matter of fashion, but necessity, which compelled the Roman emperors and the Roman ladies to go about in equipages drawn by mules

—a circumstance which raised the price of these animals considerably above that of horses.' But even the employment of mules was limited, because of the damage done to their feet on roads which were generally so badly made, if made at all, that travelling on them was only possible for short distances. It was, doubtless, in a great measure to obviate these inconveniences that the Romans constructed their wonderful *strata*. On such paved roads, cavalry or horses drawing light vehicles would probably travel a number of days without shoes; and it may be that heavy loads in carriages were transported on them for some distance by long teams of mules, as observed by Martial, in the beginning of our era: 'Longæ mulorum mandræ.'

Beyond these roads, however, quadrupeds were scarcely available for drawing heavy weights; and human strength, together with the ingenuity of the Roman engineers, was enlisted to convey, by means of rollers, levers, and various other appliances, the materials destined for building or other purposes. Even in Rome, and in many other cities built before shoeing had become general, the main thoroughfares were too narrow to permit carriages laden with bulky articles to pass. The object of this was probably to make them shady, and protect them from the sweeping winter winds, as well as to impede an enemy should he attempt to enter. All transport, therefore, must have been accomplished at an immense sacrifice of manual labour, which to us now would appear appalling. In the north of China, where horses are numer-

---

¹ ' Ego faxim muli, pretio qui superare equos
Sicut villores Gallicis cantheriis.'—*Plautus*.

ous, and their feet shod, carriages are largely employed, and the streets of the towns are wide—Peking, for example. In the south, however, where horses are extremely scarce and water-carriage convenient, as at Canton, the streets are very narrow and unfit for the passage of wheeled vehicles, and all the land transport has to be performed by men.

With the introduction of shoeing, a gradual revolution in the social economy of nations, especially those of a commercial tendency, commenced, and benefits began to be derived equivalent to the employment of a power ful moving machine, capable of being utilized as never machine was before. The many important uses for which the horse was adapted duly developed themselves; long distances could be quickly travelled, day after day, without injury to those hitherto vulnerable organs, the feet; and roads, slowly and expensively made, often wrung out of the enforced labour of slaves, were not now required to save the hoofs of horses. Heavy loads could be transported almost continuously by the same team at an accelerated pace, without demanding the tedious intervention of the levers and rollers of not long before; the horse's powers were also increased by this simple means to a degree that nothing else ever devised could have done; while its strength was husbanded, and the painfulness of its oftentimes onerous duties was perhaps rendered less acute.

Land-traffic, where shoeing is not resorted to, and where few other animals besides the horse or mule are employed, is generally at a low ebb, because everything must be carried on their backs; and as, without some covering for the feet, the weight each can carry is but small, the price of merchandise must be proportionally high, while the risks incurred are greater.   If it be true that commerce is increased in proportion as means are afforded for facilitating communication between different parts of the same country, or between kingdoms, then it must be as true that nail-shoeing has conferred a benefit on mankind of no mean character.   For whenever it had been ascertained that carriages could be con stantly made serviceable in conveying merchandise for long distances by horse-power, and without inflicting any injury on the horses, then commercial relations became vastly extended: roads of every construction, not so much required to preserve the hoofs as to aid the wheels, began to be thrown open everywhere, and the arts and manufactures received a potent stimulus, and one quite as beneficial, if we consider the age, as railways and steam-ships have conferred in modern days.

Since the realization of the increased power which shoeing conferred on the horse species, a wonderful result appears in the increase of varieties or *breeds* to meet the many requirements sought for in horses for draught or riding.

The horse, in the earlier periods of its domestication, and in nearly every country, may be supposed to have had a tolerable uniformity of proportion adapted to the purposes for which it was trained—those of carrying lightly equipped troops, and drawing small chariots containing few people.   The enterprise of Western nations, however, and the skill they have for so many centuries shown in modifying or adapting the natural capabilities of the domestic animals for various purposes, led to a gradual increase of size in the horse, in order to procure the greatest results compatible with convenience, and to save trouble and expense by reducing the number needed to draw a heavy load by at least one-half or one-third. That this result has been achieved, I need only point to the size and weight of the London dray-horse—or perhaps, better still, to the massive elephantine proportions of the Manchester or Liverpool waggon-horse, and the enormous power it can exert in moving and transporting loads which would have required two, three, or even four horses of the middle ages to stir. And this transformation could not have been brought about had the art of shoeing been unknown. The hoofs of these mammoth creatures, thick and large though they be, are not nearly strong enough to support their ponderous weight for very long, even when not in draught. But when their great strength is put forth in propelling some five or six tons in one of our streets, and halting and backing repeatedly with this load, it is easy to see that the unshod hoofs must quickly succumb to the strain imposed upon them, and the excessively developed animal would be then only a helpless mass of bone and muscle, and as useless as a railway engine off the rails, or with its wheels broken. Some idea of the great weight and attrition imposed upon the extremities of a horse of this description may be inferred from the fact, that shoes weighing from four to six pounds each are sometimes quite worn out within a month.

Intermediate between these tardy giants of busy cities, whose utility, nay, even existence, depends upon shoeing, and the original small-sized horse, the breeders display other triumphs of their skill in rearing animals, useful not only because of their strength, but also for speed in various degrees, combined with endurance when in draught; and to these shoeing is almost as essential as to the larger class, for without it, in a very brief space, they would also be inefficient. Examples might be cited *ad infinitum*, all tending to exhibit the many boons this modest handicraft has conferred on modern civilization, in enlarging the trade relations between different countries, forming, as it does, one of the chief instruments in maintaining the integrity of animal power, whether used in agriculture and commerce, or in aiding the arts and sciences to be developed. Had it not been introduced at an early age, as a matter of necessity, it must have been invented at a later period; for we can scarcely imagine a state of affairs in which our favourite and invaluable servants and companions would be so helpless after a few days' riding or driving, as to require rest or temporary slippers, until the over-worn hoofs had regained their strength.

We have seen that ancient history often speaks of the serious mishaps befalling armies when on service, through the want of some protection to the hoofs of their cavalry, lightly armed and equipped as it was; and it likewise tells us of the care bestowed on these organs, so as to keep them in the best condition to withstand wear. I have ventured to hint, that it was probably owing to their being able to shoe the great masses of cavalry composing their irresistible armies, that the barbarian races surrounding Rome were able to sweep down so rapidly and overwhelm her.

It is worthy of notice how very quickly after the

value of shoeing had become generally known, the art of war became altered, not only as regards the increased mobility of armed bodies of men, and the certain efficiency of cavalry, but as concerning tactics and equipment. Always of the greatest moment, it was only when about to commence a campaign, or when really engaged in it, that the generals of antiquity devoted so much of their attention to the preservation of their horses' hoofs; and when these began to give way, defeat was often not very far distant. Consequently, the movements of large armies were generally constrained as to rapidity, and the horsemen were armed and equipped as lightly as possible, to diminish the chances of embarrassment from this source. It may have been from their ignorance of shoeing, that the Greeks considered cavalry rather as auxiliaries than as principals in battle,[1] and that it was not employed in the Trojan war. To this circumstance, also, may we not account for the warriors in the time of Homer having two horses each, upon which they rode alternately, in order to relieve the hoofs as much as possible?[2] Alexander the Great, undoubtedly, had a large force of men who fought both on horseback and on foot (διμαχαι),[3] but Diodorus mentions how these were rendered useless, by their horses becoming hoof-worn when on service.

In the early ages, armour had its origin in the cunning or effeminacy of Asiatic nations; but the more open and dauntless European despised every device except the shield, until brought into contact with the mail-covered enemy, when he also was obliged to adopt this protection. In the

---

[1] *Müller.* Dorians, ii. 259.   [2] Iliad, v. 679, 684.
[3] *Pollux,* i. 6, 10.

time of Constantine the Great, the horses of the Cata-
phracti, or heavy-armed cavalry, were covered with defensive materials, consisting either of scale-armour, or of
plates of metal which had different names, according to
the parts of the body they protected. This corps of
cavalry was only formed in the later days of the Roman
empire, when the discipline of the legions had been destroyed, and the chief dependence began to be placed
upon horsemen. The Roman cavalry before this time
had worn metal breastplates, or loricæ. This weighty
armour, while it defended the warrior and his steed,
necessarily impeded cavalry manœuvres, and increased the
tendency to foot-lameness in the horses from want of
shoeing. It is about this period that we find extempor-
aneous devices to protect the hoofs most frequently mentioned. The cumbrous protection, however, appears to
have been soon given up; for we find Vegetius wondering
by what fatality it happened, that the Romans, after having used heavy armour so late as the time of the Emperor
Gratian (A.D. 376), should, by laying aside their breast-
plates and helmets, put themselves on a level with the barbarians, who were now commencing to sap the foundations
of the empire. May not the reason for the apparent dis-
regard of armour, which causes this writer to wonder, be
found in the circumstance, that the great weight imposed
upon the unshod hoofs, together with the rapidity of movement necessary to enable them to contend with such agile
and unencumbered foes, rendered it imperative that this
extra load should be dispensed with, in order to spare their
horses as much as possible, and to follow or attack on
more equal terms those whom we have assumed to possess

the advantages afforded by nail-shoeing — advantages hitherto overlooked, or but partially resorted to, by the Romans?

From this time until the general adoption of iron shoes, we are led to infer that horsemen were as lightly clad and armed as was compatible with the services sought from them. But after the downfall of the Roman empire, and when the horse had by this hoof-defence been converted into a more perfect animal—when it could, without prejudice, be put to the most varied uses on all kinds of ground, and in all seasons, with but a small amount of care, so far as its feet were concerned, a new era was inaugurated in the art of war, from which we may date modern improvements. For it was about the time when, as we have seen, the fashion of protecting the lower surface of the horse's foot by a rim of iron, became general, that the benefits of the feudal system introduced by the people who shod their horses, began to be experienced, and a perceptible change in tactics and equipment became noticeable.

From this system sprang the age of chivalry, when the feudal knight and the feudal tenant, heavily armed and heavily caparisoned, horse and rider closely covered with invulnerable masses of iron, and bearing clumsy weapons, sallied out to the battle-field or the tournament, or travelled great distances to the rendezvous of their superiors, there to be trained or prepared for the contests which, unhappily, were of too frequent occurrence.

Riding double was unknown to the Romans. ' Do you think that two can sit upon one horse?' asks Martial. Suetonius even describes messages being conveyed in haste by men on two horses, each horse being relieved by the rider vaulting on the other. But in the middle ages, two riding upon one horse was not unusual. Servants frequently rode behind their masters; knights took up the wounded; and altogether two persons on horseback appears to have become a common practice. In the 'Tactica' of the Emperor Leo, who first speaks of nailed shoes, we read of horsemen named *deputati*, who were appointed to carry off the wounded behind them, and for this object they had an additional stirrup hanging to the end of the saddle.

So it is, that unless horses had hoofs of a more endurable quality than they now possess, it is quite impossible they could have sustained, for many hours even, the great additional strain imposed on them, not only by the ponderous iron-shell enveloping horse and rider, but by the peculiar nature of the warfare which was introduced, and in which collisions with heavy lances had to be borne in great part by the supporting or propelling feet of the horses engaged. Shoeing was then an art of the first importance, for without it these iron-clad men and horses could never have been serviceable in war. Cuirasses and helmets would not have been so generally adopted, neither would they have become an important feature in military law; and in all probability the noble and glorious institution of knighthood would have been unknown, or would have decayed soon after its establishment, and history would have been deprived of some of its most brilliant chapters. To the art, therefore, to which they owed so much, kings and knights did not disdain to offer homage by acquiring its rudiments, and learning with their own hands to fashion and affix the garniture which made their highly-prized chargers proof against the wear of the roads; for, burthened as they were, and workmen being so scarce, a short time only was necessary to render unarmed hoofs quite unserviceable.

In later times, though the practice of the art has been confined solely to special workmen, and few above these care about, or are acquainted with its most trifling details, yet in armies the organization of the farriers' department is considered, and justly, as of much importance; for without shoes on the horses' feet, a modern army would be reduced to a most helpless state of inefficiency, and provided there was no other means of transport or defence, would be on the verge of disaster. Indeed, without this protection to the hoofs of troop, artillery, and waggon-horses, no expedition could be undertaken.

In consequence of the care always manifested in this respect, examples of loss occasioned by its neglect are few. The Russian campaign of 1812, however, furnishes an instance of the need there is for providing armies not only with shoes to protect the hoofs, but appliances which will make them independent of the seasons in northern climates. I give the notice of this example from Thiers:[1] 'Napoleon left Doroboug on the 6th of November. The whole of the army followed on the 7th and 8th. The cold had become more perceptible, and once more gave rise to painful regrets at having forgotten to provide winter clothing; and another neglect yet more baffling — that of procuring frost-nails for the shoes of the horses. The season in which the army had left, and the belief that it

[1] Hist. au Consulate, et de l'Empire, vol. xiv.

being able to guard themselves against a temperature of 9° or 10° (Reaumur); and at each ascending portion of the road, the artillery horses, even when the usual number required was doubled and trebled, were unable to drag the guns of the smallest calibre. Flogged until they were covered with blood, and their knees torn with frequent falling, they were found incapable of overcoming ordinary obstacles, through loss of strength and want of means to prevent their slipping on the ice. The ammunition waggons were abandoned, and scarcely any ammunition was saved. Soon after, the guns had to be surrendered as trophies to the Russians, but not without pain and shame to our brave artillery. The carriages were thus greatly diminished in number, and every day saw the losses augmented, and the horses expiring on the road.'

Another example—the most striking, perhaps, because the most recent—is to be found in the *Times'* Correspondent's [1] account of the Danish retreat from Schleswig to Sonderburg, on the night of the 5th February, 1865. Immediately after it had been determined that the Danes should effect a hurried retrograde movement, bad weather set in with great violence. 'The snow thickened and hardened on the ground, the road became smooth and bright as glass ; horses and men slipped dreadfully, and fell at almost every step. Not one horse in the whole Danish army was rough-shod that night; on the

[1] The Times, February 18th, 1865.

contrary, the shoes both of saddle and draught horses were worn smooth by the last five or six days' incessant march on muddy ground, and the progress of the army met with terrible hindrance at the outset. . . . . It was not long before our march began to exhibit, on a small scale, some of the horrors of the famous retreat of the French from Moscow. The night was dark—the cold terrible; the thermometer, I dare say, did not mark more than four or five degrees below the freezing-point—but the chill in our veins told a very different tale, and the slipperiness of the road was perfectly awful. The snow, which was falling thick and fast at frequent intervals, lay in the fields three or four inches deep, and fringed the trees in the forests with the most picturesque fretwork; but it was trodden to the thinnest layer by all the feet, hoofs, and wheels of a whole host, till it glistened like ice in the occasional gleam of some pale star, as one or two peeped out in the sky through the gaps opened in the mass of clouds by the fitful blast. Dragoons, artillerymen—all who travel on saddle—were dismounted; even led horses were put to the direst exertions to keep their footing; draught-horses had to be held up—and cannon, caissons, and ammunition or luggage waggons to be dragged by the sheer strength of men, whose tread was no steadier. The falling of men and of beasts, the cracking of wheels and axletrees, was prodigious. It took us full nine hours to go over the first Danish mile and a half (less than seven English miles) of ground. Morning broke upon us long before we were half way between Schleswig and Fensburg, and we reached the latter place about four o'clock. P.M., on Saturday, having accom-

plished the whole distance of twenty-two English miles
in eighteen hours. . . . . We had not gone half-a-mile
from Schleswig before we found a very heavy piece of
siege artillery forsaken on the road. The eight horses
which dragged it had become, owing to the state of the
roads, as powerless as so many new-littered kittens, and
all the efforts of the men to share the work with them
were unavailing. In the same manner, as we advanced
on our dismal march, we, who were in the rear, came
up with broken carriages, dismounted caissons, and horses
fallen never to rise. The obstruction to our progress
was indescribable.'

These examples will, perhaps, be sufficient to illus
trate the influence this art has in maintaining the efficiency
of armies, and what grave calamities may ensue when,
for lack of foresight, or through carelessness, its most
essential details are neglected, and the chief part of an
expedition is left helpless at the most trying emergencies.
For what, asks M. Bouley, can be more discouraging or
painful to an army in retreat, than to leave behind its
weak, sick, and wounded men, and its guns, ammunition,
baggage, and provisions, to be destroyed by the weather,
or to fall into the hands of perhaps a merciless enemy,
when some simple device, suitable to the occasion, would
have saved all ?

It is fortunate that, in modern times, instances of
public inconvenience occasioned by want of shoeing
are remarkably rare in the annals of civil life, for it does
not require much to prove how greatly the every-day
routine of commerce is dependent upon horses, and
therefore upon horse-shoes. Only think for a moment

that if all the horses in our large cities—such as London, Manchester, or Liverpool—were deprived of their hoof-armature, in two or three days at most they would, if worked, be all footsore; and then attempt to realize the stagnation that would take place in the movement and business of these thronging marts! A feeble illustration is afforded in what took place in Paris in 1830, when, after the revolution, coalitions of trades commenced, and, with others, when the farriers struck for more wages. As a consequence, all the shoeing-forges in Paris were closed at the same time, and remained so for about six weeks. During this period, according to the statement of M. Bouley, it was curious to note the changes that took place in the various branches of trade or pleasure-making which depended on the services of horses. Of course, at first the farriers' contumacy did not produce any very marked results, because for some days the shoes then on the hoofs sufficed to preserve them from injury. But as these became worn out day after day, and as there were no means of renewing them, the number of animals unfit for work and kept in their stables gradually became more and more numerous, until in from three to four weeks, an almost complete cessation of horse-labour had taken place. At this period, the absence of horses and carriages from the streets, and the unusual stillness reigning throughout, seemed quite perplexing, and the city looked desolate. Trade had suffered very seriously; and the public service, as well as the necessary communication between the capital and the other cities and towns of France, was sadly deranged; for as at that time railways had not been introduced, all inland conveyance of letters, despatches, passengers, and merchandise, was intrusted to the *malles-poste*, the *diligences*, and other conveyances, and as these could not be horsed, business and travelling were in abeyance.

An amicable arrangement was come to at this crisis, however, and the inconvenient state of affairs brought to a close, but not before the utility of the art, and its direct influence on the welfare of modern civilization, had been amply demonstrated. Without it, even at the present time, when railways, telegraphs, and steam-ships have usurped a large share of the work formerly performed by couriers, coaches, waggons, and canal-boats drawn by horses, there would be an amount of inconvenience which it would severely task modern ingenuity to overcome. The most useful servant ever possessed by man would be nothing else than a powerful living machine, whose forces could not be perfectly developed or satisfactorily utilized. The withdrawal of our hackney coaches from their accustomed duties is inconvenient enough, but this is a comparatively small matter when compared to the entire cessation of all horse-labour in our cities.

CHAPTER XV.

PROGRESS OF THE ART OF FARRIERY. FUTILE ATTEMPTS TO IMPROVE IT. DISADVANTAGES OF SHOEING. FUNCTIONS OF THE FOOT TO BE STUDIED. ADVANTAGES OF THE ANCIENT SYSTEM. GERMAN SHOEING AND HOOP-PARING. ITS EVIL RESULTS. TRADITIONAL SHOEING. ROUTINE. ERRONEOUS THEORIES. MALTREATMENT OF THE HORSE'S FOOT. LAFOSSE'S TEACHING. REQUIREMENTS OF GOOD SHOEING. STRUCTURE AND FUNCTIONS OF THE HOOF. BAD SHOEING. RULES TO BE OBSERVED. BEST FORM OF SHOE, AND METHOD OF APPLICATION. HEREDITARY DISEASES. SHOEING IN AMERICA AND ARABIA. EFFECTS OF EUROPEAN SHOEING. DANGERS OF IMPROPER SHOEING. SCIENTIFIC APPLICATION OF THE FARRIER'S ART. AN APPEAL TO HORSEMEN.

THERE are probably few arts which have been known and practised for so long a period, which have been found of such general utility, and yet have undergone so little modification or real improvement as this of horse-shoeing. The earliest model of an iron shoe we can discover differs but little in form from those now in everyday use; and perhaps there are not many arts which have attracted a larger share of attention and experiment by men who had made the subject their profound study, and others who had not, and knew but little of the theoretical principles which should govern its practice. Books have been written by scores, promulgating new methods; patents innumerable have thrown their ægis over inventions replaced by any other yet proposed. The reason for this most probably depends upon the fact, that the supposed improvements have been either too extravagant or speculative in their aim, and gave rise to disappointment after a brief trial; or they were so elaborate, or unsuited to the foot and its functions, that they could not be adopted.

The shady aspect of civilization, as regards an artificial existence, is manifested in the horse as palpably almost as in man; and of the many ills entailed upon this creature by domestication and continual employment upon made roads, none are more grievous, more frequent in their occurrence, or more difficult to remedy, than those attributed, directly or indirectly, justly or unjustly, to shoeing. Hence the avidity with which any reasonable proposal for the avoidance of these evils was jumped at, and the inevitable reaction and disappointment which ensued when they failed; until now, so firmly established has the present mode of shoeing become, the announcement of any improvement seldom obtains more notice than a smile of incredulity, or a hesitating and often prejudiced trial.

The truth consists in this, that it is not so much new-fangled notions or devices, which have really no practical bearing, and are usually founded on error, that are wanted, but careful attention to the anatomical and physiological teachings which the study of the limb and foot alone can give, and simple adherence to well-established principles which have their foundation in these. A neglect, or want of a just appreciation of the value of the facts which the above sciences furnish, have been fruitful sources of false doctrine in this respect, and have caused much suffering to the unfortunate horse, and loss to his owner.

For a period extending over very many centuries, it would appear that the horse's foot was regarded and treated pretty much as if it were a block of wood exposed to attrition, and that the sole aim and purpose of shoeing was to defend it from wear. Its anatomy, functions, and maladies, if it had many in primitive times, were little understood; nor, perhaps, were the less noticeable, but no less important advantages to be derived from the scientific application of farriery, thought of. As M. Megnin remarks, from the time of their invention, and during many centuries, horse-shoes were simply a narrow iron armature laid flat against the foot, with the exclusive object of protecting it from wear. This primitive idea of shoeing has its analogy in that now employed by the Arabs: an analogy which is further confirmed in the method of attaching the shoe. In both cases the nails have large heads, intended to grasp the ground; they take a short, yet strong hold of the wall of the hoof, and the points, instead of being twisted off, are simply turned round to the side of the foot. The nail-holes are circular, the necks of the nails are also round, and the shoe is light. This analogy, says Megnin, gives rise to the conviction that with the Gauls, the Gallo-Romans, the Greeks of the lower Empire, as well as with the Arabs of now-a-days, the horses' feet were scarcely pared; that they were as frequently without shoes as with them, and that the deteriorations of the horny case, and the infirmities of the inferior extremity of the limbs, were unknown to them.

The settlement of certain Germanic races in France and Britain after the departure of the Romans, and the extension of their rule, caused the gradual substitution of the German for the Celtic method of shoeing. Instead of the narrow shoes, with the flat upper surface and undulated border, heavier plates with a wider surface, and concave towards the sole of the foot, began to be introduced, and, adds M. Megnin, at this period the *boutoir*, or 'buttress,' commenced its functions, and reckless paring of the hoofs began.[1] From this time up to the present, this attendant curse of shoeing has prevailed. Cæsar Fiaschi, one of the earliest writers on farriery, gives us a long catalogue of foot diseases, directly or indirectly due to paring, and he, and all enlightened men who have succeeded him, and who have written on this subject, have protested against this wanton destruction and unmitigated cruelty. Whenever the sole began to be pared, the heels opened, and the frog mutilated, it became necessary to adopt shoes with the foot surface concave; no pressure could be borne by those parts which had been deprived of their natural protection. Therefore were the shoes *dished*—made like a

---

[1] It must not be forgotten that in the ancient laws of Wales a *paring-knife* is mentioned, as well as a 'groover' for the nail-holes.

basin—the inner border only resting on the ground, and the whole strain of the animal's weight and burden, as well as that incurred in violent exertion, was thrown entirely upon the outer margin of the foot. This could have but one result for the poor horse—disease and agony. Routine has accompanied the art from the remotest period; it haunts it now; there are but few workmen who are able or who care to reason as to its application, or its effects on the healthy functions of a most beautiful but a most complicated organ. The art of shoeing is simply traditional; and however able an artisan may prove himself in the beaver or bee-like monotony of practical detail which he has acquired by imitation from others, yet he will never advance a step beyond, unless his intelligence has been quickened by something besides the mere mechanical knowledge he has acquired by laborious but unstudied repetition. He is but a labourer or workman pursuing a useful but unscientific occupation, unless he can combine theory with practice, and extend his knowledge beyond the inert inorganic envelope, to the vital and all-important structures within, and in this way maintain them in a healthy state by his art. It is no doubt owing to this routine manner of treating the horse's foot that no progress has been made in diminishing the natural or acquired defects and diseases of this organ, which are so numerous and prove so destructive.

Previous to the beginning of the last century, it may be said that the art of shoeing was traditional; the shoes were clumsy, and, at a later period, even viciously contrived. No thought appears to have been paid to the injurious influence shoes and paring might have on the form of the hoofs, on their texture, on the true or false disposition of the limbs, or on the horse's natural movements.

And in this century, the exaggerated and mistaken notions prevailing with regard to the elastic properties of the foot have done much to perpetuate the mischief. Apparently overlooking the fact, that a large portion of the inferior part of the hoof is closely filled with inelastic bone (the os pedis); that the wings of this bone, which is of a crescent shape, extend to the very extremity of the heels, and that the inflections of the wall, termed the bars, are attached to the inner face of these wings, it has yet been stoutly maintained that this portion of the foot was largely capable of dilatation and contraction, and that these movements actually occurred during progression. The sole, too, descended and ascended, and the whole inferior surface of the horse's extremity was a wonderfully contrived resilient apparatus, whose freedom must not only be uninterrupted, but facilitated.

Paring the sole until the blood was nearly or quite oozing through, and sometimes applying extreme pressure to the frog, were the means employed to keep the foot in a natural condition; and to prevent the then extremely sensitive sole from being bruised by coming in contact with the shoe, as well as to permit its easy descent, the upper surface of the shoe was bevelled off so as to leave a wide space in this vulnerable region, and the whole strain of the weight and movement thrown on the crust or wall alone.

The result was, that the hoofs, instead of contracting and expanding, as it was erroneously believed they ought to do, only contracted; the tender horn, ruthlessly exposed by the drawing-knife to rapid desiccation and other abnormal conditions, rapidly shrank, dried, and lost its healthy properties; from this arose various disorders, such as contracted heels, fissures in the horn, wasting of the frogs, and even more deep-seated maladies of the foot. Or if the unfortunate creature was put to severe exertion, the tremendous strain thrown upon the anterior and lateral parts of the foot readily set up congestion or inflammation of the vascular textures uniting the hoof to the bone within, and flat or convex soles, deformed wall, lameness, and partial or total inefficiency was the result.

This will be rendered more apparent, perhaps, if we show a section of the anterior portion of a foot pared to 'thumb-springing,' and shod with an ordinary shoe (fig. 204).

This most injurious fashion of cutting away the sole and frog, and deeply notching the heels, is still largely in vogue in Britain; though in the army it has been for many years abolished, and the results of a rational method of shoeing are most

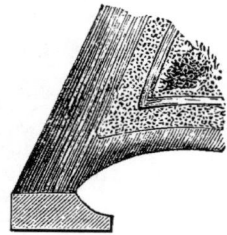

fig. 204

marked in the diminution of foot-lameness, and the maintenance of the hoofs in a natural and serviceable condition.

So far as the integrity of the foot is concerned, there can scarcely be any doubt that the primitive farriery of the early races of Gaul and Britain was preferable to that of modern days, when this excessive mutilation of the

hoof is practised. ' Although protecting the horse's foot
from exposure to undue wear, and from the injuries which
would befall it if made to undergo hardships with which it
was not naturally designed to contend, yet, unless most
judiciously employed, much that belongs to shoeing is a
serious evil; and the skill of man ought therefore to be
directed to the diminution or suppression of those prejudicial tendencies.   For example, the employment of nails
to fasten on the shoe, however carefully managed, is to a
certain extent a source of injury to the hoof; but when
used indiscreetly, is positively ruinous to the animal.
No invention yet proposed has succeeded in retaining the
shoe so firmly as nails, and the many failures that have
resulted when other fastenings have been tried, leads to
the belief that no means at once so convenient and so
efficacious will readily be substituted for them.   Again,
different models of shoes have been devised to meet
wants, real or imaginary, and to guard against the casualties incidental to the employment of the ordinary shoe,
but without success; for one after another they have all
been discarded, and the simple shoe, with all its defects,
and but slightly modified to suit particular cases, has
outlived them all.   So that there appears but little
chance that anything more simple, useful, or less injurious than the ordinary shoe, when properly applied, will
ever stand the same prolonged test, or gain such universal
favour.

But knowing the structure and uses of the several
parts of the hoof and its contents, as well as the physiology and just proportions of the limbs, the skilful artisan,
taught by the veterinary surgeon, should be able to

obviate many of the disadvantages which usually attend the use of nails and shoes, and reduce others to comparative harmlessness.

The principal object in arming the hoof with a rim of metal is to protect it from the effects of wear. This was the intention of the inventor, and to-day it is our chief aim. To prevent the outer margin of the hoof from being broken and worn, by the simplest means in our power, is the cardinal problem with regard to the preservation of the horse's foot; and nothing appears to be easier to accomplish. Before our interference with that organ, its beautiful structures were contrived to meet every demand, and its manifold functions were freely and vigorously maintained. On soft or uneven soil, the entire lower border of the wall, the sole, bars, and frog came into con tact with the ground: nature intended them to meet the ground, and there to sustain the animal's weight as well as the force of its impulsive powers. On hard or rocky land with a level surface, only the dense tough crust and bars, the thick portion of sole surrounded by them, and the resilient retentive frog meet the force of the weight and movement; and in both cases, not only with impunity, but with advantage to the interior of the foot, as well as the limb. The horn, in addition to its being a slow con ductor of heat, is dense, tough, and elastic to a degree varying with different parts of the foot, while its fibres are not only admirably disposed to support weight, secure a firm grasp of the ground, and aid the movements of the limb, but are also an excellent medium for modifying concussion or jar to the sensitive and vascular structures in their vicinity. Nature has done her best to make these

structures, perfect and suitable in every way to the requirements of limb and foot.

In the fore limb, which is chiefly concerned in sustaining weight, the crust or wall of the hoof is formed of
fibres running continuously from above, where they are
secreted, to below, where they are worn, and following the
same direction as the wall itself. As we examine them
from within to without—from the surface where they are
in contact with the living tissues, we find that they are at
first loose and soft in texture, and easily penetrated, while
they can be readily dispossessed of their moisture, and then
shrivel up into thin, brittle fragments. As we recede from
this surface and approach the external fibres, we notice
that, like the cells of the human epidermis, they grow
more resisting and dense, are smaller, packed closer and
more cohesively together, until near the outer face of the
wall, when they become rapidly harder, stronger, and
more whale-bone like, and though porous, yet appear
destitute of moisture. In this respect they resemble the
fibres of an ordinary cane, and further than this are, as in
the cane, entirely covered with a delicate, translucent,
varnish-like secretion, intended to prevent the too rapid
evaporation of moisture from the fibres, and to guard
against their shrinking and splitting. The bars are
similarly formed, and are secreted, like the wall, from the
large projecting, elastic mass, the coronary ring, that
lies in a wide concavity around the upper and inner aspect
of the crust, and has an important share in supporting the
weight, and preventing the sole being unduly pressed
upon by the bone resting upon it. The crust being
always, in an unshod condition, exposed to wear, is con-

tinually growing downwards from this coronary cushion to meet the demands of attrition ; and if hindered from coming into contact with the earth, would increase to an indefinite length. The fibres of the horny sole follow exactly the same direction as those of the wall, and are destined, like them, to come more or less in contact with the ground, and support the weight of the body. They vary in length, being shortest towards the middle of the sole, and longest at their junction with those of the wall. At this part the sole is equal to the wall in thickness. Unlike the wall fibres, however, those of the sole only attain a certain length, when the horny matter of which they are composed dries and fractures like the human hair. By this means the sole seldom, if ever, becomes abnormally thick in a state of nature, and the loose flakes that are continually forming are not only active agents in retaining the moisture necessary for maintaining the elasticity and proper development of horn, but also play the part of so many pliant defences to guard the plantar surface of the hoof from injury by extraneous substances, with which it is always coming in contact.

The frog is a most important organ. It is analogous to the elastic pads on the foot of the dog, cat, camel, elephant, and other creatures. It is designed, like these pads, to meet the ground, diminish the jar to which the limb would otherwise be subjected, especially during violent exertion, and, by its india-rubber-like properties, prevent slipping. In conjunction with the admirably constructed vascular cushion, or 'sensitive frog,' lying above it, and contained between the wings of the pedal bone, it acts as a protection and support to the large flexor tendon in its passage over the navicular bone and at its insertion into the os pedis. This function was pointed out by Lafosse in 1754: 'The frog serves as a cushion to the tendon of Achilles . . . it is composed of soft and compact horn . . . of a spongy nature . . . it ought to bear on the ground, as much for the *facilité* as for the safety of the horse in progression . . . it is the natural *point d'appui* of the flexor tendon.'

In aiding the movements of the internal parts of the foot, its influence on the lateral expansion of the hoof may be said to be *nil,* or at any rate extremely trifling; and notwithstanding all that has been imagined and written on the subject of this lateral expansion, it may with confidence be asserted that the lower margin of the horny case, from the toe to the heels, if perhaps not perfectly immovable under all circumstances, after the animal has attained maturity, yet is, in the unmutilated foot, practically so. With the unpared hoof, it may also be asserted that the sole does not descend; the descent of this portion of the foot, and its lateral expansion at the heels to any very appreciable degree, would be incompatible not only with the functions, but also with the anatomy of that organ. The elasticity required to assist in the movements of the horse and to prevent injury, is to be found in other parts of the foot and limb. Such is the result of daily observation, every variety of experiment possible to devise, and a long and attentive study of the anatomy and physiology of this wonderful structure. I have before expressed my opinion that the lateral expansion and sole descent theory has proved a sad one for the horse, and has caused him years of untold suffering and inconvenience.

The support afforded by the horny frog and plantar cushion to the flexor tendons is not without its counterpart in other regions of the body. We find cushions of fat, for example, placed in various situations to act as a pad, and particularly in maintaining the structures surrounding joints in close approximation to these, especially in the anterior and posterior extremities; but there the enveloping muscles play the part that ground pressure does on the frog.

It may be noted that the wall or crust of the fore foot is thickest at the front part, or toe, and gradually diminishes in substance, as it does in depth, towards the heels, the inside quarter and heel being the thinnest and straightest, while the outside quarter is stronger, wider, and more circular. The hind foot, on the contrary, is strongest and widest towards the quarters and heels, and is deeper there than the fore one; the frog is also smaller, and the sole more concave.

In the unshod fore foot, a large portion of the plantar surface comes into contact with the ground, even when this is in a hard condition. If we place a fresh hoof that has never been shod—I mean one that has not been trimmed and dressed by the farrier, and that belonged to an animal with no hereditary defect in this respect—on a table, we will find that the crust, bars, and a considerable portion of the posterior part of the frog are on the same plane, and must have sustained wear together. The outer surface of the crust looks shining, tough, and solid; the sole is wonderfully thick, and the horn beneath the flakes, if there are any, is moist, flexible, and easily cut; while the frog, if it be a fore foot, extends well towards the toe, and is full, round, and solid, with perhaps a few loose shreds in process of exfoliation, and the cleft extending to a very slight depth. In consistence it resembles a piece of india-rubber, if in a moist condition; but if dry, then it is harder and less vulnerable. This is the condition in which the hoof should be studied by every horseman and every farrier; as it is the condition in which it should and can be maintained by careful management and shoeing.

I much regret that I cannot in this work enter more fully into the anatomy and physiology of this important region of the horse's body; to give anything like an adequate idea of these would require a larger space than I now have at my command, and indeed is a proper subject for a special treatise.

As my object here is merely to show the use and abuse of shoeing, I may have said sufficient to show that in the unshod foot of an animal that has not been improperly reared, and has descended from sound stock, we find a perfect organ adapted to meet all natural requirements.

Domestication, and the necessities of man, however, are apt, unless carefully guarded against, to change the character and healthy condition of this and other organs. In our climate and state of civilization, the horse taken from pasture to share in the artificial existence of his master cannot long travel without protection to the hoofs. Travelled for a short distance only on hard roads during wet weather, the crust of the hoof at the toe and quarters is worn and broken away, and the sole becomes diminished in thickness; the frog resists wear better than either.

Knowing this, before the animal is put to any service, the precaution is taken to have it shod. Indeed, usually long before this period arrives, the creature has to submit to the unreasonable routine which is for ever after to dominate its life of slavery. The farrier is repeatedly called in to trim and dress the young creature's hoofs, to rasp and cut them in an unmeaning fashion, so as to keep them in a good form for shoeing. When at last shoes are applied, the foot has to submit to an amount of alteration, cutting, rasping, and beautifying, which might cause us to exclaim with Snout, 'O Bottom (or rather foot), thou art changed! what do I see on thee?' The hoof has been brought into a shape conformable to the prevailing fashion.

> Coutumes, opinion, reines de notre sort,
> Vous réglez des mortels et la vie et la mort.

So writes Voltaire, and if he had been an observing horseman, he would doubtless have included horses with mortals. By dint of knife and rasp, the dimensions of the organ, the foundation of the edifice, have been greatly reduced, and the animal rests on a narrower basis. The sole has been carefully denuded of its protecting horn until the thin pellicle of newly secreted material is exposed and readily yields to the thumb. The frog is 'scientifically' reduced on every side, the heels or commissures are well opened up, the bars are reduced in size and fantastically delineated, and the portion of the sole between them and the crust—the seat of corn—is carefully carved out à la Miles. The plantar surface of the foot altogether is much more concave than it was previously, and it looks like a masterpiece of workmanship. It may present something like the following shape, when prepared for the shoe (fig. 205). A shoe is then fitted to the foot; in all probability it is too small; it has a wide, flat ground-surface, the foot-surface has a narrow plane border on which the crust rests, and the remainder is bevelled to avoid contact with the abnormally thin sole. When this metallic plate is fastened on the hoof, and the horse once more rests on the limb, the foot has no longer its natural bearing. The whole weight of the horse, as well as any other weight he may have to sustain on his back, is borne by the crust of the foot alone. The frog is elevated above the ground, and the sole dare not come near it. In fact, the shoe has a very wide surface or web to protect the sole of the poor mutilated foot from the injury likely to be inflicted by stones on the roads: injury that, before shoeing, could have been resisted far better by nature's protection.

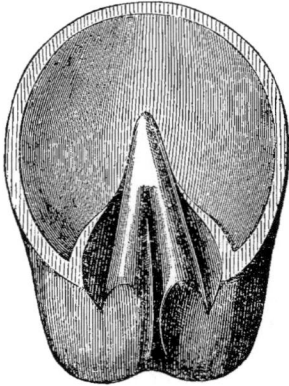

fig 205

The shoe, as we have seen, was too small; or rather, the farrier imagined the plantar surface which supported the weight and strain so admirably in a natural condition to be too large. So when the metal plate has been securely attached, a large portion of the hoof hangs over it—the best and strongest portion; and this has to be removed with the rasp or toe-knife. The nails have been driven to a certain height in the wall, and as their extremities must be riveted or clenched, these clenches must not be disturbed. The overhanging crust between them and the shoe, however, is rasped away, and the face of the foot presents a rounded or knobbed appearance very unlike its natural outline. In all probability, the whole external surface up to the coronet is tastefully rasped and polished, the varnish-like covering nature had spread over it is carefully removed,[1] and the fibres beneath are more or less damaged, are exposed to desiccation, and shrink; while below the clenches they have been entirely destroyed, and nothing is left to support the nails holding on the shoe but the thin soft fibres, as fragile almost as the pith of a rush, and which were never intended by nature to be exposed. Consequently, they lose their moisture, wither, chip, crack, and break off, and frequently the shoe is lost, and with it a large portion of the hoof.

The same process goes on with the sole and frog. The young horn, prematurely exposed, cannot resist the effects of evaporation, and shrinks in the same way. At each shoeing the same routine is followed by the farrier, and the horn is often so hard that artificial means must be adopted to soften it, in order to get off a sufficient quantity to allow the sole to spring under the thumb.

In this we cannot altogether blame the farrier; he is only carrying out the ideas of men who have published books on shoeing. Can we wonder that it soon becomes necessary to adopt every means to supply artificially that which has been removed so indiscreetly. Heavy iron shoes with plenty of cover to defend the morbidly sensitive horn of the soles, which may have been thinned till the blood

[1] So valuable is this protection, and so easily is it removed, that the groom or stableman, when washing the horse's hoofs, should never allow his water-brush to pass along the face of the crust. This part should be cleaned with a soft sponge.

was oozing through, before these cumbrous shields were applied. Words cannot describe the agony a horse must experience when he chances to put his foot on a sharp, or even a blunt stone. And yet the writers who have counselled this mutilation of the foot, have laid this tenderness—the limping gait, and falls with broken knees—to the nails of the shoe preventing expansion! Plates of leather covering the delicate frog and sole, and layers of tar and tow, are brought into requisition to compensate—though such is not confessed—for the loss of the horn; but with very small results. In a brief time, the whole of the foot becomes dwarfed; the frog, deprived of its natural function, like the muscles of a paralyzed arm, becomes atrophied, diseased, and almost disappears, the sole becomes still more concave and hard, and the foot towards the heels narrower, as in figure 206.

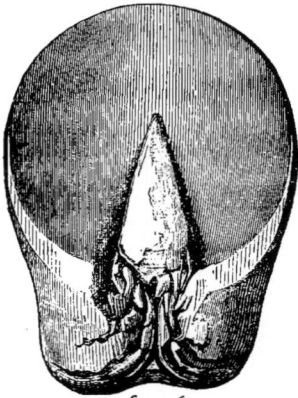

fig. 206

At the same time the unfortunate creature begins to move as if in pain; the flexor tendon, on its course over the navicular bone, has lost its support, and has from the first shoeing been acting at a very serious disadvantage. The mutilation of the hoof, by removing the best portion of its horn, at the very time it was most required, has inflicted serious injury on it and the bone over which it has to play during its arduous task of flexing the foot and limb; while the heavy iron shoe, and the increase of concussion it engenders on artificial roads, all tend to hasten the ruin of the animal—and sooner or later, depending on circumstances, we have either acute or chronic navicular disease, acute or chronic laminitis, or a host of other maladies of a more or less serious character. I am of course always speaking of the anterior extremities.

This evil of paring and rasping must be looked upon as the greatest and most destructive of all that pertains to shoeing, or even to our management of the horse. Nine-tenths of the workmen who resort to this practice cannot explain its object, and those who have written books in defence of it, say it is to allow the descent of the sole and facilitate the lateral expansion of the hoof.

Fancy our gardeners cutting and rasping the bark off our fruit-trees to assist them in their natural functions, and to improve their appearance! And yet the bark is of no more vital importance to the tree than the horn of the sole, wall, and frog is to the horse's foot.

Bracy Clark has admirably delineated the changes the hoof undergoes in a short course of modern shoeing; though, always haunted by the expansion phantom, he wrongly attributed this alteration to the nails confining the lateral movements of the heels. The same transformation from health to disease can be noted in the feet of young horses whose soles are pared and hoofs embellished at some forge where shoeing is practised on 'improved principles.'

Not only is this unscientific practice injurious to the hoof and its contents, but it indirectly reacts upon the whole limb. If the foot suffers, this must share to a greater or less extent. We have but to cast our eyes on the horses passing to and fro in large cities, to discover how many, at a comparatively early age, are limb-worn and crippled; and, though we must attribute much of this to excessive and premature toil, yet we cannot over look the effects of the hoof-mutilation and unreasonable shoeing, and are compelled to lay a large share of blame to their account.

In briefly noticing the rules which ought to guide our practice in shoeing the horse's foot, we will again glance at the most prominent and common errors in the farrier's art which occasion and perpetuate such grave evils.

The limb and hoof of the unshod horse should be attentively studied, as both are beautifully adapted for their functions, and our care should be to interfere as little as possible with these; in fact, we ought, in shoeing, to adapt to the feet shoes which will preserve the regular-ity and just direction of the limbs, maintain the integrity of the hoof in form and texture, allow freedom to those movements of which it is capable, while shielding the horn from the effects of undue wear. They should also aid the animal in retaining a firm and solid grasp of the ground or pavement, as well as assist in the impulsive efforts required in the performance of certain duties.

In a normal state of the foot, the crust or wall grows from the coronet at an equal rate at all points, and in a degree generally sufficient to compensate for the wear sustained at its lower or ground margin. When this wear is regular, and the foot may be said to stand in har-monious relations with the other parts of the member, the angle of inclination of the front of the hoof depends on the formation of the limb to a certain extent, but may be set down at from 50 to 60 degrees. This part of the hoof is longer than the heels by one-third. The crust grows to an indefinite length when prevented from sustaining wear through accident, or the application of the shoe. This growth appears to be greatest at the front of the foot, and least at the heels. This is only apparent, however, and may be accounted for by the attrition that takes place between the shoe and foot, from the last nails to the heel, where there is an amount of play which wears down the horn almost as quickly as it grows, and is evidenced by the deep furrows observed towards the heels of the shoe. This is an important fact to remember, as the continual increase in length of the toe is one of the unavoidable evils of shoeing. Every hour the balance of the limb is being altered as the foot grows forward, and more strain is thrown on the back parts of it. In a state of nature, growth and wear would be continually balancing each other. At each shoeing, the abnormal length of the foot is certainly remedied by the skilful farrier, who reduces it to its natural proportions; but he has no sooner applied his shoe than the same process of growth again slowly, but surely, alters the *aplomb*. This is, to a certain extent, irremediable. But it is not a very great evil; and it is in reducing the wall of the hoof to its proper length that a workman is known. The amount of growth varies in different animals, according to circumstances. If it is active in the shod horse, then the shoes must be more frequently removed to reduce the redundancy, and restore the lower part of the limb to its natural position. We will hereafter notice how this should be done.

The second rule—to maintain the integrity of the hoof in form and texture, and allow freedom to those move ments of which it is capable, is one of vital importance to the well-being of the animal. To indicate in a general manner how it should be enforced, I cannot do better, I think, than enumerate the various steps in the operation of shoeing, as they have been inculcated by me for several years. The directions are applicable for all kinds of horses, and even for every description of foot, and are those I give to the farriers under my supervision. It will be perceived that what we may term hygienic shoe- ing is reduced to a few simple lessons, which any one may learn and readily practise, or see carried out on their own horses; and that it has nothing of the pain- fully elaborate carving, rasping, nailing, and filing at- tending the usual method of shoeing, and which demands much skill, much labour, and after all entails grave injury on the horse.

Shoeing, as it is termed, is required either when the armature has been worn out, the hoofs have grown too long, or the wear and growth have both reached a stage when the intervention of the farrier is needed. The length of wear of the shoe will depend upon the material of which it is made, its weight, and the attrition to which it has been subjected. It is generally better that it should wear for a long than a short period; frequent shoeing, requiring frequent nailing, damages the crust by piercing its fibres and splitting them.

The shoe is said to be 'worn out' when it has lost a portion of its substance at the toe—where the greatest amount of wear usually occurs, or when it has become very thin either over the whole surface, or in one of its branches. When the shoe lasts for a long period—six weeks or two months—without being removed, the hoof usually becomes unnaturally long, widens at its under surface, and the iron being carried forward with the growth becomes buried within the crust. The horse moves awkwardly, stumbles, goes on his heels, and an undue strain is thrown on the flexor tendons and the posterior regions of the limb.

The period during which a shoe ought to wear, or be allowed to remain on the foot, depends upon circumstances. Unless in very exceptional circumstances, it should not be suffered to remain longer than four or five weeks, and neither should a horse be shod more frequently than once in three weeks or a month. It must be always remembered, that an excess of growth is far less injurious than too frequent shoeing.

It is easy to distinguish when the shoe is worn out· though some people, whenever the outer margin of the iron at the toe is worn away—and though the horse may not have been shod the full period—become alarmed, and have the animal re-shod.

So long as the shoe remains firmly attached, this wear is of little importance. If the horse has not been shod a month, I allow him to go until the plate nearly or quite breaks through at the point of wear, as he only removes that horn from the front of the hoof which must be taken away by the rasp in the operation of shoeing. This enables me to order lighter shoes to be worn.

Some horses have naturally long feet, and when they rest on the ground they appear to require 'shortening.' If a foot is raised, it will be at once seen whether this is the case—that is, if the sole has not been mutilated by the drawing-knife in the previous shoeing. If it is in its natural condition, this will be some distance from the shoe, and the latter will have lost its proper seat on the foot. This is because the crust grows indefinitely, while the sole always maintains a regular thickness.

Whether the shoes be worn out, or only require removal when the crust has obtained an excess in length, it is necessary that the farrier's assistance be called in. Before the shoes are taken off, the direction of the limb and foot should be studied, both while the horse is standing and when it is moving. This is seldom, if ever, done by the farrier; and yet it ought to be an important object to maintain or regulate the direction of the leg and hoof, which can be done by ascertaining whether in front or in profile they are in line—whether the toe, the side of the hoof, or heel, incline too much inwards or outwards—whether the heels of the hoof are too low or too high—the toe too long or too short—and if there are any traces of 'brushing' or 'cutting' on the inner sides of the hoofs, fetlocks, or knees. Seeing the horse walk or trot indicates the nature of his action — whether high or low — or if the movement of the limbs is false or irregular—and whether any fault which may exist can be rectified by shoeing.

These are very essential points to observe, as they all come within the domain of the art; and the intelligent workman can do much to modify or rectify natural or acquired defects, as well as preserve perfect form and action, and in this way carry out our first rule.

Then the shoe is removed. This is a very simple operation, and yet it requires tact and care: tact, that the horse's limb and foot be not twisted by violently wrenching off the shoe; and care, that no nails or clenches are allowed to remain in the crust, and that the latter be not broken. It is better, after cutting the clenches clean off, to spring the shoe gently at the inner or outer heel by means of the pincers, prizing them softly forward, and then across the foot—never outward—and withdrawing the nails one by one. A glance is sufficient to show the state of the sole and frog. The next step is to reduce the hoof to its proper dimensions—and this is no trifling matter. On this operation depends the true or false direction of the limbs, and it is in this respect that grave errors are often committed. It may be accepted as a truth, that the ground-surface of the foot ought to be directly transverse to the direction of the pastern, no matter how defective the limb may be; and it is in maintaining or restoring this relation, and keeping the length of the toe in harmony with that of the heels, that care and skill are required.

This is accomplished by reducing the crust. If the pastern is perpendicular to the shank-bone, and the two sides of the lower margin of the foot are directly transverse to the line passing down from these, the crust has only to be lowered equally on each side; but if the pastern deviates to the outside or inside, then more horn must be taken away from one margin than the other, to regulate this deviation. This operation, says M. Guyon, ought to be accomplished with mathematical exactitude, as a difference in height between the sides of the foot of some fractions of an inch determines considerable oscillations of the weight.

A just relation may be said to exist between the height of the toe and that of the heels, when the latter is about two-thirds that of the former. This is the natural form; though, through improper shoeing, and perhaps defective organization, it may vary. To lower the heels more than the toe, is to lengthen the foot; and to shorten the toe, and leave the heels untouched, is to raise the latter.

The amount of horn to be removed from the crust, as well as the manner of removing it, is another important consideration. As before mentioned, the heels usually wear themselves tolerably low against the extremities of the branches of the shoe; but where the latter has been firmly fixed to the crust, this up-and-down friction does not take place, and the posterior parts of the foot are proportionally long. As a general rule, however, the heels require little or no alteration, and the toe needs shortening. With the hoofs of saddle or carriage horses, this shortening is best and most safely accomplished with the rasp. Heavy draught-horses, whose hoofs may have grown excessively long, and which have more horn to spare, are oftener trimmed with the toe-knife.

If the horse is to be shod with a shoe reaching to the points of the heels, the horn of the wall at this region, if necessary, is to be removed to the degree prescribed above. Under all circumstances, every fragment of loose horn incapable of supporting the shoe, ought to be taken away, so as to reach sound material. This may be done by passing the rasp evenly along the ground-surface of the crust, gradually removing a larger amount as the toe is reached, and inclining the instrument in a sloping manner on the outer edge, so as to cut off the external fibres shorter than the internal ones. At the toe, the crust should be cut down to the level of the sole. Here the knife may be used, and the remainder of this part removed until the white or yellow line marking the junction of sole and wall is reached. This is only to take place around the toe, and no more of the sole must be taken away than is absolutely necessary to give a level bed to the shoe; or, as Osmer says, 'in order to obtain a smooth and even surface, so far as the breadth of the shoe reaches, and no farther.' In the majority of cases I never allow the knife to be used for this purpose; causing all the work to be done by the rasp. The object in cutting off the external fibres at an angle from the quarters to the toe, is to give the edge of the hoof a rounded appearance, while it equalizes its thickness, and prevents it from splitting and breaking. *The sole, frog, and bars must on no account, or under any conditions — unless those of a pathological nature — be interfered with in any way by knife or rasp.* I have already shown the urgent necessity there exists for preserving these important parts of the plantar surface in their full natural strength. As certainly as they are interfered with, and their substance reduced, so surely will the hoof be injured. Nature has made every provision for their defence. They will support the contact of hard, soft, rugged, or even sharp bodies, if allowed to escape the terrible drawing-knife; while hot, cold, wet, or dry weather has little or no influence on the interior of the foot, or on the tender horn, if man does not step in to beautify them, by robbing them of their protection — perhaps merely to please the fancy of an ignorant groom or coachman.

The custom of paring the sole until it yields to the pressure of the thumb is a barbarous one.   Fortunately for those who recommend it, its evil effects are not immediately apparent; a horse with his soles denuded of their horn until the blood oozes through them, may not manifest any great suffering, and even go sound on a level pavement; though, if he chances to put his foot on a pebble or sharp stone, his agony may be so acute as to cause him to fall.

If we closely examine the upper surface of the sole of a hoof that has been separated from its contents by maceration, we will find it perforated everywhere by myriads of minute apertures, which look as if they had been formed by the point of a fine needle.   If we also look at the vascular parts of the foot that have been in contact with this horny surface, it will be observed that they are closely studded with exceedingly fine, yet somewhat long filaments, as thickly set as the pile of the richest Genoa velvet.   These are the ' villi,' or ' papillæ,' which enter the horny cavities, and, fitting into them like so many fingers into a glove, constitute the secretory apparatus of the frog as well as the sole.   Each of these filaments forms a horntube or fibre, and passes to a certain depth in the protecting canal, whose corneous wall it builds.   When injected with some coloured preparation, one of them makes a beautiful microscopial object, appearing as a long tapering network of blood-vessels surrounding one or two parent trunks, and communicating with each other in the most wonderful manner. These filaments are also organs of tact, each containing a sensitive nerve destined to endow the foot with the attributes of a tactile organ.

This disposition will enable us to realize, to some extent, the amount of injury done by paring. The horn thrown out for their defence and support being removed by the farrier's knife, and perhaps the ends of these villi cut through, the meagre pellicle remaining rapidly shrivels up, the containing cavity of each vascular tuft as quickly contracts on the vessels and nerves, which, in their turn, diminish in volume, disappear, or become morbidly sensitive through this squeezing influence. The feet of a horse so treated are always hot, the soles look dry and stony, and become unnaturally concave; the animal goes 'tender' after each shoeing, and it is not until the horn has been regenerated to a certain extent, that he steps with anything like ease. Until the new material has been formed, each 'papilla' experiences the same amount of inconvenience and suffering that the human foot does in a new tight boot. This tenderness is usually ascribed to the nails, and other causes; and the horse in the stable rests one foot after another, as if he suffered uneasiness or pain.

The process of deterioration is comparatively slow, however, and the culprits who cause this mischief evade their responsibility. Their utmost skill, however, is racked to protect artificially the parts they have robbed and are gradually destroying. Shoes with a wide cover carefully kept from contact with the sole—for that would infallibly cause lameness—are put on the mutilated feet, and even leather soles and bolsters of tow steeped in pine-tar are stuck between the foot and shoe, with the intention of shielding the surface that has been, through ignorance, rendered morbidly sensitive and defective. What is called the excessive growth, or exuberant horn, was intended to protect the lower surface of the foot from wounds and bruises, to maintain the elasticity of the young horn beneath, and to aid the crust in sustaining the weight and impulsive efforts, at the same time strengthening the latter at its point of union, and preventing its being broken or worn away too readily.

These remarks, which we can scarcely too much insist upon noticing, apply with equal force to all horses, from the dray mammoth, to the fleet race-horse or diminutive Dartmoor pony.

Indeed, they are perhaps more applicable to the case of race-horses and hunters than to any other class. With these animals, it is of the utmost importance that the feet, especially the fore ones, be accurately levelled on both sides or ground face, according to the rule laid down, so as to obviate the risk of sprains and dislocations during rapid and energetic movements, particularly lateral twists of the lower joints. By leaving the sole, bars, and frog intact, the foot is not only strengthened, but muscular fatigue is wonderfully diminished, especially in traversing heavy ground. When the sole has been thinned and hollowed out into a cup-like shape, the foot readily penetrates to a greater depth than if it were flat, and is also more difficult to withdraw, because there is a larger extent of surface in contact with the tenacious soil. In proportion to the width of cover in the shoe, and the space between it and the sole, there is a still greater amount of adhesion, and consequent loss of speed and power, as well as diminution of stability.

For the reasons before given, the frog should remain untouched by the knife, unless it be to remove some flakes which are all but detached; though this should always be done under supervision, as the drawing-knife has no conscience. It is scarcely necessary to say that the barbarous and destructive operation of opening the heels should be sternly reprobated. The 'commissures' of the bars and frogs may be scraped out by some blunt instrument, merely to free them from soil or gravel that may have lodged at the bottom.

This is all the preparation any kind of foot usually requires for the shoe, and may be summed up in a few words: levelling the crust in conformity with the direction of the limb and foot, and removing as much of its margin as will restore it to its normal length, rounding its outer edge at the same time; and leaving the sole, frog, bars, and heels in all their natural integrity. Such is the treatment of the hoofs of the horses under my care; and so strong are they—such massive solid blocks of horn do they appear, that should a shoe by some rare chance be lost on a journey, there is no danger whatever in marching a horse for ten, twenty, or even thirty miles without another. Horses are never pricked in nailing, and foot-diseases are, I may say, scarcely known. Nearly every hoof is a model, and as perfect as before the animal was first shod.

With hoofs of this description, the kind of shoe employed is of secondary importance. I need not say that the armature needed to protect the crust and maintain the integrity of the foot will vary with the requirements of the animal, i. e. with the services demanded from him. For instance, we would not shoe a race-horse like one for draught, or a hunter like one for carriage-work; the shoes must be varied more or less in form and weight, to suit different purposes and degrees of wear. It will be understood that no fixed shape, size, or weight can be determined for all horses. It may be laid down as a rule, however, that the properties of a good shoe, no matter for what service, must be lightness and durability—opposite qualities which require skill to combine, but which are nevertheless of some moment, more particularly with horses required to move quickly, and for long periods, over paved roads.

One of the great evils that has accompanied the art of farriery for many centuries, in addition, and in immediate relation, to the mutilation of the hoof, has been the excessive weight of the shoes attached to the feet. The most primitive specimens of shoes were only a narrow band of iron, plane on both faces, and were, in all probability, fastened on uncut hoofs. With the introduction of the paring fallacy, more iron was necessary to cover the parts made tender and sensitive by being robbed of their horn, and the lateral expansion and sole-descent theory perpetuated, if it did not exaggerate, the mischief. Not only is a wide surface of metal urgently required to shield the greater part of the sole, as we see in Mr Miles's directions, but it is regarded by only too many men, who ought to know better, that in addition to width, shoes should also possess a good thickness, to *protect the foot from jar*. The absurdity of this plea does not need demonstration; it may be sufficient to

remark that the flexible horn is the best modifier of concussion, and that as the thickness of metal increases, so
does the jar.

But this supposed jar is the least of the ills attending
the use of heavy shoes. The difference in the muscular
fatigue of a limb, after carrying at its extremity for a long
distance a clumsy mass of iron, weighing, perhaps, two
pounds, and afterwards another of one or one and a half
pounds, is astonishing. I cannot, perhaps, do better than
quote the remarks of Professor Bouley, when discussing
this subject in Paris a short time ago. He says, speaking
of the omnibus horses: 'If, at the termination of a day's
work, we calculate the weight represented by the mass of
heavy shoes that a horse is condemned to carry at each
step, we will arrive at a formidable array of figures, and
in this way be able to estimate the amount of force use-
lessly expended by the animal, in raising the shoes that
surcharge his feet. The calculation I have made possesses an eloquence that dispenses with very long commentaries. Suppose that the weight of a shoe is 1000
grammes; it is not excessive to admit that a horse trots at
the rate of one step every second, or sixty steps a minute.
In a minute, then, the limb of a horse whose foot carries
1 kilogramme makes an effort necessary to raise, kilogramme after kilogramme, a weight of 60 kilogrammes.
For the four limbs, this weight in a minute is represented
by 60 × 4 = 240 kilogrammes; for the four feet during
an hour the weight is 14,000 kilogrammes; and for four
hours, the mean duration of a day's work in these omni-
buses, the total amount of weight raised has reached the
respectable figure of 57,000 kilogrammes. But the move-

ment communicated to these 57,000 kilogrammes repre
sents an expenditure of power employed by the motor
without any useful result; and as the motor is a living
one, this expense of strength represents an exhaustion, or
if you like it better, a degree of fatigue, proportioned to
the effort necessary for its manifestation. This calculation is most simple and readily understood. It is to be
noted, nevertheless, that I have omitted a considerable
fact: which is, that the weights I have tabulated are situated at the extremities of the limbs, and that the arms of
the levers on which the muscles act to raise them, being
infinitely shorter than those of the physiological resistance
to which these weights are added, the intensity of their
action ought, therefore, to be singularly increased. But
to measure this intensity of action would require a mathematical aptitude which I do not possess. I will not, therefore, dwell on this point, notwithstanding its importance,
and am content to signalize it. Otherwise, the figures I
present speak for themselves, and tell us that the diminu
tion in the weight of horse-shoes is not an accessory consideration, so far as the useful application of the horse's
strength goes.'

It will be seen that this question of weight at the
lower end of the limb is a serious one; the power moving
it acting at the upper extremities, and having but short
leverage. We can readily imagine what a difference in
power must be required to move a pound at the fore-arm
or knee, and at the lower surface of the foot, and how
much the lightening of a shoe by one or two ounces
must affect the motion of the limb.

In shoeing, this important consideration has been

carefully kept out of sight, or altogether overlooked; and yet we cannot forget that it has a great influence on the wear of the muscles, tendons, ligaments, and joints. It is the fashion to say that a horse always travels better in his old shoes, and to attribute this to the fact that he is not pinched in them. Ascribing something to this circumstance, though if the horse's hoofs had not been mutilated by the knife and rasp, he would probably, or rather ought not to feel pinched, we must also take into account that a good portion of the superfluous and fatiguing weight has been got rid of by wear.

It is worth noting the changes that take place on the ground-face of a heavy shoe on the foot of a riding-horse during a long day's journey. How in the morning we have the indications of muscular freshness and activity,— the agile step and due flexure of the articulations, putting their impress on a certain part of the metal; towards midday a change of bearing and point of friction testifying to muscular fatigue and heavier attrition; and in the afternoon, unmistakable symptoms of dragging the feet and leg-weariness.

So that in hygienic shoeing, we have a perfect right to insist that not a grain of iron more than is absolutely necessary to protect the crust from undue wear, or serve a useful purpose, be applied to the foot. Every particle beyond this is not only unnecessary, but injurious. Nature, in constructing the animal-machine, and enduing it with powers to sustain the ordinary requirements of organization, and even certain extraordinary demands, could scarcely have been expected to provide the large additional amount of energy necessary to swing backwards and forwards several ounces, or even pounds, attached to the extremity of each limb at every step.

Lightness and durability can only be attained by employing the best material. If the sole of the foot is not mutilated, it does not require to be covered by the shoe, as nature has furnished an infinitely better protection. Wide-surfaced shoes can therefore be at once dispensed with, and a narrow rim, fabricated from the very toughest and best iron, and adapted for travelling on slippery roads, while aiding foot and limb, and sufficient to sustain wear for four or five weeks, is all that is required. Here again the skilful artisan is needed, and science steps in to aid him. We have seen that the sole was destined, particularly at its junction with the crust, to sustain weight, if not cut away by the drawing-knife. We also know that it is advantageous to the whole foot and limb to give the sole as wide and general a bearing as possible; so that the one part may relieve the other—the sole coming to the aid of the crust, and the frog interposing to share the strain imposed upon both, as well as to relieve the strain on the posterior parts of the foot, flexor tendon, and limb, and keep a firm grasp of the ground by its resilient and adhesive properties.

It would, then, appear to be indicated, that the shoe applied to the foot should have its upper or hoof surface plane, in order that it might sustain the crust, and as much of this strong part of the sole as its width permitted. This is contrary to the usual practice, which only allows the crust to rest on a narrow level surface, and bevels off the remainder of the shoe to prevent contact with the sole. But the sole in these cases is mutilated, and in this unnatural condition would suffer injury if anything came in contact with it. Many years' experience of this plane foot-surfaced shoe, in various regions of the globe, and on feet of every kind and quality, have proved the soundness of this view. The foot is brought as near to a state of nature when the greater part of its plantar surface supports the weight of the body, as man can hope to achieve while submitting the horse to an artificial state of existence.

From what has been said, it will be understood that in speaking of a light shoe, a narrow and thin plate of iron was meant. The narrowness of the metal insures a good foot-hold—in this respect imitating the crust,—while its thinness brings the sole, frog, and bars in closer approximation to the ground.

It is a most difficult matter to devise a shoe that will meet every requirement. The heavy draught-horse, doomed to bring into play every muscle while endeavouring to move and drag along an enormous load, must have his feet differently armed to the hunter or race-horse, in which speed is the chief requisite. Taking into account the different character of the horny textures, it is none the less true that the same rule holds good in all with regard to the sole and frog sustaining weight, though in the slow-moving animal it is of less importance, perhaps, than in the lighter and more fleet ones. The massive draught-horse requires toe-and-heel projections on the ground-surface of the shoes to economize his locomotive powers and to aid his impulsive efforts; though his hoofs none the less require the observance of those conservative principles which have been so strongly insisted upon, but

which are so seldom applied.   To give the greatest amount
of strength and foothold to the shoes of the heavy
draught-horse, with the least amount of weight, should
always be kept in view in fabricating them.   But with
this animal the preservation of the crust is the principal
object; and to effect this, the sole and frog ought, if
possible, to be preserved intact.

The form of the shoe should, in outline, resemble the
shape of the ground surface of the hoof.   It has been
decided that its upper or sole surface must be flat from the
outer to the inner margin.   For horses other than those
of heavy draught, its width will of course vary; but it
must be an advantage to have it as narrow as is compatible, in relation to its thickness, with the amount of
wear required from it.   After what we have said, it will
perhaps be well to remember that it is better to have a
thin wide shoe than a narrow thick one—so far as the
foot surface is concerned.

The ground face of the shoe is the next point for
consideration.   This should always, if possible, be parallel
with its plantar face; that is, the shoe ought to be plane
on both surfaces, and of the same thickness on its outer
margin at least, both for hind and fore feet.   This insures
the foot and limb being kept in a natural position.   What
are termed calkins, on one or both heels, are very objectionable, for the simple reason that they raise the posterior
part of the foot higher than the anterior, and disturb the
aplomb of the limb ; and unless the hoof meets the ground
in its natural direction, some part of the leg will be certain
to experience the evil effects.   On the fore foot, calkins
are far more objectionable than on the hind one, and

their use on either is but temporary; projecting beyond the surface of the shoe, and opposing but a limited surface to the ground, their duration is limited, and when they are worn off, the foot, though in a better position, has nothing to prevent it from slipping on pavement.

For very many years inventors have endeavoured to remedy the defects of calkins in various ways. Indeed, the very earliest specimens of hoof-armature show us that the primitive farriers were no mean adepts in providing their steeds with a 'biting' foot-hold. The nails that fastened on the shoes had large semicircular heads that projected beyond the lower face of the metal on a level with the calkin, and were supported in the oval cavities of the shoe; forming, together with the calks, no less than eight catches—all powerful aids in aiding progression under certain circumstances, and guaranteeing a secure support.

Fiaschi and Blundevil give us more modern examples in their way; the 'catches' of which they speak, however, being notches in a raised welt on the border of the shoe. In this century, many plans have been adopted; the iron or steel employed being, in a number of instances, rolled by machinery, and generally channelled into grooves or concavities. The most successful of these attempts to fabricate shoes to prevent slipping appears to be that adopted by Mr Gray, of Sheffield. The bars of iron and steel from which his shoes are made are grooved up the middle by either one or two cavities, or notched in various ways. These ridges and teeth are extremely hard, the shoes being tempered after they are forged; consequently they can be made lighter than Rodway's shoes, which were also made from rolled bars.

With a plane ground-surfaced shoe, a great object to be gained in attempting to prevent slipping, and affording a grasp of the ground, is the diminution of the wide surface of metal, without interfering with the wear of the shoe but as little as possible. The simplest method of doing this, is merely changing the bevel on the foot surface of the ordinary shoe to its ground surface—making what is now concave plane, and the flat slippery ground surface concave. The effect is almost magical, in the security it gives the animal during progression, and is best exemplified in the case of the hunter, which is shod with shoes of this kind. Here we are imitating nature again, in following the concavity of the sole. There can be no doubt whatever as to the advantages to be gained in employing shoes of this description. The sole is partly supported, as well as the whole of the crust, by the wider surface of metal, while the narrower surface towards the ground affords security of tread. For ordinary wear by carriage or saddle horses, the English hunting-shoe, on unmutilated hoofs, is excellent. The hind shoes, however, should have no calkins; neither should hind or fore shoes be thickened towards the heels: this is a very bad practice.

For hunting or other purposes, a slight modification of this form of shoe can be made, which gives it a still firmer hold, especially on grass land. Besides the concave sole and frog in the unshod foot being of the greatest utility in affording a secure grasp of the ground, the angle formed by the bar and crust at the termination of the heel must also be looked upon as a useful agent in this way, and particularly in preventing the extremity of the limb from slipping forward. Some time ago, I devised a shoe something in this form, which has been employed on the road and in the hunting-field, on fore and hind feet, and with most satisfactory results ' (fig. 207).

Instead of the bevel on the ground surface gradually becoming shallower as it approaches the heels, as in the ordinary hunting-shoe, in my shoe it is rather shallow at the toe (*a*); and as it passes backwards gets deeper, until, within

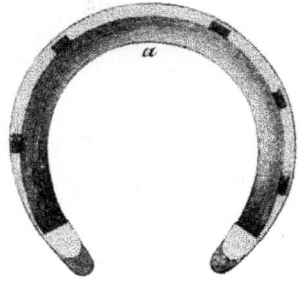

fig 207

an inch or so of the extremity of the shoe, it has cut down through the thickness of the inner border and abruptly stops, leaving a sharp catch (*b*), that, like the inflexion

' Though for ages it has been known that the sole, especially at its margin, will sustain the pressure of the shoe, I put my own method of shoeing to a practical test during the hot weather in September last. It is certain that long journeys on hard roads during the summer months, on horses whose feet are pared, and armed with the ordinary seated shoe, is likely to cause inflammation of these organs. Starting from Chatham, my wife riding an *A*rab horse, and myself mounted on an Irish mare, the first day we rode to St Albans, about 56 miles, and in three days and a forenoon reached *A*therstone, Warwickshire, a distance of about 150 miles. The horses' hoofs remained quite cool, and there was not the least symptom of tenderness during the whole journey. We returned to Chatham by another route a short time afterwards, travelling a distance of 200 miles in five days. At no time was the temperature of the feet increased beyond the normal degree. This experiment is only corroborative of what has been observed on ship-board with horses shod in a similar manner. It certainly appeared to give very different results to the journeys mentioned in some of the authors we have quoted, who speak of the poor horses lying down with painful feet the moment they were put in a stable, after a journey of some twenty or thirty miles.

of the crust at this part, gives an excellent grip that lasts until the shoe is quite worn out. With a contrivance of this kind, three important objects are secured: 1. The plane upper surface resting flat on the crust and unpared sole, leaves no space in which foreign bodies—as clay, stones, or gravel—may lodge, and in heavy ground suction is obviated. 2. The metal is only removed from the parts where it can best be spared, and where there is least wear; consequently the shoe is lightened without being weakened. 3. The level border and extremities of the branches afford an equal bearing for the foot, while the gradually deepening bevel, with its sudden check, secures a permanent and powerful catching surface. The shoe is easily made by any farrier, differing as it does so slightly from the usual hunting hoof-armature; and there is no difference between the fore and hind shoe, except in the shape—the former being more circular than the latter, which is somewhat oval. For carriage and saddle horses, each shoe should have a clip at the middle of the toe, except in special cases, when a clip at each side of the toe of the hind shoe may be necessary. Horses used for hunting should wear a clip on each side of their hind-feet shoes, the sharp edges being carefully removed from the toes and the inner branches, to prevent wounds from over-reaching, cutting, or treading. Horses have been hunted without slipping with shoes of this description, each weighing about eight or nine ounces, and they have worn a month and five weeks over all kinds of country, but particularly grass-land; and I am not aware of any shoes having been lost, or any tread or over-reach occurring during the whole time they have been in trial.

We have remarked how important it is that the shoes worn by horses should be as light as possible. It is generally a most judicious plan, if a horse wears his shoes more at one part than another, so that they do not last a sufficient time, to weld in a small piece of steel at that place, instead of thickening the shoe, and consequently making it heavier. The latter method, which is that generally adopted to save time, most frequently defeats its purpose—the increased weight causing the animal to drag his feet heavily along the ground, instead of lifting them freely

The position and shape of the nail-holes, as well as their number, is the next point to be considered. The shoe ought to be attached by nails to those parts of the crust where the horn is strongest and toughest. In the fore-foot these are in front and along the sides to the quarters, where the horn becomes thin, and nails find less support and are nearer to the living textures; this is more particularly the case towards the heel.

In the hind-foot, the crust is generally strongest towards the quarters and heels. These facts at once give us an indication as to the position of the nail-holes. In the fore-foot, nails can be driven through the crust around the toe, as far as the inside quarter, and a trifle nearer the heel on the outside. In the hind-foot, they can be driven around the toe, and even up to the points of the heels, with impunity.

The form of the nail-holes is of secondary importance. The fullering or groove of the English shoe, though artistic-looking, is a mistake; it is a waste of labour, weakens the shoe, and is of no service. The stamped shoe is in every way preferable. The square cavity, wide at the top and tapering to the bottom, gives a secure and solid lodgment to the nail-head, which of course should be of the same shape; it does not weaken the shoe, is easily made, can be placed nearer the outer or inner margin as required, and when filled with the nail is as capable of resisting wear as any other part. It is usually better to have the nail-holes stamped 'coarse;' that is, at some distance from the outer margin of the shoe, and neither inclining outwards nor inwards.

The number of nail-holes through which nails are to be driven should be as few as possible. Every nail penetrating the crust may be looked upon as a source of injury to it; and with a shoe bedded in a solid manner on the crust and sole, as I have recommended, and diminished in weight to the utmost degree compatible with endurance for a certain period, it is astonishing what a small number of nails is needed. The ordinary heavy seated-shoe is damaging to the foot, not only because it rests on such a narrow basis, but also because its weight and instability necessitates its being attached by a large number of long thick nails which do great harm to the crust. For shoes worn by medium-sized draught-horses, I never allow more than six nails in the fore and seven in the hind feet; more frequently the fore shoes are retained by five nails—three outside and two inside, and the hind ones by three on each side. The nails are comparatively small.

For carriage and saddle horses, as well as hunters, four and five small nails are employed for the fore, and generally five and six for the hind shoes. It must always be remembered, that the retention of a shoe for a sufficient time does not so much depend upon the number of nails attaching it, as upon its exact coaptation and solid bearing on the crust and sole.

The immense number of nails needed to retain the shoes of the last four or five centuries, and as we see exemplified in figure 189, was not so much in consequence of their weight and clumsiness, as the absence of level bearing on the crust, the whole strain being sustained on the extreme outer margin of the torturing encumbrance. It should be laid down as a rule, that where there is a clip there should be no nail; the one is likely to act injuriously on the other. It is scarcely necessary to say, that when so few nails are employed, they should be of the very best quality and judiciously prepared.

We have now prepared our imaginary hoof, and laid down principles to guide us in the manufacture of our shoe. The next step is to fit it. This is also an important one.

The part of the hoof intended to be protected by the iron rim has been made as level as possible by the rasp, aided a little perhaps by the knife; the surface of the shoe destined to rest on this horny bed has also been made perfectly level and smooth, particularly towards the clip or clips. It only remains now to fit the shoe and put it on. After the evidence I have adduced, and so far as my own practical experience in the matter is concerned, I need not say that fitting the shoe cold is only to be justified when it cannot be fitted hot; and that it will not be nearly so quickly, conveniently, or satisfactorily performed, nor will the shoe be so secure. The red-hot shoe at once disposes of those inequalities which cannot be discovered or removed by tools, and it shows the workman at a glance the bearing of the iron. The whole surface of the shoe intended to be in contact with the horn should be distinctly imprinted on the contour of the hoof, so as to insure the closest and most accurate intimacy between the two; and this carbonized surface should not be interfered with on any account, except by the rasp, which is employed to remove any sharpness of the edge of the crust that may have been caused in this fitting. No harm can arise from this mode of adapting the shoe. Usually a small portion of the margin of the wall has to be removed to imbed the clip; this is done with the knife.

By this hot-fitting, the shoe is made to fit the hoof; with the cold-fitting, it is the contrary. It would be departing from the object of the brief sketch I have here laid down to describe how the shoe ought to fit every foot; suffice it to say, that it should be wide enough at the quarters and heels to support the whole of the crust, but yet not wide or long enough to endanger the opposite limbs by striking them, or run the chance of being torn off by the other feet treading upon it; and it should not impinge upon the frog, neither prevent that organ from playing its part in the physiology of the foot.

The shoe, dressed round its edges with a file (my shoes are usually made in a tool, and finished off with a file on their concavity, especially towards the 'catch,' or 'sunk calkin'), is then nailed on. Every nail should pass through sound horn, and a short thick hold of the wall is better than a long thin one. A foot allowed to grow

strong in the manner I have described, will suffer no inconvenience in having the nails driven well home in the
shoe. Every nail should form a part of the shoe, and
scarcely project above it; and when all have been firmly
wedged in, they should be tightly 'drawn up' by hammer and pincers. Nothing then remains to be done but
to bend down, or 'clench,' the small portion of the nail
that remains on the outer face of the crust, after the point
has been twisted off. This should be accomplished by
shortening the fragment with the rasp, so as to leave just
enough to turn over; then with the slightest touch of the
knife or the edge of the rasp, the small barb of horn immediately beneath it is cut away—no notch or trench must
be made, and the clench laid down flush with the general
face of the crust. No more rasping or cutting should be
permitted on any account.

It is usually recommended that the wall should not
be rasped above the clenches; they who give this re
commendation are ignorant of the fact, that as much, if
not more, harm is done by rasping below than above
these rivets. Those who study what I have said concerning the structure of the crust of the hoof will readily
enough understand how this happens. Over the whole
external surface of this part, it has been shown that a
beautifully fine translucent horn or varnish was spread,
to prevent undue desiccation of the horn, and consequent brittleness. Immediately beneath this are the
dense resisting fibres, which are intended to resist wear,
and are most capable of supporting a shoe, through the
medium of the nails; in fact they are the fibres which
ought to perform this duty, as beneath them, towards

the inner aspect of the wall, the horn rapidly becomes soft, spongy, and more like the pith of a rush than horn fibres. What is the usual treatment this region of the hoof receives in, I will be bold to say, nearly every forge in this country, and on the continent, perhaps, as well? The farrier, obeying those whom he has reason to believe know better than himself, respects, it may be, the upper part of the crust, but certainly is not required to do as much for the lower. Owing to his having neglected to rasp away a sufficient amount from its ground border, when preparing the foot for the shoe, or having nailed on one which is too small, a large piece of hoof projects beyond the edge of the shoe, particularly in the front part. This is torn away by the rasp, after the clenches have been made; and by the time the shoer on improved principles has finished his task, what do we see? The wall of the foot, instead of coming down from the coronet to the shoe in all its integrity and evenness of slope, as soon as it reaches the clenches, is chopped abruptly down wards and rounded over like an ill-shaped roll, giving the foot a stump-like appearance, and greatly diminishing the extent of its bearing surface. The greatest evil, however, is in the loss of the strong tough horn, whose presence is so necessary to protect the lower margin of the hoof, and to afford support and hold to the nails. In consequence of its removal, these have nothing to depend upon but the thin, soft horn, and this being exposed to influences it was never intended to meet, quickly desiccates, shrivels, becomes brittle, and breaks away. Then we have a hoof which requires the greatest care in shoeing; the operation of rasping being repeated each time increases the evil, and should a shoe chance to come off on the road, an accident, as we may infer, extremely likely to happen, great damage will be done to the pared sole and the thin, brittle, split-up crust, and in all probability the animal will be lamed. The morbid desire to make fine work of shoeing when the horse first began to be shod, ends in the greatest amount of skill and labour being required to continue it, and keep the animal fit for service, though with deformed feet, seriously damaged horn, and perhaps great suffering. When the coachman or groom's fancy compels the farrier to carry his rasp to the top of the hoof, and make that organ far better fitted for exhibition on a sportsman's table than to meet the rude contact of the ground, or withstand the influences of weather and frequent shoeings, then the injury is greatly increased.

The so-called ' coronary frog-band,' or cuticular prolongation that extends in a wide, whitish-coloured band around the upper part of the hoof, and which is often so scrupulously destroyed in shoeing, is intended by nature to protect the fibres of the wall from the effects of heat and dryness while they are being secreted or so immature as to be incapable of resisting these influences; for it will be remembered that the wall is formed at the coronet, and this covering guarantees not only the integrity of the newly-made horn-tubes, but also maintains the secreting vessels that enter them in a healthy condition, and competent to supply fresh material for wear. Its destruction induces ' sandcrack,' and other morbid conditions of the crust.

After the clenches have been evenly laid down on the wall of the hoof, no more should be done, unless it be to

43

round a little more the edge of the small fragment of horn that may project on each side of the clip, and thus prevent its liability to split. The angle of the face of the hoof should never be interrupted after the shoe is nailed on, but should be the same from top to toe, as in the natural foot. This is a matter of vital importance. Too much stress cannot be laid upon the conservation of the horn of the foot; and no amount of rasping can give the hoof the beautiful polish it has in its natural state.

To diminish the weight, and permit one portion of the posterior part of the foot to come in direct contact with the ground along with the frog, a three-quarter shoe is often applied—the portion of iron extending from the inside quarter to the point of the heel being cut off, and the shoe at this part thinned a little. The horn left unprotected is never interfered with. This is an excellent shoe for saddle and carriage horses, which may be employed on the worst roads while wearing it. For feet that have suffered very much from the effects of rasping and paring, and which are liable to have bruised heels (or corns), its use is attended with the greatest benefit.

The same may be said of tips or half-shoes. An unreasonable prejudice appears to exist against the use of these short light plates; but if they are properly used, there can be no doubt whatever that they are entitled to a far larger share of attention than they have yet received. Their very limited employment hitherto may have arisen from the imperfect manner in which they have been applied. They protect those parts of the crust most liable to damage by attrition — extending around the toe and reaching no farther than the quarters; while the heels and frog, when left unpared and unrasped, are strong enough to meet all demands made upon them, at the same time they are not deprived of their physiological functions. The diminution in the weight of the shoe is a matter of some importance, in addition to these considerations. Of course these shoes are only needed for the fore-feet; the hind-feet shoes, so long as they are not over heavy, are level, and do not wound the other limbs, may be the ordinary pattern.

In describing the latest novelties in shoeing, we glanced at the method introduced by M. Charlier, and which is, to a great extent, only a modification of that recommended by Lafosse. So far as my experience has gone, I must give my testimony to its merits. The introducer asserts that it favours the elasticity, or lateral expansion, of the hoof; if any proof were needed that the lower border of the hoof does not expand it would be proved by the use of this incrusted shoe. Its great merits are its lightness, and the fact that it allows the sole, frog, and bars to participate in supporting weight and strain. This is a great object gained. But to thoroughly incrust the metal, which is scarcely the width of the wall, but is very much thicker than the ordinary shoe, a proportionate amount of horn must be removed from the best part of the foot, and when this *rainure* has been made, the hoof is seriously mutilated; the junction between the sole and crust has been considerably weakened, and this is of serious moment. The workman is in far too close proximity to the living tissues, and the greatest skill is needed to prevent the rim from encroaching on them when driven back.

43 *

This is another objection. A greater one lies in the danger of a shoe breaking or coming off when there is not another at hand to take its place. The horse could not travel very far on the sole and frog alone, and the road-side farrier would have much difficulty in attaching an ordinary shoe.

To be safe, it must not be deeply incrusted, especially in thin hoofs, and then the portion projecting above the level of the sole, from its thinness, is quickly worn. It certainly prevents slipping on pavement, but, it would appear, is not found so beneficial on ice. As a winter shoe, I fear it will be useless, as there is no means of attaching anything to it to give the horse a grip on ice; even frost-nails cannot be advantageously used. Again, as a pathological shoe, when dressings or other appliances are required for the sole, this will afford no assistance in retaining them, like the ordinary shoe. It must always be fitted hot; in this respect it is inferior to the sub-plantar shoe, which, on an emergency, can be fitted and attached without a forge.

It will not be suitable for every description of hoof, particularly one in which there is any tendency to separation between the sole and wall; neither will it altogether suffice for hunting or racing purposes. Of course, on any kind of horse, one would not think of applying it indiscriminately to the hind-feet; indeed on these there is no necessity for it. On the fore-feet of a hunter it does not afford, one would think, a sufficient grip of the ground, and appears to offer no advantages beyond its being, perhaps, a trifle lighter than the shoe I have proposed. The hunter's sole and frog, if left unpared, receive their full share of pressure with the ordinary hunting-shoe.

The Charlier shoe is difficult to make, and takes a much longer time to apply by inexperienced workmen, and the smaller and thinner the hoofs are, the more this difficulty is increased. It requires skilful artisans, who will, consequently, demand a higher price for their labour. And even when fabricated from the best iron, I have found it very liable to break at some one of the nail-holes, and one of its most objectionable tendencies is to widen at the points of the heels, owing to the lightness of the metal. This can only be remedied by making the shoe stronger, and of course heavier, or by having the last nails placed near the ends of the branches.

In the face of these obstacles, this method of shoeing can scarcely be expected altogether to supersede the sub-plantar system.

For carriage and saddle horses, condemned to travel incessantly on the pavement of large towns, and which have strong hoofs, it may be advantageous to resort to it, and particularly in cases where the heels have a tendency to contraction.

I have tried it with success in these cases, but the same result would have followed the use of 'tips.' A narrow rim of iron the length of a tip, incrusted in the wall, is an excellent pathological shoe for a contracted foot, or even for ordinary wear by light carriage or saddle horses.

Though my experience of the 'ferrure Charlier' has been in its favour, yet I would not at present venture to recommend it for general application. It is not likely to supplant the ordinary method if carried out as I have advised; but it will no doubt always remain, like the tip and three-quarter shoe, a valuable accessory mode of defending and preserving the hoof, and remedying its diseases or defects. This view would appear to be gaining ground in Paris, where it was at first employed for every purpose. Its utility has now become better known, and its use is, perhaps, much more limited than it was some time ago.

I need not enter into a discussion in this place as to the advantages or disadvantages of the French mode of *ajusture*, or curving up the toes of the shoes *en bateau*. It may be sufficient to state that, for the hind-shoes, it is a grave mistake, as the horse relies greatly on the toes of these feet in propelling himself and he cannot so well make the ground a fixed point, if the sharp edge be rounded upwards. It is scarcely more reasonable when applied to the fore-shoes.

Goodwin, followed by Miles, has founded his recommendation on a very morbid specimen of an *os pedis*. We do not require abnormal examples to guide us in devising an armature for a healthy organ. Others have pointed out the natural wear as indicated by a worn-out shoe; as well might we have our own new boots and shoes fashioned at the heels and toes exactly like those we can no longer wear. For stumbling horses, shoes of this shape may be useful, but otherwise they should not be employed. In some respects they cause a loss of power to the horse, and at all times the farrier is liable to err in giving too much curve. This not only damages the hoof, but it makes the horse's support less secure. It has been said that it diminishes the risk of sprains of the back tendons; but this is not correct, if one may judge from the number of lame horses to be seen in those countries where this adjustment is practised. It also tends to slipping.

I am satisfied that the English plane-surfaced shoe is the best in every respect.

Thus far, then, we have devoted some attention to the uses and abuses of horse-shoeing—shoeing as it ought to be practised, and shoeing as it is generally practised. Without doing more than pointing out the most salient features of the subject—all details relative to the organization of the horse's foot and the practice of farriery being reserved for another opportunity—-it will be seen that though of vital importance to the welfare of the useful creature, nothing is more easy of execution than a rational system of shoeing; and few arts are more difficult to practise than the ordinary irrational one, simply because the artisan has destroyed what he cannot repair, and must then use his best skill to protect what remains. It is the case of an imperfect art attempting to improve and beautify nature.

The subject of shoeing is an important one in another point of view. For very many years, veterinary surgeons have agreed that various diseases of the limbs have a hereditary tendency; the principal of these are splints, ossification of the lateral cartilages, ossific deposits around the pastern bones, navicular disease, and spavin in the hock. To what extent these maladies might be due at first to the influence of improper shoeing, in addition to travelling upon artificial roads, we cannot discuss in this place. Certain it is, however, that in countries where horses are unshod, these diseases are rare, if not altogether absent.

In North Carolina, for instance, at a former period, horses did not wear shoes; and it has been asserted that they did not then suffer from the diseases of the feet and legs they now do.[1]

In mentioning this, however, we must take into account the fact that unshod horses do not always perform the same amount of severe labour, or undergo such long-continued exertion, and that there are generally no hard roads.

We can understand, nevertheless, how improper shoeing may induce diseases of this kind. Look at the horse which has been shod upon 'improved principles,' whose hoofs have been pared according to the directions given in some of the standard treatises on shoeing! He is not exactly lame—he is not quite a cripple—but is only tender in his feet. His soles have been 'thumb-tested,' to prove that they were thin enough; the miserable shred of horn remaining, and into which thousands of the most beautiful sensitive villi pass, is rapidly shrinking on these minute processes; in doing so it squeezes them painfully and unrelentingly, each in its narrow tube, as in a closing vice. The surface of the sole feels hot as fire, and the animal stands resting, first one foot, and then the other, showing symptoms of general uneasiness. What would the poor brute not give to get

[1] *Darwin.* Animals and Plants under Domestication. *Brickell.* Nat. Hist. of North Carolina, 1793.

his sole and frog on the ground, just to ease them; and yet they are so tender that he would be even worse off than he is now with thick shoes on, and perhaps calkins higher at one side than the other, throwing the strain all on one side of the limb? This tenderness has been ascribed by those who believed in lateral expansion and sole descent, and consequently patronized paring to excess, to the binding action of the nails, standing on straw, being kept in stalls—indeed, everything but the right cause, and which they had themselves been guilty of inflicting. The gradual contraction of the hoof, the diseased frog, and the painful altered gait, were never ascribed to anything else than the cursed contact of the iron shoe. And yet the changed and unnatural direction of the limbs, induced by the pain in the feet, as well as by the unreasonable shoes applied to these poor tortured organs, was also producing disease in other parts of the member.

These diseases have usually been attributed to the fast paces, and concussion on the hard roads. To a certain extent this may be correct, but it must be borne in mind that we at the same time have maintained foot and limb in the worst possible condition to resist these influences.

The Arab method of shoeing is far superior to our own in this respect. The shoe rests on the wall, sole, and frog of the foot, the latter being particularly supported by the light metal plate; the nails, rough and clumsy as they are, obtain a short thick hold of the sole and crust, and are badly riveted—though it is extremely rare that a shoe comes off on a journey lasting for weeks together.

Years of shoeing in this rude fashion do not alter the shape of the Arab horse's hoofs; the longest day's ride, no matter how fast or fatiguing, whether on burning sand or on sun-baked rocky ground, will seldom, if ever, cause him to have inflamed feet. Foot diseases, so far as my experience in Turkey and Syria goes, are all but unknown; and that most formidable of all maladies—navicular disease, I could neither see nor learn anything about. And any one who has seen Turk or Arab ride, will scarcely venture to say that they, as a rule, spare their horses on a journey, or ride as if they were afraid of laming them. And yet what happens when these Eastern horses come to Europe, and instead of their own primitive farriery, are shod upon improved principles? M. Megnin, an excellent authority on this subject, when speaking of the damage done by paring and hollowing out the sole, says: 'The best proof of the inconveniences of this practice is afforded us by the horses we obtain from Africa to mount our light cavalry. These horses, had they remained in their own country, would have preserved their hoofs as models of perfect health; but they are not six months in the hands of our *maréchaux*, before they have lost their precious qualities.'[1] And elsewhere he remarks : 'A shoe, no matter how clumsily it may be placed upon an unpared foot, does not cause one-tenth the injury that a fine shoe carefully attached to a hoof pared nearly to the quick (*jusqu'à la rosée*) will do.' 'This is seen every day in our mounted corps. What are the horses which furnish the largest number of cripples with contracted feet, corns, and

[1] Op. cit., p. 154.

sandcracks? Those of the officers; and simply because they are *too carefully, too properly shod.'*

As Samson's strength was concentrated in his uncut locks of hair, so it may truly be said that the highest development of a horse's powers is intimately dependent on the integrity of the horn of his feet (which we may assert is also a mass of hairs). And just as the giant was rendered helpless by the use of a razor, at the instigation of the crafty Delilah, so is the noble soliped in a great measure deprived of his strength and graceful movements by the unjustifiable and barbarous employment of the knife and rasp. There can scarcely be any doubt that the practice of paring the soles and frogs, and raising them from contact with the ground, by which they are thrown into disuse, and waste just as the muscles of a man's arm would if the limb were tied up for years, induces a hereditary tendency to contraction and deformity of the feet, as well as the occurrence of several serious maladies which affect them.

Taking into account the amount of work horses may have to perform, and making every allowance for its effects during a lengthened period, there can be no doubt whatever that the feet will remain nearly, or quite, as perfect after twenty or thirty years' service as they were before being submitted to the farrier's care, if only a rational system of shoeing be pursued.

The indispensable art of farriery, while serving the purpose for which it was originally intended, should also, as we have so often insisted, be conservative in its relations towards the foot. The natural form and functions of this all-important organ should be maintained intact; and even when the foot, limb, or even certain regions of the body, are irregular or defective, this handicraft may be successfully utilized in regulating, or curing, these. Science now-a-days requires that it may furnish more than a simple defence for the horny case ; it must not only be a protector of nature's work, but it must also be a remedial agent when that work, from some cause or other, is deranged or imperfect so far as to be unserviceable to man. The mere mechanical workman, who sees nothing in the horse's foot but the horn, which he may cut and rasp away to suit his fancy, or through which he may recklessly drive any number of nails, and knows not how to apply the resources of this art to the many circumstances which urgently require a deviation from routine, is not the artisan who can truly minister in assisting, as well as protecting, nature.

The art of farriery, by careful study, and by the application to it of those teachings which are to be derived from anatomy and physiology, should take the rank of a science ; but even then it would, and must always, remain a science of practice and experience.

No more useful lesson can, perhaps, be read with regard to our management of the horse than that to be found in the history of horse-shoes and horse-shoeing. It is one in which humanity and utility have for many ages been, and probably always will be, deeply concerned; and it is one of the most sacred duties devolving upon us to see that, while we exact services from this noble creature which we could not obtain from any other, and which make its whole life one of slavery and toil, we do our utmost to remove from its path any pain or discomfort which this exaction may entail. I can conceive no greater torture man can inflict on this most willing servant, than that induced by ignorance or neglect in the application of shoes to its feet.

Let every one who can, strive to prevent the unscientific and ruinous mutilation of the hoofs by paring and rasping. It is a practice which is only worthy of a barbarous age, and was a fit accompaniment to the hideous fashion of cropping the horse's ears, amputating his tail, and curving the miserable stump remaining over the poor animal's back—a fashion which, though it made a burlesque of nature's handiwork, was yet far less injurious and torturing than a vicious system of shoeing.

THE END.

INDEX.

JOHN CHILDS AND SON, PRINTERS.

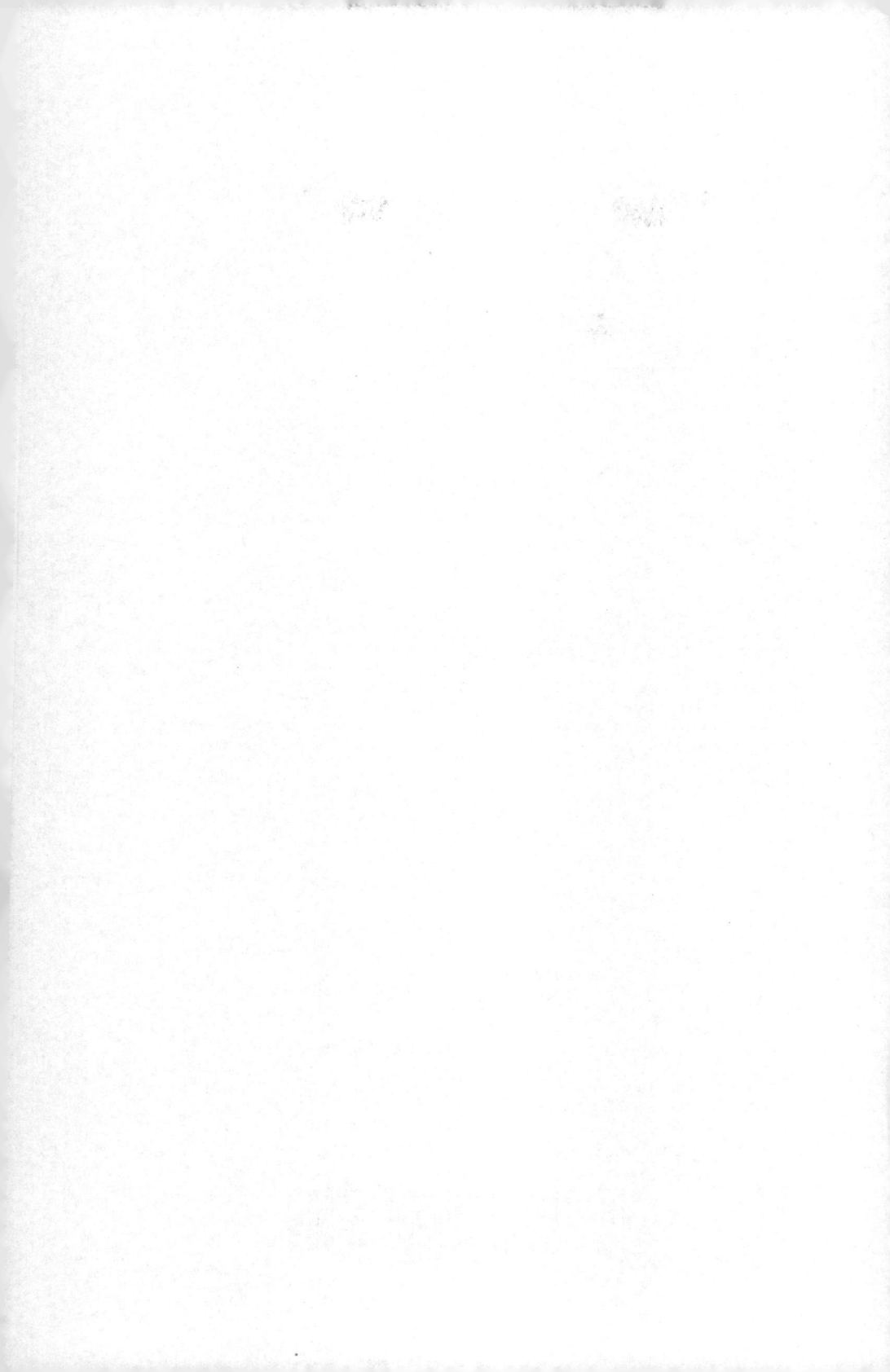

Printed in Great Britain
by Amazon